KT-368-463

Medical Statistics

Fourth Edition

A Textbook for the Health Sciences

David Machin
Division of Clinical Trials and Epidemiological Sciences, National Cancer Centre, Singapore,
Medical Statistics Group, School of Health and Related Research, University of Sheffield, UK,
Children's Cancer and Leukaemia Group, University of Leicester, UK

Michael J Campbell
Medical Statistics Group, School of Health and Related Research, University of Sheffield, UK

Stephen J Walters
Medical Statistics Group, School of Health and Related Research, University of Sheffield, UK

John Wiley & Sons, Ltd

Copyright © 2007   John Wiley & Sons Ltd, The Atrium, Southern Gate, Chichester,
West Sussex PO19 8SQ, England

Telephone (+44) 1243 779777

Email (for orders and customer service enquiries): cs-books@wiley.co.uk
Visit our Home Page on www.wileyeurope.com or www.wiley.com

All Rights Reserved. No part of this publication may be reproduced, stored in a retrieval system
or transmitted in any form or by any means, electronic, mechanical, photocopying, recording,
scanning or otherwise, except under the terms of the Copyright, Designs and Patents Act 1988 or
under the terms of a licence issued by the Copyright Licensing Agency Ltd, 90 Tottenham Court
Road, London W1T 4LP, UK, without the permission in writing of the Publisher. Requests to the
Publisher should be addressed to the Permissions Department, John Wiley & Sons Ltd, The
Atrium, Southern Gate, Chichester, West Sussex PO19 8SQ, England, or emailed to permreq@
wiley.co.uk, or faxed to (+44) 1243 770620.

Designations used by companies to distinguish their products are often claimed as trademarks. All
brand names and product names used in this book are trade names, service marks, trademarks or
registered trademarks of their respective owners. The Publisher is not associated with any product
or vendor mentioned in this book.

This publication is designed to provide accurate and authoritative information in regard to the
subject matter covered. It is sold on the understanding that the Publisher is not engaged in
rendering professional services. If professional advice or other expert assistance is required, the
services of a competent professional should be sought.

Other Wiley Editorial Offices

John Wiley & Sons Inc., 111 River Street, Hoboken, NJ 07030, USA

Jossey-Bass, 989 Market Street, San Francisco, CA 94103-1741, USA

Wiley-VCH Verlag GmbH, Boschstr. 12, D-69469 Weinheim, Germany

John Wiley & Sons Australia Ltd, 33 Park Road, Milton, Queensland 4064, Australia

John Wiley & Sons (Asia) Pte Ltd, 2 Clementi Loop #02-01, Jin Xing Distripark, Singapore
129809

John Wiley & Sons Canada Ltd, 6045 Freemont Blvd, Mississauga, Ontario, L5R 4J3, Canada

Wiley also publishes its books in a variety of electronic formats. Some content that appears in
print may not be available in electronic books.

Anniversary Logo Design: Richard J. Pacifico

Library of Congress Cataloging-in-Publication Data

Campbell, Michael J., PhD.
   Medical statistics : a textbook for the health sciences / Michael J.
Campbell, David Machin, Stephen J. Walters. – 4th ed.
     p. ; cm.
   Includes bibliographical references.
   ISBN 978-0-470-02519-2 (cloth : alk. paper)
   1. Medical statistics. 2. Medicine–Research–Statistical methods. I. Machin, David,
1939– II. Walters, Stephen John. III. Title.
   [DNLM: 1. Biometry–methods. 2. Research Design. 3. Statistics. WA 950 C189m 2007]
   R853.S7C36 2007
   610.72′7–dc22
WEST SUFFOLK NHS FOUNDATION TRUST
LIBRARY & INFORMATION CENTRE
British Library Cataloguing in Publication Data

A catalogue record for this book is available from the British Library
ISBN 978-0-470-02519-2 5.2.14 ·

Typeset in 10.5/12.5 Times by SNP Best-set Typesetter Ltd., Hong Kong
Printed and bound in Singapore by Markono Print Media Pte Ltd
DATE

VENDOR 8 2013   Tomlinsons

CLASSMARK   WA 900 HA29
                    CAM

PRICE   £ 26·95

Contents

Preface to the Fourth Edition

Revised editions of books are often only minor departures from previous editions. In this edition, however, with the aid of a new co-author we have attempted a total revamp of our previously successful textbook. We did this because not only have twenty years passed but the statistical requirements of medical journals are now more rigorous and there has been an increasing demand for the newer statistical methods to meet new scientific challenges. Despite this, we have retained the popular approach of explaining medical statistics with as little technical detail as possible, so as to make the textbook accessible to a wide audience. In general, we have placed the, sometimes unavoidable, more technical aspects at the end of each chapter. We have updated many of the examples to give a more modern approach, but have retained a few classics from the earlier editions, because they so well illustrate the point we wish to make.

To aid the individual learner, exercises are included at the end of each chapter, with answers provided at the end of the book. We have concentrated the design issues into three chapters, concerning the design of observational studies, randomised clinical trials and sample size issues. Many health scientists will have to validate their methods of measurement, and a new feature in this book is a chapter on reliability and validity.

Students of the health sciences, such as medicine, nursing, dentistry, physiotherapy, occupational therapy, and radiography should find the book useful, with examples relevant to their disciplines. The aim of training courses in medical statistics pertinent to these areas is not to turn the students into medical statisticians but rather to help them interpret the published scientific literature and appreciate how to design studies and analyse data arising from their own projects.

We envisage the book being useful in two areas. First, for *consumers* of statistics who need to be able to read the research literature in the field with a critical eye. All health science professionals need to be able to do this, but for many this is all they will need. We suggest that Chapters 1–7 would form the basis of a course for this purpose. However, some (perhaps trainee) professionals will go on to design studies and analyse data from projects, and so, secondly, the book will be useful to *doers* of statistics, who need relatively straightforward methods that they can be confident of using. Chapters 8–15 are aimed at this audience, though clearly they also need to be familiar with the earlier chapters. These students will be doing statistics on computer packages, so we have given 'generic' output which is typical of the major packages, to aid in the interpretation of the results.

We thank Lucy Sayer from Wiley for her patience, for what initially was simply a revision, but is now essentially a new textbook.

David Machin
Singapore and Sheffield and Leicester, UK

Michael J Campbell
Sheffield, UK

Stephen J Walters
Sheffield, UK

November 2006

1 Uses and abuses of medical statistics

Medical Statistics Fourth Edition, David Machin, Michael J Campbell, Stephen J Walters
© 2007 John Wiley & Sons, Ltd

Summary

Statistical analysis features in the majority of papers published in health care journals. Most health care practitioners will need a basic understanding of statistical principles, but not necessarily full details of statistical techniques. Medical statistics can contribute to good research by improving the design of studies as well as suggesting the optimum analysis of the results. Medical statisticians should be consulted early in the planning of a study. They can contribute in a variety of ways at all stages and not just at the final analysis of the data once the data have been collected.

1.1   Introduction

Most health care practitioners do not carry out medical research. However, if they pride themselves on being up to date then they will definitely be consumers of medical research. It is incumbent on them to be able to discern good studies from bad; to be able to verify whether the conclusions of a study are valid and to understand the limitations of such studies. Evidence-based medicine (EBM) or more comprehensively evidence-based health care (EBHC) requires that health care practitioners consider critically all evidence about whether a treatment works. As Machin and Campbell (2005) point out, this requires the systematic assembly of all available evidence followed by a critical appraisal of this evidence.

A particular example might be a paper describing the results of a clinical trial of a new drug. A physician might read this report to try to decide whether to use the drug on his or her own patients. Since physicians are responsible for the care of their patients, it is their own responsibility to ensure the validity of the report, and its possible generalisation to particular patients. Usually, in the reputable medical press, the reader is to some extent protected from grossly misleading papers by a review process involving both specialist clinical and statistical referees. However, often there is no such protection in the general press or in much of the promotional literature sponsored by self-interested parties. Even in the medical literature, misleading results can get through the refereeing net and no journal offers a guarantee as to the validity of its papers.

The use of statistical methods pervades the medical literature. In a survey of original articles published in three UK journals of general practice; *British Medical Journal* (*General Practice Section*), *British Journal of General Practice* and *Family Practice*; over a 1-year period, Rigby et al (2004) found that 66% used some form of statistical analysis. It appears, therefore, that the majority of papers published in these journals require some statistical knowledge for a complete understanding.

Statistics is not only a discipline in its own right but it is also a fundamental tool for investigation in all biological and medical science. As such, any serious investigator in these fields must have a grasp of the basic principles. With modern computer facilities there is little need for familiarity with the technical details of statistical calculations. However, a health care professional should understand when such calculations are valid, when they are not and how they should be interpreted.

1.2 Why use statistics?

To students schooled in the 'hard' sciences of physics and chemistry it may be difficult to appreciate the variability of biological data. If one repeatedly puts blue litmus paper into acid solutions it turns red 100% of the time, not most (say 95%) of the time. In contrast, if one gives aspirin to a group of people with headaches, not all of them will experience relief. Penicillin was perhaps one of the few 'miracle' cures where the results were so dramatic that little evaluation was required. Absolute certainty in medicine is rare.

Measurements on human subjects rarely give exactly the same results from one occasion to the next. For example, O' Sullivan et al (1999), found that systolic blood pressure in normal healthy children has a wide range, with 95% of children having systolic blood pressures below 130 mmHg when they were resting, rising to 160 mmHg during the school day, and falling to below 130 mmHg at night.

This variability is also inherent in responses to biological hazards. Most people now accept that cigarette smoking causes lung cancer and heart disease, and yet nearly everyone can point to an apparently healthy 80-year-old who has smoked for 60 years without apparent ill effect.

Although it is now known from the report of Doll et al (2004) that about half of all persistent cigarette smokers are killed by their habit, it is usually forgotten that until the 1950s, the cause of the rise in lung cancer deaths was a mystery and commonly associated with diesel fumes. It was not until the carefully designed and statistically analysed case–control and cohort studies of Richard Doll and Austin Bradford Hill and others, that smoking was identified as the true cause. Enstrom and Kabat (2003) have now moved the debate on to whether or not passive smoking causes lung cancer. This is a more difficult question to answer since the association is weaker.

With such variability, it follows that in any comparison made in a medical context, differences are almost bound to occur. These differences may be due to real effects, random variation or both. It is the job of the analyst to decide how much variation should be ascribed to chance, so that any remaining variation can be assumed to be due to a real effect. This is the art of statistics.

1.3   Statistics is about common sense and good design

A well-designed study, poorly analysed, can be rescued by a reanalysis but a poorly designed study is beyond the redemption of even sophisticated statistical manipulation. Many experimenters consult the medical statistician only at the end of the study when the data have been collected. They believe that the job of the statistician is simply to analyse the data, and with powerful computers available, even complex studies with many variables can be easily processed. However, analysis is only part of a statistician's job, and calculation of the final 'p-value' a minor one at that!

A far more important task for the medical statistician is to ensure that results are comparable and generalisable.

Example from the literature: Fluoridated water supplies

A classic example is the debate as to whether fluorine in the water supply is related to cancer mortality. Burke and Yiamouyannis (1975) considered 10 fluoridated and 10 non-fluoridated towns in the USA. In the fluoridated towns, the cancer mortality rate had increased by 20% between 1950 and 1970, whereas in the non-fluoridated towns the increase was only 10%. From this they concluded that fluoridisation caused cancer. However, Oldham and Newell (1977), in a careful analysis of the changes in age–gender–ethnic structure of the 20 cities between 1950 and 1970, showed that in fact the excess cancer rate in the fluoridated cities increased by only 1% over the 20 years, while in the unfluoridated cities the increase was 4%. They concluded from this that there was no evidence that fluoridisation caused cancer. No statistical significance testing was deemed necessary by these authors, both medical statisticians, even though the paper appeared in a statistical journal!

In the above example age, gender and ethnicity are examples of confounding variables as illustrated in Figure 1.1. In this example, the types of individuals exposed to fluoridation depend on their age, gender and ethnic mix, and these same factors are also known to influence cancer mortality rates. It was established that over the 20 years of the study, fluoridated towns were more likely to be ones where young, white people moved away and these are the people with lower cancer mortality, and so they left behind a higher risk population.

Any observational study that compares populations distinguished by a particular variable (such as a comparison of smokers and non-smokers) and ascribes the differences found in other variables (such as lung cancer rates) to the first variable is open to the charge that the observed differences are in fact due to some other, confounding, variables. Thus, the difference in lung

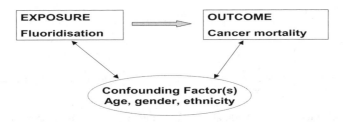

Figure 1.1 Graphical representation of how confounding variables may influence both exposure to fluoridisation and cancer mortality

cancer rates between smokers and non-smokers has been ascribed to genetic factors; that is, some factor that makes people want to smoke also makes them more susceptible to lung cancer. The difficulty with observational studies is that there is an infinite source of confounding variables. An investigator can measure all the variables that seem reasonable to him but a critic can always think of another, unmeasured, variable that just might explain the result. It is only in prospective randomised studies that this logical difficulty is avoided. In randomised studies, where exposure variables (such as alternative treatments) are assigned purely by a chance mechanism, it can be assumed that unmeasured confounding variables are comparable, on average, in the two groups. Unfortunately, in many circumstances it is not possible to randomise the exposure variable as part of the experimental design, as in the case of smoking and lung cancer, and so alternative interpretations are always possible. Observational studies are further discussed in Chapter 12.

1.4 Types of data

Just as a farmer gathers and processes a crop, a statistician gathers and processes data. For this reason the logo for the UK Royal Statistical Society is a sheaf of wheat. Like any farmer who knows instinctively the difference between oats, barley and wheat, a statistician becomes an expert at discerning different types of data. Some sections of this book refer to different data types and so we start by considering these distinctions. Figure 1.2 shows a basic summary of data types, although some data do not fit neatly into these categories.

Example from the literature: Risk factors for endometrial cancer

Table 1.1 gives a typical table reporting baseline characteristics of a set of patients entered into a case–control study which investigated risk factors for endometrial cancer (Xu et al, 2004). We will discuss the different types of data given in this paper.

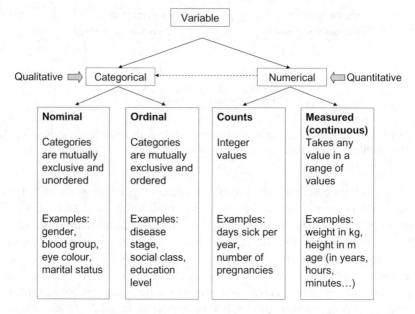

Figure 1.2   Broad classification of the different types of data with examples

Categorical or qualitative data

Nominal categorical data   Nominal or categorical data are data that one can *name* and put into categories. They are not measured but simply counted. They often consist of unordered 'either–or' type observations which have two categories and are often know as *binary*. For example: Dead or Alive; Male or Female; Cured or Not Cured; Pregnant or Not Pregnant. In Table 1.1 having a first-degree relative with cancer, or taking regular exercise are binary variables. However, categorical data often can have more that two categories, for example: blood group O, A, B, AB, country of origin, ethnic group or eye colour. In Table 1.1 marital status is of this type. The methods of presentation of nominal data are limited in scope. Thus, Table 1.1 merely gives the number and percentage of people by marital status.

Ordinal data   If there are more than two categories of classification it may be possible to order them in some way. For example, after treatment a patient may be either improved, the same or worse; a woman may never have conceived, conceived but spontaneously aborted, or given birth to a live infant. In Table 1.1 education is given in three categories: none or elementary school, middle school, college and above. Thus someone who has been to middle school has more education than someone from elementary school but

Table 1.1   Demographic characteristics and selected risk factors for endometrial cancer. Values are numbers (percentages) unless stated otherwise

Characteristic	Cases	Controls
Number of women (n)	832	846
Mean (SD) age (years)	55.3 (8.60)	55.7 (8.58)
Education		
No formal education or just elementary school	204 (24.5)	234 (27.7)
Middle school	503 (60.5)	513 (60.6)
College and above	125 (15.0)	99 (11.7)
Marital status		
Unmarried	14 (1.7)	10 (1.2)
Married or cohabiting	724 (87.0)	742 (87.7)
Separated, divorced, or widowed	94 (11.3)	94 (11.1)
Per capita income in previous year (yuan)		
≤4166.7	230 (27.7)	244 (28.9)
4166.8–6250.3	243 (29.2)	242 (28.6)
6250.4–8333.3	57 (6.9)	50 (5.9)
≥8333.3	301 (36.2)	309 (36.6)
No of pregnancies		
None	62 (7.5)	35 (4.1)
1	137 (16.5)	109 (12.9)
2	199 (23.9)	208 (24.6)
3	194 (23.3)	207 (24.5)
4	141 (17.0)	157 (18.6)
≥5	99 (11.9)	130 (15.4)
Cancer among first degree relatives	289 (34.7)	228 (27.0)
Oral contraceptive use	147 (17.7)	207 (24.5)
Regular exercise	253 (30.4)	287 (33.9)
Age at menarche*	14 (13 to 16)	15 (13 to 16)
Age at menopause (among postmenopausal women)*	50.1 (48.6 to 52.5)	49.4 (47.1 to 51.1)
Body mass index*	25.1 (22.7 to 27.9)	23.7 (21.4 to 26.3)

From Xu et al (2004). Soya food intake and risk of endometrial cancer among Chinese women in Shanghai: population-based case–control study. *British Medical Journal*, **328**, 1285–1291: reproduced by permission of the BMJ Publishing Group.
*Median (25th to 75th centile).

less than someone from college. However, without further knowledge it would be wrong to ascribe a numerical quantity to position; one cannot say that someone who had middle school education is twice as educated as someone who had only elementary school education. This type of data is also known as *ordered categorical data*.

Ranks   In some studies it may be appropriate to assign ranks. For example, patients with rheumatoid arthritis may be asked to order their preference for four dressing aids. Here, although numerical values from 1 to 4 may be assigned to each aid, one cannot treat them as numerical values. They are in fact only codes for best, second best, third choice and worst.

Numerical or quantitative data

Count data   Table 1.1 gives details of the number of pregnancies each woman had had, and this is termed count data. Other examples are often counts per unit of time such as the number of deaths in a hospital per year, or the number of attacks of asthma a person has per month. In dentistry, a common measure is the number of decayed, filled or missing teeth (DFM).

Measured or numerical continuous   Such data are measurements that can, in theory at least, take any value within a given range. These data contain the most information, and are the ones most commonly used in statistics. Examples of continuous data in Table 1.1 are: age, years of menstruation and body mass index.

However, for simplicity, it is often the case in medicine that continuous data are *dichotomised* to make nominal data. Thus diastolic blood pressure, which is continuous, is converted into hypertension (>90 mmHg) and normotension (≤90 mmHg). This clearly leads to a loss of information. There are two main reasons for doing this. It is easier to describe a population by the proportion of people affected (for example, the proportion of people in the population with hypertension is 10%). Further, one often has to make a decision: if a person has hypertension, then they will get treatment, and this too is easier if the population is grouped.

One can also divide a continuous variable into more than two groups. In Table 1.1 per capita income is a continuous variable and it has been divided into four groups to summarise it, although a better choice may have been to split at the more convenient and memorable intervals of 4000, 6000 and 8000 yuan. The authors give no indication as to why they chose these cut-off points, and a reader has to be very wary to guard against the fact that the cuts may be chosen to make a particular point.

Interval and ratio scales

One can distinguish between *interval* and *ratio* scales. In an *interval* scale, such as body temperature or calendar dates, a difference between two measurements has meaning, but their ratio does not. Consider measuring temperature (in degrees centigrade) then we cannot say that a temperature of 20°C is twice as hot as a temperature of 10°C. In a *ratio* scale, however, such as body weight, a 10% increase implies the same weight increase whether expressed in kilograms or pounds. The crucial difference is that in a ratio scale, the value of zero has real meaning, whereas in an interval scale, the position of zero is arbitrary.

One difficulty with giving ranks to ordered categorical data is that one cannot assume that the scale is interval. Thus, as we have indicated when discussing ordinal data, one cannot assume that risk of cancer for an individual educated to middle school level, relative to one educated only to primary school level is the same as the risk for someone educated to college level, relative to someone educated to middle school level. Were Xu et al (2004) simply to score the three levels of education as 1, 2 and 3 in their subsequent analysis, then this would imply in some way the intervals have equal weight.

1.5 How a statistician can help

Statistical ideas relevant to good design and analysis are not easy and we would always advise an investigator to seek the advice of a statistician at an early stage of an investigation. Here are some ways the medical statistician might help.

Sample size and power considerations

One of the commonest questions asked of a consulting statistician is: How large should my study be? If the investigator has a reasonable amount of knowledge as to the likely outcome of a study, and potentially large resources of finance and time, then the statistician has tools available to enable a scientific answer to be made to the question. However, the usual scenario is that the investigator has either a grant of a limited size, or limited time, or a limited pool of patients. Nevertheless, given certain assumptions the medical statistician is still able to help. For a given number of patients the probability of obtaining effects of a certain size can be calculated. If the outcome variable is simply success or failure, the statistician will need to know the anticipated percentage of successes in each group so that the difference between them can be judged of potential clinical relevance. If the outcome variable is a quantitative measurement, he will need to know the size of the difference between the two groups, and the expected variability of the measurement. For example, in a survey to see if patients with diabetes have raised blood pressure the medical statistician might say, 'with 100 diabetics and 100 healthy subjects in this survey and a possible difference in blood pressure of 5 mmHg, with standard deviation of 10 mmHg, you have a 20% chance of obtaining a statistically significant result at the 5% level'. (The term 'statistically significant' will be explained in Chapter 7.) This statement means that one would anticipate that in only one study in five of the proposed size would a statistically significant result be obtained. The investigator would then have to decide whether it was sensible or ethical to conduct a trial with such a small probability of success. One option would be to increase the size of the survey until success (defined as a statistically significant result if a difference of 5 mmHg or more does truly exist) becomes more probable.

Questionnaires

Rigby et al (2004), in their survey of original articles in three UK general practice journals, found that the most common design was that of a cross-sectional or questionnaire survey, with approximately one third of the articles classified as such.

For all but the smallest data sets it is desirable to use a computer for statistical analysis. The responses to a questionnaire will need to be easily coded for computer analysis and a medical statistician may be able to help with this. It is important to ask for help at an early stage so that the questionnaire can be piloted and modified before use in a study. Further details on questionnaire design and surveys are given in Chapter 12.

Choice of sample and of control subjects

The question of whether one has a representative sample is a typical problem faced by statisticians. For example, it used to be believed that migraine was associated with intelligence, perhaps on the grounds that people who used their brains were more likely to get headaches but a subsequent population study failed to reveal any social class gradient and, by implication, any association with intelligence. The fallacy arose because intelligent people were more likely to consult their physician about migraine than the less intelligent.

In many studies an investigator will wish to compare patients suffering from a certain disease with healthy (control) subjects. The choice of the appropriate control population is crucial to a correct interpretation of the results. This is discussed further in Chapter 12.

Design of study

It has been emphasised that design deserves as much consideration as analysis, and a statistician can provide advice on design. In a clinical trial, for example, what is known as a double-blind randomised design is nearly always preferable (see Chapter 13), but not always achievable. If the treatment is an intervention, such as a surgical procedure it might be impossible to prevent individuals knowing which treatment they are receiving but it should be possible to shield their assessors from knowing. We also discuss methods of randomisation and other design issues in Chapter 13.

Laboratory experiments

Medical investigators often appreciate the effect that biological variation has in patients, but overlook or underestimate its presence in the laboratory. In dose–response studies, for example, it is important to assign treatment at random, whether the experimental units are humans, animals or test tubes. A statistician can also advise on quality control of routine laboratory measurements and the measurement of within- and between-observer variation.

Displaying data

A well-chosen figure or graph can summarise the results of a study very concisely. A statistician can help by advising on the best methods of displaying data. For example, when plotting histograms, choice of the group interval can affect the shape of the plotted distribution; with too wide an interval important features of the data will be obscured; too narrow an interval and random variation in the data may distract attention from the shape of the underlying distribution. Advice on displaying data is given in Chapters 2 and 3.

Choice of summary statistics and statistical analysis

The summary statistics used and the analysis undertaken must reflect the basic design of the study and the nature of the data. In some situations, for example, a median is a better measure of location than a mean. (These terms are defined in Chapter 3.) In a matched study, it is important to produce an estimate of the difference between matched pairs, and an estimate of the reliability of that difference. For example, in a study to examine blood pressure measured in a seated patient compared with that measured when he is lying down, it is insufficient simply to report statistics for seated and lying positions separately. The important statistic is the change in blood pressure as the patient changes position and it is the mean and variability of this difference that we are interested in. This is further discussed in Chapter 8. A statistician can advise on the choice of summary statistics, the type of analysis and the presentation of the results.

1.6 Further reading

Swinscow and Campbell (2002) is an introductory text, which concentrates mainly on the analysis of studies, while Bland (2000) and Campbell (2006) are intermediate texts. Altman (1991) and Armitage et al (2002) give lengthier and more detailed accounts. Machin and Campbell (2005) focus on the design, rather than analysis, of medical studies in general.

1.7   Exercises

1. Consider a survey of nurses' opinions of their working conditions. What type of variables are: (i) length of service (ii) staff grade (iii) age (iv) salary (v) number of patients seen in a day (vi) possession of a degree.
2. What differences do you think are there in a discrete measurement such as shoe size, and a discrete measurement such as family size?
3. Many continuous variables are dichotomised to make them easier to understand e.g. obesity (body mass index $>30 \text{kg/m}^2$) and anaemia (haemoglobin level $<10 \text{g/dl}$). What information is lost in this process? If you were told that a patient was anaemic, what further information would you want before treating the patient? How does a label, such as anaemia, help?

2 Describing and displaying categorical data

Medical Statistics Fourth Edition, David Machin, Michael J Campbell, Stephen J Walters
© 2007 John Wiley & Sons, Ltd

Summary

This chapter illustrates methods of summarising and displaying binary and categorical data. It covers proportions, risk and rates, relative risk, and odds ratios. The importance of considering the absolute risk difference as well as the relative risk is emphasized. Data display covers contingency tables, bar charts and pie charts.

2.1   Summarising categorical data

Binary data are the simplest type of data. Each individual has a label which takes one of two values. A simple summary would be to count the different types of label. However, a raw count is rarely useful. Furness et al (2003) reported more accidents to white cars than to any other colour car in Auckland, New Zealand over a 1-year period. As a consequence, a New Zealander may think twice about buying a white car! However, it turns out that there are simply more white cars on the Auckland roads than any other colour. It is only when this count is expressed as a *proportion* that it becomes useful. When Furness et al (2003) looked at the proportion of white cars that had accidents compared to the proportion of all cars that had accidents, they found the proportions very similar and so white cars are not more dangerous than other colours. Hence the first step to analysing categorical data is to count the number of observations in each category and express them as proportions of the total sample size. Proportions are a special example of a *ratio*. When time is also involved (as in counts per year) then it is known as a *rate*. These distinctions are given below.

Ratios, proportions, percentages, risk and rates

A *ratio* is simply one number divided by another. If we measure the weight of a person (in kg/) and the height (in metres), then the ratio of weight to height^2 is the *Body Mass Index*.

Proportions are ratios of counts where the numerator (the top number) is a subset of the denominator (the bottom number). Thus in a study of 50 patients, 30 are depressed, so the proportion is 30/50 or 0.6. It is usually easier to express this as a percentage, so we multiply the proportion by 100, and state that 60% of the patients are depressed. A proportion is known as a *risk* if the numerator counts events which happen prospectively. Hence if 300 students start nursing school and 15 drop out before finals, the *risk* of dropping out is 15/300 = 0.05 or 5%.

Rates always have a time period attached. If 600000 people in the UK die in one year, out of a population of 60000000, the death *rate* is 600000/600000000 or 0.01 deaths per person per year. This is known as the *crude death rate* (crude because it makes no allowance for important factors such as age). Crude death rates are often expressed as deaths per thousand per year, so the crude death rate is 10 deaths per thousand per year, since it is much easier to imagine 1000 people, of whom 10 die, than it is 0.01 deaths per person! We will discuss these issues in more details in Section 12.2.

Illustrative example: Special care baby unit

Simpson (2004) describes a prospective study, in which 98 preterm infants were given a series of tests shortly after they were born, in an attempt to predict their outcome after 1 year. We will use this example in this chapter and in Chapter 3 where we discuss quantitative data. One categorical variable recorded was the type of delivery. in five categories as displayed in Table 2.1. The first column shows category names, whilst the second shows the number of individuals in each category together with its percentage contribution to the total.

In addition to tabulating each variable separately, we might be interested in whether the type of delivery is related to the gender of the baby. Table 2.2 shows the distribution of type of delivery by gender; in this case it can be said that delivery type has been *cross-tabulated* with gender. Table 2.2 is an example of a *contingency* table with five rows (representing type of delivery) and two columns (gender). Note that we are interested in the distribution of modes of delivery within gender, and so the percentages add to 100 down each column, rather than across the rows.

Table 2.1 Type of delivery for 98 babies admitted to a special care baby unit (Simpson, 2004)

Type of delivery	Frequency	Percentage
Standard vaginal delivery	38	39
Assisted vaginal delivery	10	10
Elective caesarean section	8	8
Emergency caesarean section	13	13
Emergency caesarean section/ not in labour	29	30
Total	**98**	**100**

Reproduced by permission of AG Simpson.

Table 2.2   Type of delivery and gender of 98 babies admitted to a special care baby unit (Simpson, 2004)

Type of delivery	Gender	
	Male n (%)	Female n (%)
Standard vaginal delivery	15 (33)	23 (43)
Assisted vaginal delivery	4 (9)	6 (11)
Elective caesarean section	4 (9)	4 (8)
Emergency caesarean section	6 (13)	7 (13)
Emergency caesarean section/not in labour	16 (36)	13 (25)
Total	**45 (100)**	**53 (100)**

Reproduced by permission of AG Simpson.

Table 2.3   Example of 2×2 contingency table with a binary outcome and two groups of subjects

Outcome	Treatment group	
	Test	Control
Positive	a	b
Negative	c	d
	$a + c$	$b + d$

Labelling binary outcomes

For binary data it is common to call the outcome 'an event' and 'a non-event'. So having a car accident in Auckland, New Zealand may be an 'event'. We often score an 'event' as 1 and a 'non-event' as 0. These may also be referred to as a 'positive' or 'negative' outcome or 'success' and 'failure'. It is important to realise that these terms are merely labels and the main outcome of interest might be a success in one context and a failure in another. Thus in a study of a potentially lethal disease the outcome might be death, whereas in a disease that can be cured it might be being alive.

Comparing outcomes for binary data

Many studies involve a comparison of two groups. We may wish to combine simple summary measures to give a summary measure which in some way shows how the groups differ. Given two proportions one can either subtract one from the other, or divide one by the other.

Suppose the results of a clinical trial, with a binary categorical outcome (positive or negative), to compare two treatments (a new test treatment versus a control) are summarised in a 2×2 contingency table as in Table 2.3. Then the results of this trial can be summarised in a number of ways.

The ways of summarising the data presented in Table 2.3 are given below.

Summarising comparative binary data: Differences in proportions, and relative risk

From Table 2.3, the proportion of subjects with a positive outcome under the active or test treatment is $p_{\text{Test}} = \dfrac{a}{a+c}$ and under the control treatment is $p_{\text{Control}} = \dfrac{b}{b+d}$.

The difference in proportions is given by

$$d_{\text{prop}} = p_{\text{Test}} - p_{\text{Control}}.$$

In prospective studies the proportion is also known as a risk. When one ignores the sign, the above quantity is also known as the *absolute risk difference* (ARD), that is

$$ARD = |p_{\text{Control}} - p_{\text{Test}}|,$$

where the symbols |·| mean to take the absolute value.

If we anticipate that the treatment to reduce some bad outcome (such as deaths) then it may be known as the *absolute risk reduction* (ARR). The risk ratio, or relative risk *(RR)*, is

$$RR = p_{\text{Test}} / p_{\text{Control}}.$$

A further summary measure, used only in clinical trials is the *number needed to treat/harm*. This is defined as the inverse of the ARD. We will discuss it further in Chapter 13, where we will consider clinical trials in more detail.

Each of the above measures summarises the study outcomes, and the one chosen may depend on how the test treatment behaves relative to the control. Commonly, one may chose an absolute risk difference for a clinical trial and a relative risk for a prospective study. In general the relative risk is independent of how common the risk factor is. Smoking increases one's risk of lung cancer by a factor of 10, and this is true in countries with a high smoking prevalence and countries with a low smoking prevalence. However, in a clinical trial, we may be interested in what reduction in the proportion of people with poor outcome a new treatment will make.

Example: Importance of considering both absolute risk reduction and relative risk

Women aged 15–45 not on the contraceptive pill have a risk of deep vein thrombosis (DVT) of about 20 per 100 000 women per year. Consider a contraceptive pill which increases the risk to 40 per 100 000 per year. The relative risk of DVT for the new pill is 2, which would seem a large risk. However, the increase in risk is 20/100 000 = 0.00002, or an additional 2 women with DVTs in 10 000 years of exposure. This risk is very small and hence may be considered worthwhile, when balanced against other factors such as cost or convenience. Also, it is worth mentioning that a pregnant woman has a risk of a DVT of about 80 per 100 000 per year. When one reads in the papers about a new risk to health that has been discovered, often only the relative risk is quoted, but one should ask about the absolute risk difference, which is often negligible. If you are at very low risk, then you will remain at very low risk even when exposed to a hazard, unless the relative risk for the hazard is enormous!

Example: Summarising results from a clinical trial – smoking cessation

Table 2.4 shows the results of a randomised controlled trial conducted by Quist-Pauslen and Gallefoss (2003) to determine whether a nurse-led smoking cessation intervention can improve smoking cessation rates in patients admitted for coronary heart disease. There are two study groups: the control group (randomised to receive usual care) and the experimental or intervention group (randomised to receive a booklet and which emphasised the health benefits of quitting smoking after a coronary event). The main outcome measure was smoking cessation rates at 1 year determined by self-report and biomedical verification.

The proportion of patients who stopped smoking in the Intervention group is 57/100 = 0.57 and in the Control group 44/118 = 0.37 or a difference of 0.20 or 20%. If we started with 100 women in each arm we would expect 20 fewer patients smoking in the intervention arm compared to the control at the end of the study.

The Relative Risk is 0.57/0.37 = 1.5. This is the risk of stopping smoking (a good thing) with the intervention compared to the control group. Thus patients with coronary heart disease are 1.5 times more likely to stop smoking in the intervention group than the control group.

Table 2.4 Smoking cessation rates at one year in patients with coronary heart disease

Stopped Smoking	Intervention		Control	
	n	%	n	%
Yes	57	57	44	37
No	43	43	74	63
	100	100	118	100

From Quist-Paulsen and Gallefoss (2003). Randomised controlled trial of smoking cessation intervention after admission for coronary heart disease. *British Medical Journal*, **327**, 1254–1257: reproduced by permission of the BMJ Publishing Group.

Summarising binary data – odds and odds ratios

A further method of summarising the results is to use the odds of an event rather than the probability. The odds of an event are defined as the ratio of the probability of occurrence of the event to the probability of non-occurrence, that is, $p/(1 - p)$.

Using the notation of Table 2.3 we can see that the odds of an outcome for the test group to the odds of an outcome for control group is the ratio of odds for test group to the odds for control group:

The odds ratio (OR) is

$$\left(\frac{p_{Test}}{1 - p_{Test}} \right) \Bigg/ \left(\frac{p_{Control}}{1 - p_{Control}} \right).$$

The odds ratio (OR) from Table 2.3 is

$$OR_{Test/Control} = \left(\frac{a}{c} \right) \Bigg/ \left(\frac{b}{d} \right) = \frac{ad}{bc}.$$

When the probability of an event happening is rare, the odds and probabilities are close, because then a is much smaller than c and so $a/(a + c)$ is approximately a/c and b is much smaller than d and so $b/(b + d)$ is approximately b/d. Thus the OR approximates the RR when the successes are rare (say with a maximum incidence less than 10% of either p_{Test} or $p_{Control}$) Sometime the odds ratio is referred to as 'the approximate relative risk'. The approximation is demonstrated in Table 2.5.

Why should one use the odds ratio?

The calculation for an odds ratio (OR) may seem rather perverse, given that we can calculate the relative risk directly from the 2×2 table and the odds ratio is only an approximation of this. However, the OR appears quite often in the literature, so it is important to be aware of it. It has certain mathematical properties that render it attractive as an alternative to the RR as a summary measure. Indeed, some statisticians argue that the odds ratio is the

Table 2.5 Comparison of RR and OR for different baseline rates

p_{Test}	$p_{Control}$	RR	OR	RR and OR
0.05	0.1	0.5	0.47	Close
0.1	0.2	0.5	0.44	Close
0.2	0.4	0.5	0.38	Not close
0.4	0.2	2	2.66	Not close
0.2	0.1	2	2.25	Close
0.1	0.05	2	2.11	Close

Table 2.6 Results of study on cannabis use and psychosis (Henquet et al, 2005)

Psychosis	Cannabis use		Total
	Yes	No	
Yes	82	342	424
No	238	1775	2013
Total	320	2117	2437

natural parameter and the relative risk merely an approximation. The OR features in logistic regression (see Section 9.6) and as a natural summary measure for case–control studies (see Section 12.8).

Example from the literature: Cohort study – psychosis and cannabis

Henquet et al (2005) took a random sample of 2437 normal adolescents and questioned them about their use of cannabis. They followed them up 4 years later and asked about psychotic symptoms. The results are summarised in Table 2.6.

The risk of psychosis for non-cannabis users is $342/2117 = 0.16$, while the risk of psychosis for cannabis users is $82/320 = 0.26$. Thus the relative risk of psychosis for cannabis smokers is $0.26/0.16 = 1.625$ or an increased risk of 62.5%.

The odds ratio of psychosis for cannabis smokers is $(82 \times 1775)/(342 \times 238) = 1.79$, which is close to the relative risk. This is because the chance of getting psychosis is still reasonably small. This is the result quoted by Henquet et al (2005), who used ORs because they analysed the data using logistic regression (see Section 9.6).

One point about the OR that can be seen immediately from the formula is that the OR for Failure as opposed to the OR for Success in Table 2.3 is given by $OR = bc/ad$. Thus the OR for Failure is just the inverse of the OR for Success.

Thus in the cannabis and psychosis study, the odds ratio of *not* developing psychosis for the cannabis group is $1/1.79 = 0.56$. In contrast the relative risk of *not* developing psychosis is $(1 - 0.26)/(1 - 0.16) = 0.88$, which is not the same as the inverse of the relative risk of developing psychosis for the cannabis group which is $1/1.625 = 0.62$.

This symmetry of interpretation of the OR is one of the reasons for its continued use.

2.2 Displaying categorical data

Categorical data may be displayed using either a *bar chart* or a *pie chart*. Figure 2.1 shows a bar chart of type of delivery for the 98 babies in the

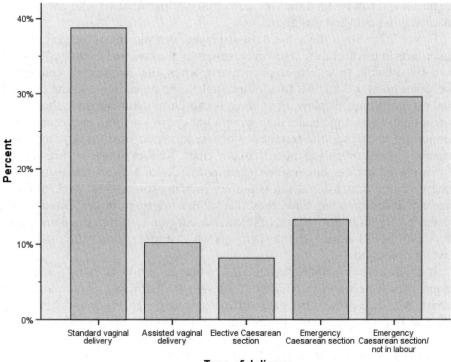

Figure 2.1 Bar chart showing type of delivery for 98 babies admitted to a special care baby unit (Simpson, 2004). Reproduced by permission of AG Simpson

(a) Without three-dimensional effects   (b) With three-dimensional effects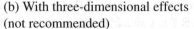
                                               (not recommended)

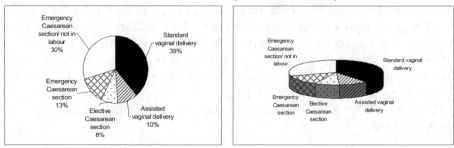

Figure 2.2   Pie chart showing type of delivery for 98 babies admitted to a special care baby unit (Simpson, 2004). Reproduced by permission of AG Simpson

Simpson (2004) study. Along the horizontal axis are the different delivery categories whilst on the vertical axis is percentage. Each bar represents the percentage of the total population in that category. For example, examining Figure 2.1, it can be seen that the percentage of participants who had a standard vaginal delivery was about 39%.

Figure 2.2a shows the same data displayed as a pie chart. One often sees pie charts in the literature. However, generally they are to be avoided as they can be difficult to interpret particularly when the number of categories becomes greater than five. In addition, unless the percentages in the individual categories are displayed (as here) it can be much more difficult to estimate them from a pie chart than from a bar chart. For both chart types it is important to include the number of observations on which it is based, particularly when comparing more than one chart. Neither of these charts should be displayed in three dimensions (see Figure 2.2b for a three-dimensional pie chart). Three-dimensional charts feature in many spreadsheet packages, but are not recommended since they distort the information presented. They make it very difficult to extract the correct information from the figure, and, for example in Figure 2.2b the segments which appear nearer the reader are over emphasised.

If the sample is further classified into whether or not the baby is a boy or a girl then it becomes impossible to present the data as a single pie or bar chart. We could present the data as two separate pie charts or bar charts side by side but it is preferably to present the data in one graph with the same scales and axes to make the visual comparisons easier.

In this case we could present the data as a *clustered* bar chart as shown in Figure 2.3. This clearly shows that there is a difference in the type of delivery experienced by mothers with male babies compared to female babies. Mothers with a female baby were more likely to have a normal vaginal delivery than mothers with a male baby. If we had used the actual counts on the vertical

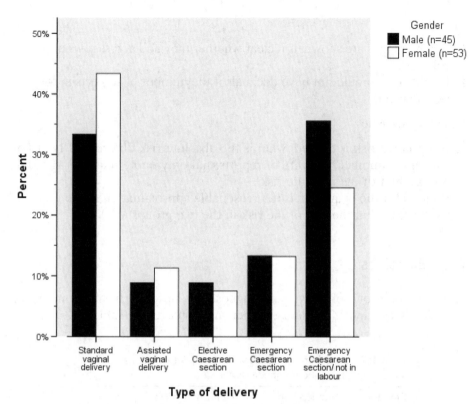

Figure 2.3 Clustered bar chart showing type of delivery by gender for 98 babies admitted to a special care baby unit (Simpson, 2004). Reproduced by permission of AG Simpson

axis, then because of the different sizes of the two groups, here, 45 male and 53 female babies, this difference in frequencies of type of delivery between the two groups may not have been as obvious.

If you do use the relative frequency scale as we have, then it is recommended good practice to report the actual total sample sizes for each group in the legend. In this way, given the total sample size and relative frequency (from the height of the bars) we can work out the actual numbers of mothers with the different types of delivery.

2.3 Points when reading the literature

In figures:

1. Is the number of subjects involved clearly stated?
2. Are appropriate axes clearly labelled and scales indicated?
3. Do the titles adequately describe the contents of the tables and graphs?

In tables:

1. If percentages are shown, is it clear whether they add across rows or down columns.
2. Percentages should not have decimals if the number of subjects in total is less than 100.

Summary statistics:

1. If a relative risk is quoted, what is the absolute risk difference? Is this a very small number? Beware of reports that only quote relative risks and give no hint of the absolute risk!
2. If an odds ratio is quoted, is it a reasonable approximation to the relative risk? (Ask what the size of the risk in the two groups are.)

2.4 Exercises

1. The blood group of 55 women diagnosed as suffering from thromboembolic disease and 145 healthy women are displayed in Table 2.7.

Table 2.7 Blood group distribution for healthy women and those with thromboembolic disease

Blood group	Women with thromboembolic disease	Healthy women	Total
A	32	51	83
B	8	19	27
AB	6	5	11
O	9	70	79
Total	55	145	200

   (i) Display the blood group data for the 55 thromboembolic women as a bar chart.
   (ii) Display the blood group data for the 55 thromboembolic women and 145 healthy women using a clustered bar chart. Can you see if there is a difference in the blood groups between the thromboembolic women and healthy women?

2. Ninety-nine pregnant women, with dystocia (difficult childbirth or labour), were allocated at random to receive immersion in water in a birth pool (Intervention group: Labour in water 49 women) or standard augmentation for dystocia (Control group: Augmentation 50 women) in a

randomised controlled trial to evaluate the impact of labouring in water during the first stage of labour (Cluett et al, 2004). The main outcome was use of epidural analgesia at any stage of labour. The results are shown in Table 2.8.

Table 2.8 Epidural analgesia data from a randomised controlled trial of labouring in water compared with standard augmentation for management of dystocia in first stage of labour (Cluett et al, 2004)

Epidural analgesia at any stage of labour	Intervention (Labour in water)	Control (Augmentation)
Yes	23	33
No	26	17
Total	49	50

(i) What is the proportion of women that had an epidural in each of the two groups?

(ii) What is the relative risk of the use of an epidural for the Labour in water women compared with the Augmentation women?

(iii) Calculate the OR of epidural for the Labour in water women compared with Augmentation women. Compare this estimated OR with the RR estimate from part ii: what do you notice?

(iv) Find the absolute risk difference for the use of an epidural for Labour in water compared to Augmentation.

3. A newspaper headline states that a new drug for early stage breast cancer reduces the risk of recurrence of the disease by 50%. What other information would you like before deciding to take the drug?

3 Describing and displaying quantitative data

Medical Statistics Fourth Edition, David Machin, Michael J Campbell, Stephen J Walters
© 2007 John Wiley & Sons, Ltd

Summary

This chapter discusses the choice and method of calculation of measures of location and variation. We cover means, medians, modes, range, standard deviation and inter-quartile range. We also illustrate methods of graphical and tabular display for continuous data.

3.1   Summarising continuous data

A quantitative measurement contains more information than a categorical one, and so summarizing these data is more complex. One chooses summary statistics to condense a large amount of information into a few intelligible numbers, the sort that could be communicated verbally. The two most important pieces of information about a quantitative measurement are 'where is it?' and 'how variable is it?' These are categorised as measures of location (or sometimes 'central tendency') and measures of spread or variability.

Measures of location

Mean or average   The arithmetic mean or average of n observations $\bar{x}$ (pronounced x bar) is simply the sum of the observations divided by their number; thus:

$$\bar{x} = \frac{\text{Sum of all sample values}}{\text{Size of sample}} = \frac{\sum_{i=1}^{n} x_i}{n}.$$

In the above equation, x_i represents the individual sample values and $\sum_{i=1}^{n} x_i$ their sum. The Greek letter 'Σ' (sigma) is the Greek capital 'S' and stands for 'sum' and simply means 'add up the n observations x_i from the 1st to the last (nth)'.

Example: Calculation of the mean – birthweights

Consider the following five birthweights in kilograms recorded to 1 decimal place selected randomly from the Simpson (2004) study of low birthweight babies which is described in more detail in Chapter 2.

$$1.2, 1.3, 1.4, 1.5, 2.1$$

The sum of these observations is $(1.2 + 1.3 + 1.4 + 1.5 + 2.1) = 7.5$. Thus the mean $\bar{x} = 7.5/5 = 1.50\,\text{kg}$. It is usual to quote 1 more decimal place for the mean than the data recorded.

The major advantage of the mean is that it uses all the data values, and is, in a statistical sense, efficient. The mean also characterises some important statistical distributions to be discussed in Chapter 4. The main disadvantage of the mean is that it is vulnerable to what are known as outliers. Outliers are single observations which, if excluded from the calculations, have noticeable influence on the results. For example if we had entered '21' instead of '2.1' in the calculation of the mean, we would find the mean changed from 1.50 kg to 7.98 kg. It does not necessarily follow, however, that outliers should be excluded from the final data summary, or that they result from an erroneous measurement.

If the data are binary, that is nominal data that can only have two values which are coded 0 or 1, then $\bar{x}$ is the proportion of individuals with value 1, and this can also be expressed as a percentage. Thus, in Simpson's data, if 15 out of 98 babies were very low birthweight (<1 kg) and if this is coded as a '1' in the data set, and a '0' coded for those above 1 kg, then the mean of this variable is 0.15 or 15%.

Median   The median is estimated by first ordering the data from smallest to largest, and then counting upwards for half the observations. The estimate of the median is either the observation at the centre of the ordering in the case of an odd number of observations, or the simple average of the middle two observations if the total number of observations is even.

Example: Calculation of the median – birthweights

Consider the following five birthweights in kilograms selected randomly from the Simpson (2004) study.

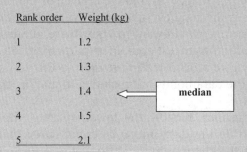

Rank order	Weight (kg)
1	1.2
2	1.3
3	1.4
4	1.5
5	2.1

If we had observed an additional value of 3.5 kg in the birthweight the median would be the average of the 3rd and the 4th observation in the ranking, namely the average of 1.4 and 1.5, which is 1.45 kg.

The median has the advantage that it is not affected by outliers, so for example the median in the data would be unaffected by replacing '2.1' with '21'. However, it is not statistically efficient, as it does not make use of all the individual data values.

Mode   A third measure of location is termed the mode. This is the value that occurs most frequently, or, if the data are grouped, the grouping with the highest frequency. It is not used much in statistical analysis, since its value depends on the accuracy with which the data are measured; although it may be useful for categorical data to describe the most frequent category. However, the expression 'bimodal' distribution is used to describe a distribution with two peaks in it. This can be caused by mixing two or more populations together. For example, height might appear to have a bimodal distribution if one had men and women in the population. Some illnesses may raise a biochemical measure, so in a population containing healthy individuals and those who are ill one might expect a bimodal distribution. However, some illnesses are *defined* by the measure of, say obesity or high blood pressure, and in these cases the distributions are usually unimodal with those above a given value regarded as *ill*.

Example from the literature: Mean, median and mode

In the study by Xu et al (2004) described in Chapter 1, the mean age of the 832 cases with cancer was 55.3 years, their median BMI was 25.1 and the modal marital status is the combined category 'married or cohabiting'.

Measures of dispersion or variability

Range and interquartile range   The range is given as the smallest and largest observations. This is the simplest measure of variability. For some data it is very useful, because one would want to know these numbers, for example in a sample the age of the youngest and oldest participant. However, if outliers are present it may give a distorted impression of the variability of the data, since only two of the data points are included in making the estimate.

Quartiles   The quartiles, namely the lower quartile, the median and the upper quartile, divide the data into four equal parts; that is there will be approximately equal numbers of observations in the four sections (and exactly equal if the sample size is divisible by four and the measures are all distinct). The quartiles are calculated in a similar way to the median; first order the data and then count the appropriate number from the bottom. The interquartile range is a useful measure of variability and is given by the difference of the lower and upper quartiles. The interquartile range is not vulnerable to outliers, and whatever the distribution of the data, we know that 50% of them lie within the interquartile range.

Illustrative example: Calculation of the range, quartiles and interquartile range

Suppose we had 10 birthweights arranged in increasing order from the Simpson (2004) study.

Order	Birthweight (kg)
1	1.51
2	1.55
3	1.79
4	2.10
5	2.18
6	2.22
7	2.37
8	2.40
9	2.81
10	2.85

3 ⟸ Lower quartile (25th percentile)

5 / 6 ⟸ Median (50th percentile)

Inter quartile range

8 ⟸ Upper quartile (75th percentile)

The range of birthweights in these data is from 1.51 kg to 2.85 kg (simply the smallest and largest birthweights).

The median is the average of the 5th and 6th observations $(2.18 + 2.22)/2 = 2.20$ kg. The first half of the data has five observations so the first quartile is the 3rd ranked observation, namely 1.79 kg, and similarly the third quartile would be the 8th ranked observation, namely 2.40 kg. So the interquartile range is from 1.79 to 2.40 kg.

Standard deviation and variance   The standard deviation (*SD* or *s*) is calculated as follows:

$$SD = s = \sqrt{\frac{\sum_{i=1}^{n}(x_i - \bar{x})^2}{n-1}}.$$

The expression $\Sigma_{i=1}^{n}(x_i - \bar{x})^2$ may look complicated, but it is easier to understand when thought of in stages. From each x value subtract the mean $\bar{x}$, square this difference, then add each of the n squared differences. This sum is then divided by $(n - 1)$. This expression is known as the *variance*. The variance is expressed in square units, so we take the square root to return to the original units, which gives the standard deviation, s. Examining this expression it can be seen that if all the x's were the same, then they would equal $\bar{x}$ and so s would be zero. If the x's were widely scattered about $\bar{x}$, then s would be large. In this way s reflects the variability in the data. The standard deviation is vulnerable to outliers, so if the 2.1 was replaced by 21 we would get a very different result.

Illustrative example: Calculation of the standard deviation

Consider the five birthweights (in kg): 1.2, 1.3, 1.4, 1.5, 2.1. The calculations to work out the standard deviation are given in the following table.

Subject	Weight (kg) x_i	Mean Weight (kg) $\bar{x}$	Differences from mean $x_i - \bar{x}$	Square of differences from mean $(x_i - \bar{x})^2$
1	1.2	1.5	−0.30	0.09
2	1.3	1.5	−0.20	0.04
3	1.4	1.5	−0.10	0.01
4	1.5	1.5	0.00	0.00
5	2.1	1.5	0.60	0.36
Totals (Sum)	7.5		0	0.50 kg^2
Mean	1.50		Variance	0.13 kg^2
n	5		Standard	
$n-1$	4		deviation	0.35 kg

Variance = 0.50/4

SD = square root of the Variance

We first find the mean to be 1.5 kg, then subtract this from each of the five observations to get the 'Differences from the mean'. Note that the sum of this column is zero. This will always be the case: the positive deviations from the mean cancel the negative ones.

A convenient method of removing the negative signs is by squaring the deviations, which is given in the next column, which is then summed to get 0.50 kg^2. Note that the bulk of this sum (72%) is contributed by one observation, the value 2.1 from subject 5, which is the observation furthest from the mean. This illustrates that much of the value of an SD is derived from the outlying observations. We now need to find the average squared deviation. Common sense would suggest dividing by n, but it turns out that this actually gives an estimate of the population variance which is too small. This is because we use the estimated mean $\bar{x}$ in the calculation in place of the true population mean. In fact we seldom know the population mean so there is little choice but for us to use its estimated value, $\bar{x}$, in the calculation (see Chapter 6). The consequence is that it is then better to divide by what are known as the *degrees of freedom*, which in this case is $n - 1$, to obtain the SD.

Why is the standard deviation useful? From Simpson's data, the mean and standard deviation of the birthweight of the 98 babies are 1.31 kg and 0.424 kg, respectively. It turns out in many situations that about 95% of observations will be within two standard deviations of the mean. This is known as a *reference interval* and it is this characteristic of the standard deviation which makes it so useful. It holds for a large number of measurements commonly made in medicine. In particular it holds for data that follow a Normal distribution (see Chapter 4). For this example, this implies that the majority of babies will weigh between 0.46 and 2.16 kg.

Standard deviation is often abbreviated to SD in the medical literature.

Example from the literature: Interquartile range and standard deviation – age of menopause

Xu et al (2004) gave the median of the age of menopause for cases as 50.1 years and the interquartile range is 48.6 to 52.5. Thus we know that 50% of women experienced the menopause within a 4-year age range.

It is somewhat unfortunate that although they follow good practice and give the interquartile range for age at menarche and age at menopause, which will both have non-Normal distributions, they give the $SD = 8.60$ for the age of cases at the time of study, although this too is likely to have a non-Normal distribution.

Means or medians?   Means and medians convey different impressions of the location of data, and one cannot give a prescription as to which is preferable; often both give useful information. If the distribution is symmetric, then in general the mean is the better summary statistic, and if it is skewed then the median is less influenced by the tails. If the data are skewed, then the median will reflect a 'typical' individual better. For example if in a country median income is £20 000 and mean income is £24 000, most people will relate better to the former number.

It is sometimes stated, incorrectly, that the mean cannot be used with nominal, or ordered categorical data but, as we have noted before, if nominal data are scored 0/1 then the mean is simply the proportion of 1's. If the data are ordered categorically, then again the data can be scored, say 1, 2, 3, etc., and a mean calculated. This can often give more useful information than a median for such data, but should be used with care, because of the implicit assumption that the change from score 1 to 2, say, has the same meaning (value) as the change from score 2 to 3, and so on.

3.2   Displaying continuous data

A picture is worth a thousand words, or numbers, and there is no better way of getting a 'feel' for the data than to display them in a figure or graph. The general principle should be to convey as much information as possible in the figure, with the constraint that the reader is not overwhelmed by too much detail.

Dot plots

The simplest method of conveying as much information as possible is to show all of the data and this can be conveniently carried out using a dot plot.

Example: Dot plot – birthweights

The data on birthweight and type of delivery are shown in Figure 3.1 as a dot plot. This method of presentation retains the individual subject values and clearly demonstrates differences between the groups in a readily appreciated manner. An additional advantage is that any outliers will be detected by such a plot. However, such presentation is not usually practical with large numbers of subjects in each group because the dots will obscure the details of the distribution.

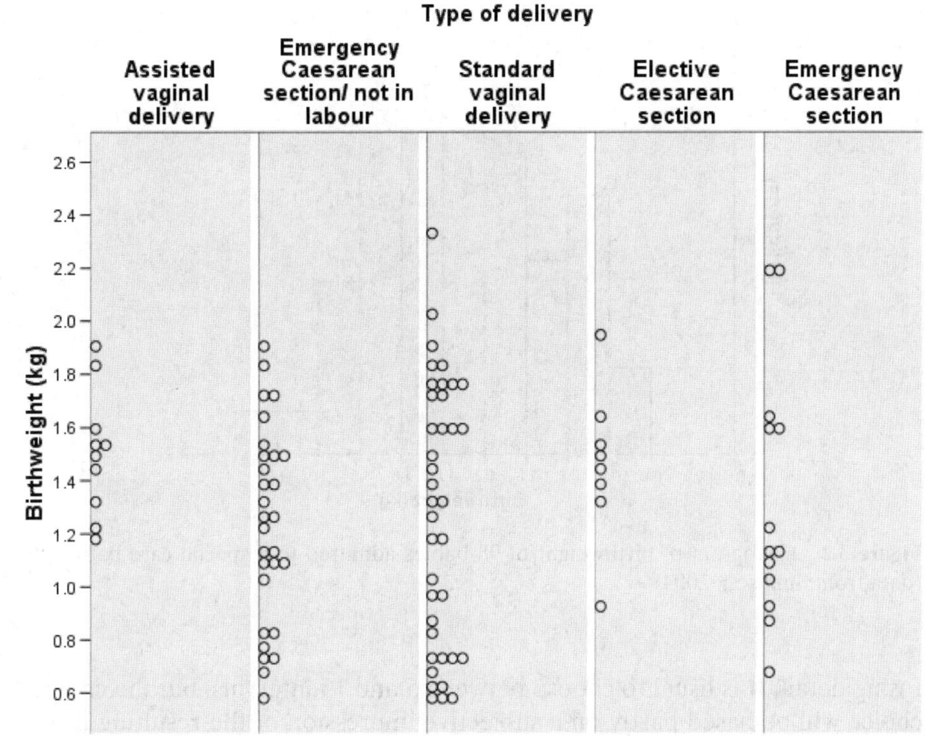

Type of delivery

Figure 3.1   Dot plot showing birth weight by type of delivery for 98 babies admitted to a special care baby unit (data from Simpson, 2004)

Histograms

The patterns may be revealed in large data set of a numerically continuous variable by forming a histogram with them. This is constructed by first dividing up the range of variable into several non-overlapping and equal intervals, classes or bins, then counting the number of observations in each. A histogram for all the birthweights in the Simpson (2004) data is shown in Figure 3.2. In this histogram the intervals corresponded to a width of 0.2 kg. The area of each histogram block is proportional to the number of subjects in the particular birthweight category concentration group. Thus the total area in the histogram blocks represents the total number of babies.

Relative frequency histograms allow comparison between histograms made up of different numbers of observations which may be useful when studies are compared.

The choice of the number and width of intervals or bins is important. Too few intervals and much important information may be smoothed out; too many intervals and the underlying shape will be obscured by a mass of con-

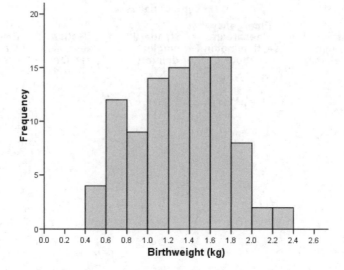

Figure 3.2   Histogram of birthweight of 98 babies admitted to a special care baby unit (data from Simpson, 2004)

fusing detail. It is usual to choose between 5 and 15 intervals, but the correct choice will be based partly on a subjective impression of the resulting histogram. Histograms with bins of unequal interval length can be constructed but they are usually best avoided.

Box-whisker plot

If the number of points is large, a dot plot can be replaced by a box-whisker plot which is more compact than the corresponding histogram.

> ### Illustrative example: Box-whisker plot – birthweight by type of delivery
>
> A box-whisker a plot is illustrated in Figure 3.3 for the birthweight and type of delivery from Simpson (2004). The 'whiskers' in the diagram indicate the minimum and maximum values of the variable under consideration. The median value is indicated by the central horizontal line while the lower and upper quartiles by the corresponding horizontal ends of the box. The shaded box itself represents the interquartile range. The box-whisker plot as used here therefore displays the median and two measures of spread, namely the range and interquartile range.

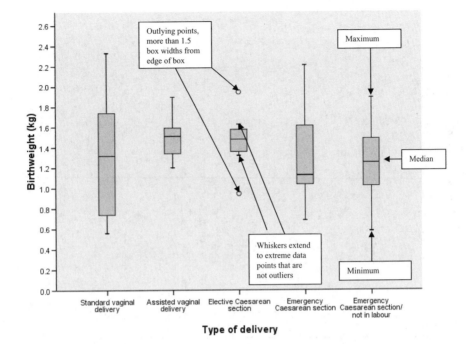

Figure 3.3 Box-whisker plot of birthweight by method of delivery for 98 babies admitted to a special care baby unit (data from Simpson, 2004)

Scatter plots

When one wishes to illustrate a relationship between two continuous variables, a scatter plot of one against the other may be informative.

Illustrative example: Scatter plot – birthweight by maternal age

A scatter plot is illustrated in Figure 3.4 for the birthweight of 98 babies against their mother's age. The sloping line is the regression line (see Chapter 9) of birthweight on maternal age.

It is clear from the almost flat or horizontal regression line that the birthweight and maternal age are not associated in this sample of babies. In theory it is possible that maternal age may have an influence on birthweight, but vice versa cannot be the case. In this case, if one variable, x, (maternal age) could cause the other, y, (birthweight) then it is usual to plot the x variable on the horizontal axis and the y variable on the vertical axis.

In contrast, if we were interested in the relationship between mothers' weight and height then either variable could cause or influence the other. In this example it would be immaterial which variable (height or weight) is plotted on which axis.

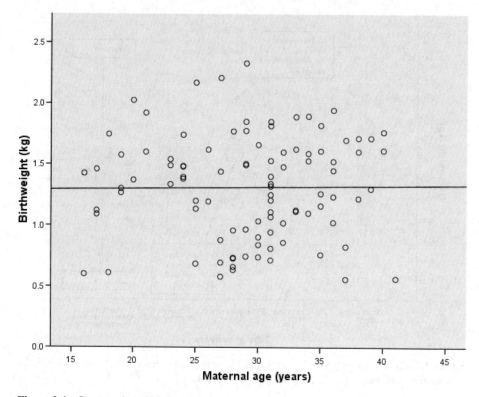

Figure 3.4   Scatter plot of birthweight by maternal age, for 98 babies admitted to a special care baby unit (data from Simpson, 2004)

Measures of symmetry

One important reason for producing dot plots and histograms is to get some idea of the shape of the distribution of the data. In Figure 3.2 there is a (slight) suggestion that the distribution of birthweight is not symmetric; that is if the distribution were folded over some central point, the two halves of the distribution would not coincide. When this is the case, the distribution is termed *skewed*. A distribution is right (left) skewed if the longer tail is to the right (left) (see Figure 3.5). If the distribution is symmetric then the median and mean will be close. If the distribution is skewed then the median and inter-quartile range are in general more appropriate summary measures than the mean and standard deviation, since the latter are sensitive to the skewness.

For Simpson's birthweight data the mean from the 98 babies is 1.31 kg and the median is 1.34 kg so we conclude the data are reasonably symmetric. One is more likely to see skewness when the variables are constrained at one end or the other. For example waiting time or time in hospital cannot be negative, but can be very large for some patients and relatively short for the majority.

Right or positively skewed   Left or negatively skewed

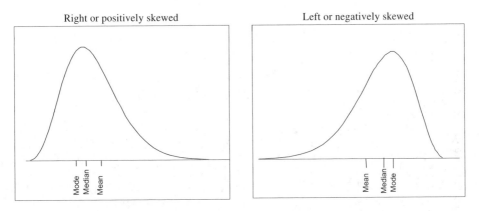

Figure 3.5 Examples of two skewed distributions

In the data from Xu et al (2004), the median age at menopause for cases is 50.1 years, but this is not exactly mid way between the first quartile and third quartiles of 48.6 and 52.5 years respectively, thus indicating a skewed rather than a symmetric distribution.

A common skewed distribution is annual income, where a few high earners pull up the mean, but not the median. In the UK about 68% of the population earn less than the average wage, that is, the mean value of annual pay is equivalent to the 68th percentile on the income distribution. Thus many people who earn more than the earnings of 50% (the median) of the population will still feel under paid!

3.3 Within-subject variability

In Figure 3.1, measurements were made only once for each baby – the subject. Thus the variability, expressed, say, by the standard deviation, is the *between-subject* variability. If, however, measurements are made repeatedly on one subject, we are assessing *within-subject* variability.

Illustrative example: Within-subject variability – resting carotid pulse rate

Figure 3.6 shows an example in which the resting carotid pulse rate, assessed by counting the beats in the neck against the second hand of a watch for 1 minute, was measured every 5 minutes for an hour. The observed pulse rate is subject to fluctuations. The subject was at rest and receiving no active therapy; nevertheless there is considerable minute-to-minute variation but little evidence of any trend over time. Such variation is termed *within-subject variation*. The *within-subject* standard deviation in this case is $SD = 2.2$ with a mean pulse rate of 63.0 beats/minute.

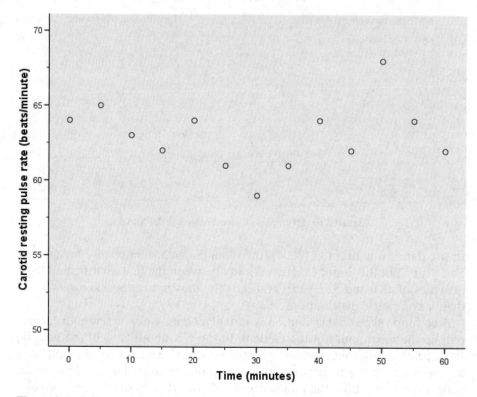

Figure 3.6 Self-assessed resting carotid pulse rate as recorded every 5 minutes for 1 minute for an hour

If another subject had also done this experiment, we could calculate their within-subject variation as well, and perhaps compare the variabilities for the two subjects using these summary measures.

Successive within-subject values are unlikely to be independent, that is, consecutive values will be dependent on values preceding them. For example, if a patient with heart disease records their pulse rate, then if pulse rate is low on one day it is likely to be low the next. This does not imply that the pulse will be low, only that it is a good bet that it will be. In contrast, examples can be found in which high values of pulse rate are usually followed by lower values and vice versa. With independent observations, the pulse rate on one day gives no indication or clue as to the pulse rate on the next.

It is clear from Figure 3.6 that the pulse rates are not constant over the observation period. This is nearly always the case when medical observations or measurements are taken over time. Such variation occurs for a variety of reasons. For example, pulse rate may depend critically on when the patient last exercised, medication, pacemakers or even on the time of day if some diurnal rhythm is influencing levels. In addition, there may be variability in the actual measurement of pulse rate, induced possibly by the patient's perception of pulse rate itself being subject to variation. There may be observer-to-observer variation if the successive pulse rates were recorded by different personnel rather than always the patient. The possibility of recording errors in the laboratory, transcription errors when conveying the results to the clinic or for statistical analysis, should not be overlooked in appropriate circumstances. When only a single observation is made on one patient at one time only, then the influences of the above sources of variation are not assessable, but may nevertheless all be reflected to some extent in the final entry in the patient's record.

Suppose successive observations on a patient taken over time fluctuate around some more or less constant pulse rate, then the particular level may be influenced by factors within the patient. For example, pulse rates may be affected by the presence of a viral infection which is unrelated to the cause of the heart disease itself. Levels may also be influenced by the severity of the underlying condition and whether concomitant treatment is necessary for the patient. Levels could also be influenced by other factors, for example, alcohol, tobacco consumption and diet. The cause of some of the variation in pulse rates may be identified and its effect on the variability estimated. Other variation may have no obvious explanation and is usually termed *random* variation. This does not necessarily imply there is no cause of this component of the variation but rather that its cause has not been identified or is being ignored.

Different patients with heart disease observed in the same way may have differing average levels of pulse rate from each other but with similar patterns of variation about these levels. The variation in mean pulse rate levels from patient to patient is termed *between-subject variation*.

Observations on different subjects are usually regarded as independent. That is, the data values on one subject are not influenced by those obtained from another. This, however, may not always be the case, particularly with subjective measures in which different patients may collaborate in recording their pulse rate.

In the investigation of total variability it is very important to distinguish within-subject from between-subject variability. In a study there may be measures made on different individuals and also repeatedly on the same individual. Between- and within-subject variation will always be present in any biological material, whether animals, healthy subjects, patients or histological sections. The experimenter must be aware of possible sources which contribute to the variation, decide which are of importance in the intended study, and design the study appropriately.

3.4 Presentation

Graphs

In any graph there are clearly certain items that are important. For example, scales should be labelled clearly with appropriate dimensions added. The plotting symbols are also important; a graph is used to give an impression of pattern in the data, so bold and relatively large plotting symbols are desirable. By all means identify the position of the point with a fine pen but mark it so others can see. This is particularly important if it is to be reduced for publication purposes or presented as a slide in a talk.

A graph should never include too much clutter; for example, many overlapping groups each with a different symbol. In such a case it is usually preferable to give a series of graphs, albeit smaller, in several panels. The choice of scales for the axes will depend on the particular data set. If transformations of the axes are used, for example, plotting on a log scale, it is usually better to mark the axes using the original units as this will be more readily understood by the reader. Breaks in scales should be avoided. If breaks are unavoidable under no circumstances must points on either side of a break be joined. If both axes have the same units, then use the same scale for each. If this cannot be done easily, it is sensible to indicate the line of equality, perhaps faintly in the figure. False impressions of trend or lack of it, in a time plot can sometimes be introduced by omitting the zero point of the vertical axis. This may falsely make a mild trend, for example a change from 101 to 105, into an apparently strong trend (seemingly as though from 1 to 5). There must always be a compromise between clarity of reproduction that is filling the space available with data points and clarity of message. Appropriate measures of variability should also be included. One such is to indicate the range of values covered by two standard deviations each side of a plotted mean.

It is important to distinguish between a bar-chart and a histogram. Bar-charts display counts in mutually exclusive categories, and so the bars should have spaces between them. Histograms show the distribution of a continuous variable and so should not have spaces between the bars. It is not acceptable to use a bar-chart to display a mean with standard error bars (see Chapter 6). These should be indicated with a data point surrounded with errors bars, or better still a 95% confidence interval.

With currently available graphics software one can now perform extensive exploration of the data, not only to determine more carefully their structure, but also to find the best means of summary and presentation. This is usually worth considerable effort.

Tables

Although graphical presentation is very desirable it should not be over-looked that tabular methods are very important (see Table 1.1). In particular, tables can give more precise numerical information than a graph, such as the number of observations, the mean and some measure of variability of each tabular entry. They often take less space than a graph containing the same information. Standard statistical computer software can be easily programmed to provide basic summary statistics in tabular form on many variables.

3.5 Points when reading the literature

1. Is the number of subjects involved clearly stated?
2. Are appropriate measures of location and variation used in the paper? For example, if the distribution of the data is skewed, then has the median rather the mean been quoted? Is it sensible to quote a standard deviation, or would a range or interquartile range, be better? In general do *not* use SD for data which have skewed distributions.
3. On graphs, are appropriate axes clearly labelled and scales indicated?
4. Do the titles adequately describe the contents of the tables and graphs?
5. Do the graphs indicate the relevant variability? For example, if the main object of the study is a within-subject comparison, has within-subject variability been illustrated?
6. Does the method of display convey all the relevant information in a study? For example if the data are paired, is the pairing shown? Can one assess the distribution of the data from the information given?

3.6 Exercises

1. The age (in years) of a sample of 20 motor cyclists killed in road traffic accidents is given below.

18	41	24	28	71	52	15	20	21	31
16	24	33	44	20	24	16	64	24	32

   (i) Draw a dot plot and histogram. Is this distribution symmetric or skewed?
   (ii) Calculate the mean, median and mode.
   (iii) Calculate the range, inter quartile range and standard deviation. Which of these is better to describe the variability of these data?

2. The table below shows the height of 12 fathers and their fully-grown sons.

Father's height (cm)	Son's height (cm)
190	189
184	186
183	180
182	179
179	187
178	184
175	183
174	171
170	170
168	178
165	174
164	165

(i) Draw a scatter plot of father's height versus son's height.

(ii) From the graph does there appear to be a relationship between the two variables?

4 Probability and decision making

Medical Statistics Fourth Edition, David Machin, Michael J Campbell, Stephen J Walters
© 2007 John Wiley & Sons, Ltd

Summary

Probability is defined in terms of either the long-term frequency of events, as model based or as a subjective measure of the certainty of an event happening. Examples of each type are given. The ideas associated with the study of probability are illustrated in the context of diagnostic tests. The two major elements associated with the clinical value of diagnostic tests are their sensitivity and their specificity. The concepts of independent events and mutually exclusive events are discussed, and the use of Bayes' theorem is demonstrated. When the result of a diagnostic test is a continuous variable, there may be difficulty in deciding an appropriate cut-off point to categorise those with and without the condition of interest, and relative operating characteristic (ROC) curves can be used to help with the decision.

4.1   Types of probability

There are three main ways of looking at probability which we are described as the 'frequency', 'model-based' and 'subjective' approaches as shown in Figure 4.1.

We all have an intuitive feel for probability but it is important to distinguish between probabilities applied to single individuals and probabilities applied to groups of individuals. Every year about 600000 people die in United Kingdom. From year to year this number is stable to an extent that surprises some people, (see Figure 4.2) and statisticians are able to predict it with better than 99% accuracy. There are about 60 million people in the United Kingdom and for a single individual, with no information about his age or state of health, the chances of him or her dying in any particular year are 600000/60000000 or about 1 in 100. This is termed the crude mortality rate as it ignores differences in individuals due, for example, to their gender or age, which are known to influence mortality. Thus the number of deaths

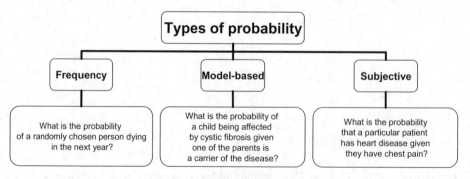

Figure 4.1   Three types of probability

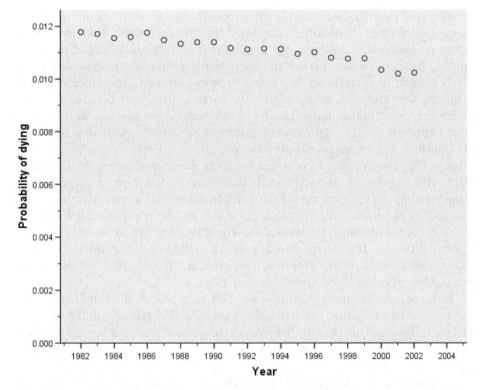

Figure 4.2 Crude mortality rates in the United Kingdom from 1982 to 2002 (from ONS, 2004). Crown copyright material is reproduced with the permission of the Controller of OPSI and the Queen's Printer

in a group can be accurately predicted but, despite this, it is not possible to predict exactly which of the individuals are going to die.

The basis of the idea of probability is a sequence of what are known as independent trials. To calculate the probability of an individual dying in 1 year we give each one of a group of individuals a trial over a year and the event occurs if the individual dies. As in the previous paragraph, the estimate of the (crude) probability of dying is the number of deaths divided by the number in the original group. The idea of independence is difficult, but is based on the fact that whether or not one individual survives or dies does not affect the chance of another individual's survival. On a very simple level and where the probability of an event is known in advance, consider tossing one coin 100 times. Each toss of the coin is a 'trial' and the event might be 'heads'. If the coin is unbiased, that is one which has no preference for 'heads' or 'tails', we would expect heads half of the time and thus say the probability of a head is 0.5.

The probability of an event is the proportion of times it occurs in a long sequence of trials. Thus, when it is stated that the probability that an unborn child is male is 0.51, we base our expectation on large numbers of previous births. Similarly, when it is stated that patients with a certain disease have a 50% chance of surviving 5 years, this is based on past experience of other patients with the same disease. In some cases a 'trial' may be generated by randomly selecting an individual from the general population, as discussed in Chapters 6 and 12, and examining him or her for the particular attribute in question. For example, suppose the prevalence of diabetes in the population is 1%. The prevalence of a disease is the number of people in a population with the disease at a certain time divided by the number of people in the population (see Chapter 12 for further details). If a trial was then conducted by randomly selecting one person from the population and testing him or her for diabetes, the individual would be expected to be diabetic with probability 0.01. If this type of sampling of individuals from the population were repeated, then the proportion of diabetics in the total sample taken would be expected to be approximately 1%.

However, in some situations we can determine probabilities without repeated sampling. For example, we know that the possibility of a '6' when throwing a die is 1/6, because there are six possibilities, all equally likely. Nevertheless we may wish to conduct a series of trials to verify this fact.

In genetics, if a child has cystic fibrosis but neither parent was affected, then it is known that each parent must have genotype cC, where c denotes a cystic fibrosis gene and C denotes a normal gene. The possibility that one of the parents is cc is discounted, as this would imply that one parent had cystic fibrosis. In any subsequent child in that family there are four possible and equally likely genotype combinations: cc, Cc, cC and CC. Only cc leads to the disease. Thus it is known that the probability of a subsequent child being affected is 1/4, and *if* the child is not affected (and so is Cc, cC or CC), the probability of being a carrier (type Cc or cC) is 2/3. These 'model based' probabilities are not based on repeated examinations of families with cystic fibrosis, but rather on the Mendelian theory of genetics.

Another type of probability is 'subjective' probability. When a patient presents with chest pains, a clinician may, after a preliminary examination, say that the probability that the patient has heart disease is about 20%. However, although the clinician does not know this yet, the individual patient either has or has not got heart disease. Thus at this early stage of investigation the probability is a measure of the 'strength of the belief' of the clinician in the two alternative hypotheses, that the patient has got heart disease. The next step is then to proceed to further examinations of the patient in order to modify the strength of this initial subjective belief so that he or she becomes more certain of which is the true situation – the patient has heart disease or the patient does not.

The three types of probability all have the following properties.

- All probabilities lie between 0 and 1.
- When the outcome can never happen the probability is 0.
- When the outcome will definitely happen the probability is 1.

4.2 Diagnostic tests

Uses of a diagnostic test

In making a diagnosis, a clinician first establishes a possible set of diagnostic alternatives and then attempts to reduce these by progressively ruling out specific diseases or conditions. Alternatively, the clinician may have a strong hunch that the patient has one particular disease and he then sets about confirming it. Given a particular diagnosis, a good diagnostic test should indicate either that the disease is very unlikely or that it is very probable. In a practical sense it is important to realise that a diagnostic test is useful only if the result influences patient management since, if the management is the same for two different conditions, there is little point in trying strenuously to distinguish between them.

Sensitivity and specificity

Many diagnostic test results are given in the form of a continuous variable (that is one that can take any value within a given range), such as diastolic blood pressure or haemoglobin level. However, for ease of discussion we will first assume that these have been divided into positive or negative results. For example, a positive diagnostic result of 'hypertension' is a diastolic blood pressure greater than 90 mmHg; whereas for 'anaemia', a haemoglobin level less than 10 g/dl is required. How to best choose these cut-off points is addressed later in this chapter.

For every diagnostic procedure (which may involve a laboratory test of a sample taken) there is a set of fundamental questions that should be asked. First, if the disease is present, what is the probability that the test result will be positive? This leads to the notion of the sensitivity of the test. Second, if the disease is absent, what is the probability that the test result will be negative? This question refers to the specificity of the test. These questions can be answered only if it is known what the 'true' diagnosis is. In the case of organic disease this can be determined by biopsy or, for example, an expensive and risky procedure such as angiography for heart disease. In other situations it may be by 'expert' opinion. Such tests provide the so-called 'gold standard'.

Example from the literature: Diagnosis of heart disease

Consider the results of an assay of N-terminal pro-brain natriuretic peptide (NT-proBNP) for diagnosis of heart failure in a general population survey in those over 45 years of age and in patients with existing diagnosis of heart failure obtained by Hobbs et al (2002) and summarised in Table 4.1. Heart failure was identified when NT-proBNP >36 pmol/l.

Table 4.1　Results of NT-proBNP assay in the general population over 45 and those with a previous diagnosis of heart failure (after Hobbs et al, 2002)

NT-proBNP (pmol/l)		Confirmed diagnosis of heart failure		
		Present	Absent	Total
		(D+)	(D−)	
>36	Positive (T+)	35 (a)	7 (b)	42
≤36	Negative (T−)	68 (c)	300 (d)	368
Total		103	307	410

We denote a positive test result by $T+$, and a positive diagnosis of heart failure (the disease) by $D+$. The prevalence of heart failure in these subjects is $(a + c)/(a + b + c + d) = 103/410 = 0.251$ or approximately 25%. Thus, the probability of a subject chosen at random from the combined group having the disease is estimated to be 0.251. We can write this as $p(D+) = 0.251$.

The *sensitivity* of a test is the proportion of those with the disease who also have a positive test result. Thus the sensitivity is $a/(a + c) = 35/103 = 0.340$ or 34%. Now sensitivity is the probability of a positive test result (event $T+$) given that the disease is present (event $D+$) and can be written as $p(T+|D+) = 0.340$, where the '|' is read as 'given'.

The *specificity* of the test is the proportion of those without disease who give a negative test result. Thus the specificity is $d/(b + d) = 300/307 = 0.977$ or 98%. Now specificity is the probability of a negative test result (event $T−$) given that the disease is absent (event $D−$) and can be written as $p(T−|D−) = 0.977$.

Since sensitivity is *conditional* on the disease being present, and specificity on the disease being absent, in theory, they are unaffected by disease prevalence. For example, if we doubled the number of subjects with true heart failure from 103 to 206 in Table 4.1, so that the prevalence was now $206/(410) = 50\%$, then we could expect twice as many subjects to give a positive test result. Thus $2 \times 35 = 70$ would have a positive result. In this case

Table 4.2 Summary of definitions of sensitivity and specificity

Test result	True diagnosis	
	Disease present	Disease absent
Positive	Sensitivity	Probability of a false positive
Negative	Probability of a false negative	Specificity

the sensitivity would be 70/206 = 0.34, which is unchanged from the previous value. A similar result is obtained for specificity.

Sensitivity and specificity are useful statistics because they will yield consistent results for the diagnostic test in a variety of patient groups with different disease prevalences. This is an important point; sensitivity and specificity are characteristics of the test, not the population to which the test is applied. Although indeed they are independent of disease prevalence, in practice if the disease is very rare, the accuracy with which one can estimate the sensitivity will be limited.

Two other terms in common use are: *the false negative rate* (*or probability of a false negative*) which is given by $c/(a + c) = 1 -$ Sensitivity, and the false positive rate (or probability of a false positive) or $b/(b + d) = 1 -$ Specificity.

These concepts are summarised in Table 4.2. In such tables it is important for consistency always to put true diagnosis on the top, and test result down the side. Since sensitivity = 1 - Probability(false **n**egative) and specificity = 1 - Probability(false **p**ositive), a possibly useful mnemonic to recall this is that 'se**n**sitivity' and '**n**egative' have '**n**'s in them and 's**p**ecificity' and '**p**ositive' have '**p**'s in them.

4.3 Bayes' Theorem

Predictive value of a test

Suppose a clinician is confronted by a patient over 45 years with symptoms suggestive of heart failure, and that the results of the study described in Table 4.1 are to hand. The doctor therefore believes that the patient has coronary artery disease with probability 0.25. Expressed in gambling terms of betting, one would be willing to bet with odds of about 0.25 to 0.75 or 1 to 3 that the patient does have heart failure. The patient then has the assay of NT-proBNP and the result is positive. How does this modify the odds?

It is first necessary to calculate the probability of the patient having the disease, given a positive test result. From Table 4.1, there are 103 subjects with a positive test, of whom 35 have heart failure. Thus, the estimate of 0.251

for the patient is adjusted upwards to the probability of disease with a positive test result which equals $35/(35 + 7) = 35/42 = 0.833$.

This gives the *predictive value of a positive test* or $p(D+|T+)$. The *predictive value of a negative test* is $p(D-|T-)$.

From Table 4.1 the predictive value of a positive NT-proBNP assay is $35/42 = 0.833$ and the predictive value of a negative assay is $300/368 = 0.815$. These values are affected by the prevalence of the disease. For example, if those with the disease doubled in Table 4.1, then the predictive value of a positive assay would then become $70/(70 + 7) = 0.909$ and the predictive value of a negative assay $300/(300 + 136) = 0.688$.

How does the predictive value $p(D+|T+)$ relate to sensitivity $p(T+|D+)$? Clearly the former is what the clinician requires and the latter is what is supplied with the test. To determine this we need some more details concerned with probability.

Multiplication rule and Bayes' Theorem

For any two events A and B, the joint probability of A *and* B, that is the probability of both A and B occurring simultaneously, is equal to the product of the probability of A given B times the probability of B, thus:

$$p(A \text{ and } B) = p(A|B) \times p(B).$$

This is known as *the multiplication rule* of probabilities.

Suppose event A occurs when the NT-proBNP assay is positive and event B occurs when heart failure is truly present. The probability of having both a positive assay and heart failure is thus $p(T+ \text{ and } D+)$. From Table 4.1, the probability of picking out one subject with both a positive assay and heart failure from the combined group of 410 subjects is $35/410 = 0.085$.

However, from the multiplication rule

$$p(T+ \text{ and } D+) = p(T+|D+) \times p(D+).$$

Now $p(T+|D+) = 0.340$ is the sensitivity of the test and $p(D+) = 0.251$ is the prevalence of heart failure and so $p(T+ \text{ and } D+) = 0.340 \times 0.251 = 0.085$, as before.

It does not matter if the labelling of disease and test had been reversed, that is adopting the convention that A occurs when heart failure is present and B occurs when the assay is positive, and so it is clear that $p(A \text{ and } B) = p(B \text{ and } A)$. From the multiplication rule it follows that

$$p(A|B)p(B) = p(B|A)p(A).$$

This leads to what is known as *Bayes' theorem* or

$$p(B|A) = \frac{p(A|B)p(B)}{p(A)}.$$

This formula is not appropriate if $p(A) = 0$, that is if A is an event which cannot happen.

Bayes' theorem enables the predictive value of a positive test to be related to the sensitivity of the test, and the predictive value of a negative test to be related to the specificity of the test. Bayes' theorem enables *prior* assessments about the chances of a diagnosis to be combined with the eventual test results to obtain an *a posteriori* assessment about the diagnosis. It reflects the procedure of making a clinical judgement.

In terms of Bayes' theorem, the diagnostic process is summarised by

$$p(D+|T+) = \frac{p(T+|D+)p(D+)}{p(T+)}.$$

The probability $p(D+)$ is the *a priori* probability and $p(D+|T+)$ is the *a posteriori* probability.

Bayes' theorem is usefully summarised when we express it in terms of the *odds* of an event, rather than the probability. Formally, if the probability of an event is p, then the odds are defined as $p/(1 - p)$. The probability that an individual has heart failure, before testing, from Table 4.1 is 0.251, and so the odds are $0.251/(1 - 0.251) = 0.335$, often written as $1:0.335$ or approximately $3:1$.

Illustrative example: Bayes' theorem NT – proBNP assay for heart failure

This example illustrates Bayes' theorem in practice by calculating the positive predictive value for the data of Table 4.1. There, $p(T+) = 42/410 = 0.102$, $p(D+) = 0.251$ and $p(T+|D+) = 0.340$ thus

$$p(D+|T+) = \frac{\text{Sensitivity} \times \text{Prevalence}}{\text{Probability of positive result}}$$
$$= \frac{p(T+|D+)p(D+)}{p(T+)}$$
$$= \frac{0.340 \times 0.251}{0.102} = 0.837.$$

Example: Positive predictive value

The prevalence of a disease is 1 in 1000, and there is a test that can detect it with a sensitivity of 100% and specificity of 95%. What is the probability that a person has the disease, given a positive result on the test?

To calculate the probability of a positive result consider 1000 people in which one person has the disease. The test will certainly detect this one person. However, it will also give a positive result on 5% of the 999 people without the disease. Thus the total positives is $1 + (0.05 \times 999) = 50.95$ and the probability is $50.95/1000 = 0.0595$. Thus,

$$p(D+|T+) = \frac{1 \times 0.001}{0.05095} = 0.02.$$

Likelihood ratio

The clear simplicity of diagnostic test data, particularly when presented as a 2×2 table, (see Table 4.1), is confounded by the many ways of reporting the results (Table 4.2). The likelihood ratio (LR) is a simple measure combining sensitivity and specificity defined as

$$LR = \frac{p(T+|D+)}{p(T+|D-)} = \frac{Sensitivity}{1 - Specificity}$$

It can be shown that Bayes' theorem can be summarised by:

Odds of disease after test = Odds of disease before test $\times$ LR.

Example: Likelihood ratio – NT-proBNP assay for heart failure

From Table 4.1, the prevalence of heart failure in these subjects is $= 103/410 = 0.251$, so the pre-test odds of disease are $0.251/(1 - 0.251) = 0.34$. The $LR = 0.340/(1 - 0.977) = 14.8$, and so the odds of the disease after the test are $14.8 \times 0.341 = 5.1$. This can be verified from the post-test probability of $p(D+|T+) = 0.833$ calculated earlier, so that the post-test odds are $0.833/(1 - 0.833) = 5.0$. This differs from the 5.1 only because of rounding errors in the calculation. So the pre-test odds of heart failure of 0.34 have changed to a post-test odds (of heart failure) of 5.0 following a positive test result.

The usefulness of a test will depend upon the prevalence of the disease in the population to which it has been applied.

Example: Predictive value and prevalence of the disease – NT-proBNP assay for heart failure

Table 4.3 gives details of the predictive values of a positive and a NT-proBNP assay test assuming the sensitivity and specificity are 0.340 and 0.977 respectively, but the prevalence of heart failure varies from 0.05 to 0.95. In this example, likelihood ratio, $LR = 0.340/0.023 = 14.8$.

In general a useful test is one which considerably modifies the pre-test probability. From Table 4.3 one can see that if the disease is very rare or very common, with a prevalence of 0.05 or 0.95 then the probabilities of disease given a positive test are reasonably close to the prevalence and the probability of a negative test is close to $(1 - \text{Prevalence})$, and so the test is of questionable value.

Example from the literature

Shaw et al (2004) compared detection of aspiration (the entry of secretions or foreign material into the trachea and lungs) by bedside examination made by a bronchial auscultation team (Speech and Language Therapist, and Physiotherapist) compared with videofluoroscopy, as the 'gold standard' in 105 patients with dysphagia (difficulty swallowing). The results for the three most commonly diagnosed conditions are given in Table 4.4.

In Table 4.4 it can be seen that sensitivity and specificity are to some extent complementary. The bedside examination made by a bronchial auscultation team is quite sensitive to the diagnosis of risk of aspiration, at the price of not being very specific. On the other hand, for the other two conditions, the bronchial auscultation team is not very sensitive, but is very unlikely to diagnose the conditions, if they are not present.

Table 4.3 Illustration of how predictive value changes with prevalence of the disease in question

Initial probability of disease (prevalence)	Predictive value of positive test	Predictive value of negative test	Useful test?
0.05	0.44	0.97	No
0.50	0.94	0.60	Yes
0.70	0.97	0.39	Yes
0.95	1.00	0.07	No

Table 4.4 Comparison of detection of aspiration by bedside examination made by a bronchial auscultation team (Speech and Language Therapist, and Physiotherapist) compared with videofluoroscopy

Diagnosis	Sensitivity	Specificity	Positive predictive value (%)
Risk of aspiration	0.87	0.37	80
Aspiration	0.45	0.88	69
Silent aspiration	0.14	0.92	22

From Shaw et al (2004). Bronchial auscultation: an effective adjunct to speech and language therapy bedside assessment when detecting dysphagia and aspiration? *Dysphagia*, **19**, 211–218: © Dysphagia Research Society, reproduced by permission of Springer Science and Business Media.

Independence and mutually exclusive events

Two events A and B are *independent* if the fact that B has happened does not influence whether A will occur, that is $p(A|B) = p(A)$, or $p(B|A) = p(B)$. Thus from the multiplication rule two events are independent if $p(A \text{ and } B) = p(A) \times p(B)$.

In Table 4.1, if the results of the NT-proBNP assay were totally unrelated to whether or not a patient had coronary heart failure, that is, they are independent, we might expect

$$p(D+ \text{ and } T+) = p(T+) \times p(D+).$$

Thus if we estimate $p(D+ \text{ and } T+) = 35/410 = 0.085$, $p(D+) = 103/410 = 0.251$ and $p(T+) = 42/410 = 0.102$, then the difference

$$p(D+ \text{ and } T+) - p(D+)p(T+) = 0.085 - (0.251 \times 0.102) = 0.059$$

This provides an estimate of whether these events are independent. It would be exactly zero in such a case were the true probabilities known. In this case, where the probabilities are also estimated, the size of the difference would suggest they are close to independence. The question of deciding whether events are or are not independent is clearly an important one and belongs to statistical inference. It is discussed in more detail in Chapter 7.

In general, a clinician is not faced with a simple question: 'Has the patient got heart failure?', but often with a whole set of different diagnoses. Usually these diagnoses are considered to be *mutually exclusive*; that is if the patient has one disease, he or she does not have any other. Similarly when a coin is tossed the event can be either a 'head' or a 'tail' but cannot be both. If two events A and B are mutually exclusive then the addition rule of mutually exclusive events applies:

$$p(A \text{ or } B) = p(A) + p(B).$$

It also follows that if A and B are mutually exclusive, they cannot occur together, and so

$$p(A \text{ and } B) = 0.$$

It is easy to confuse independent events and mutually exclusive events, but one can see from the above that mutually exclusive events cannot be independent as if you have one you cannot have the other(s).

4.4 Relative (receiver)–operating characteristic (ROC) curve

When a diagnostic test produces a continuous measurement, then a convenient diagnostic cut-off must be selected to calculate the sensitivity and specificity of the test.

Example from the literature: Sensitivity and specificity – disease severity

Johnson et al (2004) looked at 106 patients about to undergo an operation for acute pancreatitis. Before the operation, they were assessed for risk using a score known as the APACHE (Acute Physiology And Chronic Health Evaluation) II score. APACHE-II was designed to measure the severity of disease for patients (aged 16 or more) admitted to intensive care units. The complications after the operation were classified as either 'mild' or 'severe'. The authors also wanted to compare this score with a newly devised one the APACHE_O which included a measure of obesity. The convention is that if the APACHE-II is above 8 the patient is at high risk of severe complications. Table 4.5 shows the results using this cut-off value.

From Table 4.5 we obtain the sensitivity to be $22/27 = 0.81$, or 81%, and the specificity to be $8/13 = 0.62$, or 62%.

Table 4.5 Number of subjects above and below 8 of the APACHE-II score severity of complication

APACHE-II	Complication after operation		Total
	Severe	Mild	
>8	22	5	27
≤8	5	8	13
Total	27	13	40

In the above example, we need not have chosen APACHE-II = 8 as the cut-off value. Other possible values range from APACHE-II = 0 to 27 with these data. For each possibility there is a corresponding sensitivity and specificity.

We can display these calculations by graphing the sensitivity on the y-axis (vertical) and the false positive rate (1 – Specificity) on the x-axis (horizontal) for all possible cut-off values of the diagnostic test. The resulting curve is known as the relative (or receiver) operating characteristic (ROC) curve.

Example from the literature: ROC – disease severity

The ROC curves from the study of Johnson et al (2004) are shown in Figure 4.3 for the APACHE-II and APACHE_O data.

A perfect diagnostic test would be one with no false negative results (that is sensitivity of 1) or false positive results (specificity of 1) and would be represented by a line that started at the origin and went up the y-axis to a sensitivity of 1, and then across to a specificity of 0. A test that produces false positive results at the same rate as true positive results would produce a ROC curve on the diagonal line $y = x$. Any reasonable diagnostic test will display a ROC curve in the upper left triangle of Figure 4.3. When more than one laboratory test is available for the same clinical problem one can compare ROC curves, by plotting both on the same figure.

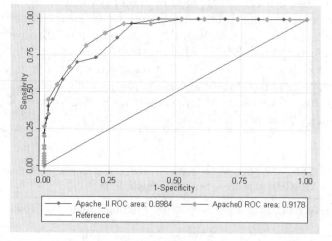

Figure 4.3 Receiver–operating characteristic curve for APACHE_O and APACHE-II data from 106 patients with acute pancreatitis. From Johnson et al (2004). Comparison of APACHE-II score and obesity score (APACHE-O) for the prediction of severe acute pancreatitis. *Pancreatology*, **4**, 1–6: reproduced by permission of Karger AG, Basel

The selection of an optimal combination of sensitivity and specificity for a particular test requires an analysis of the relative medical consequences and costs of false positive and false negative interpretations. Thus, the reason for not giving angiographs to all patients with suspected heart disease is that it is a difficult and expensive procedure, and carries a non-negligible risk to the patient. An alternative test such as the exercise test might be tried, and only if it is positive would angiography then be carried out. If the exercise test is negative then the next stage would be to carry out biochemical tests, and if these turned out positive, once again angiography could be performed.

Analysis of ROC curves

As already indicated, a perfect diagnostic test would be represented by a line that started at the origin, travelled up the y-axis to 1, then across the ceiling to an x-axis value of 1. The area under this ROC curve, termed the AUC, is then the total area of the panel; that is, $1 \times 1 = 1$. In the example of Figure 4.3, the two tests are not 'perfect' but one can see that the AUC for APACHE_O is 0.92 and is slightly bigger than for APACHE-II at 0.90. The AUC can be used as a measure of the performance of a diagnostic test against the ideal and may also be used to compare different tests.

An area of 0.90 means that a randomly selected individual from the diseased group has a laboratory test value larger than that for the randomly chosen individual from the non-diseased group for 90% of the time. Because the area under the ROC plot condenses the information of the graph to a single number, it is desirable to consider the plot as well as the area.

Further details of diagnostic studies, including sample sizes required for comparing alternative diagnostic tests, are given in Machin and Campbell (2005, Chapter 10).

4.5 Points when reading the literature

1. To whom has the diagnostic test been applied? It is possible that characteristics of the patients or stage and severity of the disease can influence the sensitivity of the test. For example, it is likely that a test for cancer will have greater sensitivity for advanced rather than early disease. Have the authors given enough information to enable us to be sure of the disease status?
2. How has the group of patients used in the analysis been selected, and in particular how has the decision to verify the test by the gold standard been made? A common error is to select patients in some manner for verification of a previous diagnosis; this usually leads to positive tests being over-represented in the verified sample and the sensitivity being inflated. It is also common for investigation to assume that unverified cases are disease-

free, which can lead to inflated specificity estimates. The best way to avoid such bias is to construct a prospective study in which all patients receive definite verification of disease status.

3. How have the investigators coped with specimens they were not able to interpret? If the reason for failure to interpret is essentially random, and is unrelated to disease status, then the test characteristics can be estimated. If it is related to disease status then these results cannot be ignored when interpreting the results. In any case, the proportion of non-interpretable results should be reported in any diagnostic test efficacy study, since it is an important consideration in the cost-effectiveness of the test.

4. Did the investigator who provided the diagnostic test result know other clinical results about the patients? Diagnostic tests are usually carried out during or, in conjunction with, the clinical examination. Where there is an element of subjectivity in a test, such as an ECG stress test, a remarkable improvement in sensitivity can be shown when the investigator is aware of other symptoms of the patient!

5. Was the reproducibility of the test result determined? This could be done by repeating the test with different operators, or at different times, or with different machines, depending on the circumstances.

6. Did the patients who had the test actually benefit as a consequence of the test?

7. How good is the gold standard? An ideal gold standard either may not exist or be very expensive or invasive and therefore not carried out. In this case, the test used as the gold standard may be subject to error, which turn will make the estimates of sensitivity and specificity problematical.

4.6 Exercises

Decide whether the answers to the following questions are true or false.

1. In a group of patients presenting to a hospital casualty department with abdominal pain, 30% of patients have acute appendicitis. Seventy per cent of patients with appendicitis have a temperature greater than 37.5°C, 40% of patients without appendicitis have a temperature greater than 37.5°C.

   (a) The sensitivity of temperature greater than 37.5°C as a marker for appendicitis is 21/49.
   (b) The specificity of temperature greater than 37.5°C as a marker for appendicitis is 42/70.
   (c) The positive predictive value of temperature greater than 37.5°C as a marker for appendicitis is 21/30.
   (d) The predictive value of the test might be different in another population.

(e) The specificity of the test will depend upon the prevalence of appendicitis in the population to which it is applied.

2. A new laboratory test is developed for the diagnosis of rectal cancer.

   (a) A sensitivity of 85% implies that 15% of patients with rectal cancer will give negative findings when tested.
   (b) A specificity of 95% implies that 5% of patients with a negative test will actually have rectal cancer.
   (c) A positive predictive value of 75% implies that 25% of patients with a positive test will not have rectal cancer.
   (d) The sensitivity of the test will depend upon the prevalence of rectal cancer in the population to which it is applied.
   (e) The predictive value of the test will depend upon the prevalence of rectal cancer in the population to which it is applied.

3. Three tests (A, B and C) for the diagnosis of breast cancer in premenopausal women were assessed against a 'gold standard' taken to be 100% accurate. Their sensitivities were A 90%, B 85%, C 80%. Their specificities were A 100%, B 90%, C 95%. All three tests carried the same cost, and none was associated with any side-effects. It follows that:

   (a) In these circumstances test A will always be preferable to test B.
   (b) In these circumstances test B will always be preferable to test C.
   (c) Test B detects a higher proportion of cases than test C.
   (d) There are no false positive results with test A.
   (e) The predictive value of test B will depend on the prevalence of disease in the population to which it is applied.

5 Distributions

Medical Statistics Fourth Edition, David Machin, Michael J Campbell, Stephen J Walters
© 2007 John Wiley & Sons, Ltd

Summary

Three theoretical statistical distributions, the Binomial, Poisson and Normal are described. The properties of the Normal distribution and its importance are stressed and its use in calculating reference intervals is also discussed.

5.1   Introduction

In the previous chapter we defined the probability that an event will happen under given circumstances as the proportion of repetitions of those circumstances in which the event would occur in the long run. For example, if we toss a coin it comes down either heads or tails. If we carry on tossing our coin, we should get several heads and several tails. If we go on doing this for long enough, then we would expect to get as many heads as we do tails. So the probability of a head being thrown is a half, because in the long run a head should occur on half the throws. The number of heads which might arise in several tosses of the coin is called a *random variable* that is a variable which can take more than one value each with given probabilities attached to them.

If we toss a coin the two possibilities; Head (H) – scored 1, or Tail (T) – scored 0, are mutually exclusive and these are the only events which can happen. If we let X be a random variable which is the number of heads shown on a single toss and is therefore either 1 or 0, then the probability distribution, for X is: Probability (Head) = ½; Probability (Tail) = ½ and is shown graphically in Figure 5.1a.

What happens if we toss two coins at once? We now have four possible events: HH, HT, TH and TT. There are all equally likely and each has probability ¼. If we let Y be the number of heads then Y has three possible values 0, 1 and 2. $Y = 0$ only when we get TT and has probability ¼. Similarly $Y = 2$ only when we get HH, so has probability ¼. However $Y = 1$ either when we get HT or TH and so has probability ¼ + ¼ = ½. The probability distribution for Y is shown in Figure 5.1b.

In general, we can think of the tosses of the coin as trials, each of which can have an outcome of success (head) or failure (tail). These distributions are all examples of what is known as the Binomial distribution. In this chapter we will discuss three distributions that are the backbone of medical statistics: the Binomial, the Poisson and the Normal. Each distribution has a formula, known as the *probability distribution function*. This gives the probability of observing an event, and the formulas are given in Section 5.7. The formulae contain certain constants, known as *parameters,* which identify the particular distribution, and from which various characteristics of the distribution, such as its mean and standard deviation, can be calculated.

5.2   The Binomial distribution

If a group of patients is given a new treatment such as acupuncture, for the relief of a particular condition, such as tension type headache, then the

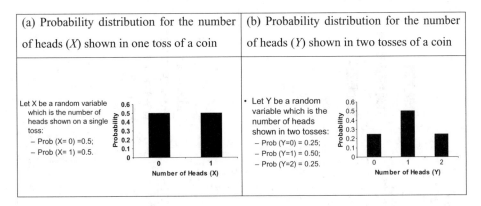

| (a) Probability distribution for the number of heads (X) shown in one toss of a coin | (b) Probability distribution for the number of heads (Y) shown in two tosses of a coin |

Figure 5.1   Examples of probability distributions

proportion p being successfully treated can be regarded as estimating the population treatment success rate π. (Here, π denotes a population value and has no connection at all with the mathematical constant 3.14159.) The sample proportion p is analogous to the sample mean $\bar{x}$, in that if we score zero for those s patients who fail on treatment, and unity for those r who succeed, then $p = r/n$, where $n = r + s$ is the total number of patients treated. The Binomial distribution is characterised by the mathematical variables n (the number of individuals in the sample, or repetitions of the trial) and π (the true probability of success for each individual, or in each trial). The formula is given as Equation 5.1 in Section 5.8.

For a fixed sample size n the shape of the binomial distribution depends only on π. Suppose $n = 5$ patients are to be treated, and it is known that on average 0.25 will respond to this particular treatment. The number of responses actually observed can only take integer values between 0 (no responses) and 5 (all respond). The binomial distribution for this case is illustrated in Figure 5.2. The distribution is not symmetric, it has a maximum at one response and the height of the blocks corresponds to the probability of obtaining the particular number of responses from the five patients yet to be treated.

Figure 5.2 illustrates the shape of the Binomial distribution for various n and $\pi = 0.25$. When n is small (here 5 and 10), the distribution is skewed to the right. The distribution becomes more symmetrical as the sample size increases (here 20 and 50). We also note that the width of the bars decreases as n increases since the total probability of unity is divided amongst more and more possibilities.

If π were set equal to 0.5, then all the distributions corresponding to those of Figure 5.2 would be symmetrical whatever the size of n. On the other hand, if $\pi = 0.75$ then the distributions would be skewed to the left.

We can use the properties of the Binomial distribution when making inferences about proportions, as we shall see in subsequent chapters.

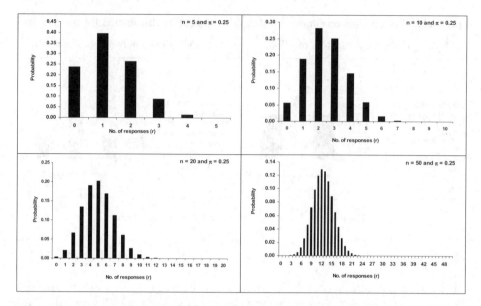

Figure 5.2 Binomial distribution for $\pi = 0.25$ and various values of n. The horizontal scale in each diagram shows the value of r the number of successes

---

Example from the literature: Acupuncture and headache

Melchart et al (2005) give the successful response rate to acupuncture treatment in 124 patients with tension type headache as 46%. From their data we have $p = 58/124 = 0.46$.

Suppose a doctor treated four acupuncture patients. What is the probability that at most one responds?

This implies that either 0 or 1 respond. We can use Equation 5.1, with $r = 0$ to give $0.54^4 = 0.0850$ and with $r = 1$ to give $4 \times (1 - 0.54) \times 0.54^3 = 0.2897$. Summing these two probabilities gives $p = 0.0850 + 0.2897 = 0.3747$.

5.3 The Poisson distribution

The Poisson distribution is used to describe discrete quantitative data such as counts that occur independently and randomly in time or space at some average rate. For example the number of deaths in a town from a particular disease per day, or the number of admissions to a particular hospital typically follows a Poisson distribution.

The Poisson random variable is the count of the number of events that occur independently and randomly in time or space at some rate, λ. The formula for a Poisson distribution is given as equation 5.2 in section 5.7.

We can use our knowledge of the Poisson distribution to calculate the anticipated number of hospital admissions on any particular day or the number of deaths from lung cancer in a year in a town. We can use this information to compare observed and expected values, to decide if, for example, the number of deaths from cancer in an area is unusually high.

Figure 5.3 shows the Poisson distribution for four different means $\lambda = 1, 4,$ 10 and 15. For $\lambda = 1$ the distribution is very right skewed, for $\lambda = 4$ the skewness is much less and as the mean increases to $\lambda = 10$ or 15 it is more symmetrical, and looks more like the Binomial distribution in Figure 5.2.

Example from the literature: Cadaveric heart-beating donors

Wight et al (2004) looked at the variation in cadaveric heart-beating organ donor rates in the UK. Heart-beating donors are patients who were seriously ill in an intensive care unit (ICU) and are placed on a ventilator. They found that they were 1330 organ donors, aged 15–69, across the UK for the two years 1999 and 2000 combined. Assuming the population of the UK is 60 million, the expected rate of donors is 0.011 donors per 1000 population. Suppose a health region served a population of 100000. What is the probability of getting no donors in a year?

With these historical data we would anticipate an average of $\lambda = 0.011 \times$ 100000/1000 = 1.1 donors per year. Using this value in equation 5.2, for r = 0, Prob(0) = exp($-\lambda$), we obtain Prob(0) = $e^{-1.1}$ = 0.3329. Thus there is a very high chance, about 1 in 3, of not getting any donors in any one year.

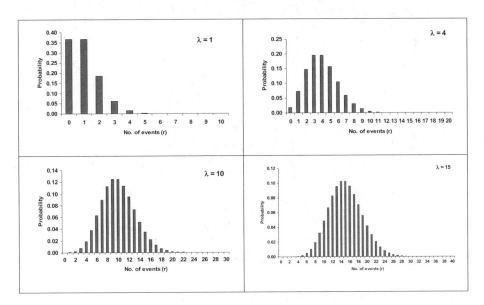

Figure 5.3 Poisson distribution for various values of λ. The horizontal scale in each diagram shows the value of r

5.4 Probability for continuous outcomes

So far we have looked at what is the probability of a particular value, for example, a success or failure on treatment, for *discrete* data. As the number of possible values increases the probability of a particular value decreases. For continuous variables, such as birth weight and blood pressure, the set of possible values is infinite (only limited by the precision of how we take the measurements). So we are more interested in the probability of the having values between certain limits rather than one particular value. For example, what is the probability of having a systolic blood pressure of 140 mmHg or higher?

The vertical scale of histograms, such as Figure 3.2, shown so far, have been frequencies and depend on the total number of observations. As an alternative we can use the relative frequency (or %) on the vertical scale. The advantage of using the relative frequency is that the scale of different histograms, with the same outcome but different sample sizes, will be the same. Such a histogram, as in Figure 5.4 can be given the rather formal name of an empirical relative frequency distribution but it is simply the observed distribution of the data in a sample.

If we imagine for the birthweight data in Figure 5.4 that we have a very large sample (many more than 98 babies) and by taking smaller and smaller intervals to classify the birth weights (much smaller than 0.2 kg) then the

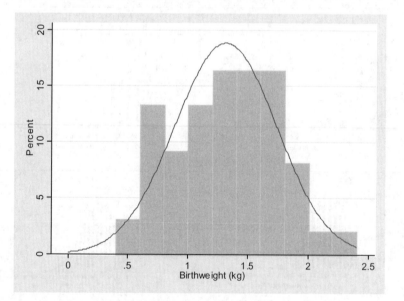

Figure 5.4 Empirical relative frequency distributions of birth weight of 98 babies admitted to special care baby unit and the associated probability distribution (data from Simpson, 2004). Reproduced by permission of AG Simpson

histogram will start to look like a smooth curve. In these circumstances the distribution of observations may be approximated by a smooth underlying curve which is also shown in Figure 5.4. This curve is called a *probability distribution* and is the theoretical equivalent of an empirical relative frequency distribution. Probability distributions are used to calculate the probability that different values will occur; for example, what is the probability of having a birthweight of 2.0 kg or less? It is often the case with medical data that the histogram of a continuous variable obtained from a single measurement on different subjects will have a symmetric 'bell-shaped' distribution.

5.5 The Normal distribution

This symmetric 'bell-shaped' distribution mentioned above is known as the Normal distribution and is one of the most important distributions in statistics. One such example is the histogram of the birthweight (in kilograms) of the 3226 newborn babies shown in Figure 5.5.

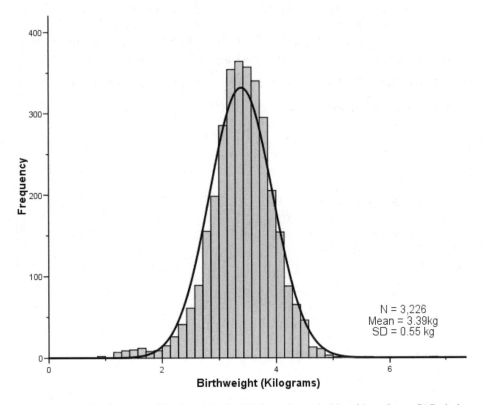

Figure 5.5 Distribution of birthweight in 3226 newborn babies (data from O'Cathain et al, 2002)

To distinguish the use of the same word in *normal* range (which we discuss later) and *Normal* distribution we have used a lower and upper case convention throughout this book.

The histogram of the sample data is an estimate of the population distribution of birth weights in newborn babies. This population distribution can be estimated by the superimposed smooth 'bell-shaped' curve or 'Normal' distribution shown. We presume that if we were able to look at the entire population of newborn babies then the distribution of birthweight would have exactly the Normal shape. The Normal distribution has properties as shown in Figure 5.6.

The Normal distribution (Figure 5.6) is completely described by two parameters: one, μ, represents the population mean or centre of the distribution and the other, σ, the population standard deviation. The formula for the Normal distribution is given as Equation 5.3 (Section 5.8). Populations with small values of the standard deviation σ have a distribution concentrated close to the centre, μ; those with large standard deviation have a distribution widely spread along the measurement axis (Figure 5.7).

There are infinitely many Normal distributions depending on the values of μ and σ. The Standard Normal distribution has a mean of zero and a variance (and standard deviation) of one and a shape as shown in Figure 5.8. The formula is given as Equation 5.4 in Section 5.8. If the random variable X has a Normal distribution with mean, μ and standard deviation, σ, then the standardised Normal deviate $z = \dfrac{X - \mu}{\sigma}$ is a random variable that has a standard Normal distribution.

Total area under the curve = 1 (or 100%). Bell shaped and symmetrical about its mean. The peak of the curve lies above the mean. Any position along the horizontal axis can be expressed as a number of SDs away from the mean. The mean and median coincide.	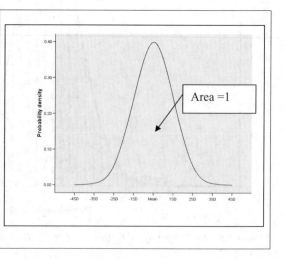

Figure 5.6   The Normal probability distribution

The areas under the standard Normal distribution curve have been tabulated (Table 5.1 and Table T1, p. 316). Table 5.1, shows that for a value of z,
that is the number of standard deviations away from the mean of zero, the
area to the left or the right of this value or the combined value. Using Figure
5.8 or Table 5.1, we can note that most of the area, i.e. 68% of the probability
is between −1 and +1 SD, the large majority (95%) between −2 and +2 SD,
and almost all (99%) between −3 and +3.

As can be seen from Table 5.1 using, z values of 1.96, that is, 1.96 SD away
from the mean) then exactly 95% of the Normal distribution lies between

$$\mu - 1.96 \times \sigma \text{ and } \mu + 1.96 \times \sigma.$$

(a) effect of changing mean ($\mu_2 > \mu_1$)   (b) effect of changing SD ($\sigma_2 > \sigma_1$)

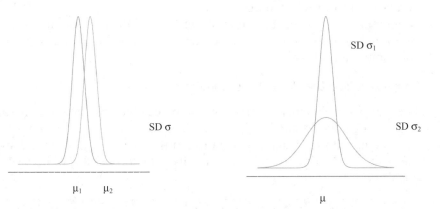

Figure 5.7   Probability distribution functions of the Normal distributions with different
means and standard deviations

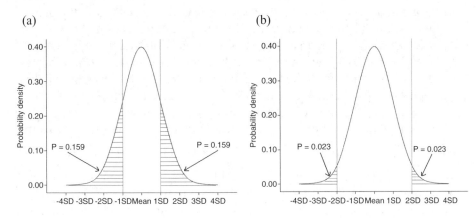

31.7% of observations lie outside the mean ± 1 SD   4.6% of observations lie outside the mean ± 2SD

Figure 5.8   Areas (percentages of total probability) under the standard Normal curve

Table 5.1   Selected probabilities associated with the Normal distribution

Standardised deviate	Probability of greater deviation	
$z = (x - \mu)/\sigma$	In either direction	In one direction
0	1.000	0.500
1	0.317	0.159
2	0.046	0.023
3	0.0027	0.0013
1.645	0.10	0.05
1.960	0.05	0.025
2.576	0.01	0.005

Changing the multiplier 1.960 to 2.576, exactly 99% of the Normal distribution lies in the corresponding interval.

In practice the two parameters of the Normal distribution, μ and σ, must be estimated from the sample data. For this purpose a random sample from the population is first taken.

How do we use the Normal distribution?

The Normal probability distribution can be used to calculate the probability of different values occurring. We could be interested in: what is the probability of being within 1 standard deviation of the mean (or outside it)? We can use a Normal distribution table which tells us the probability of being outside this value.

Illustrative example: Normal distribution – birthweights

Using the birthweight data from the O'Cathain et al (2002) study let us assume that the birthweight for new born babies has a Normal distribution with a mean of 3.4 kg and a standard deviation of 0.6 kg. So what is the probability of giving birth to a baby with a birthweight of 4.5 kg or higher?

Since birthweight is assumed to follow a Normal distribution, with mean of 3.4 kg and SD of 0.6 kg, we therefore know that approximately 68% of birthweights will lie between 2.8 and 4.0 kg and about 95% of birthweights will lie between 2.2 and 4.6 kg. Using Figure 5.9 we can see that a birthweight of 4.5 kg is between 1 and 2 standard deviations away from the mean.

First calculate, z, the number of standard deviations 4.5 kg is away from the mean of 3.4 kg, that is, $z = \dfrac{4.5 - 3.4}{0.6} = 1.83$. Then look for $z = 1.83$ in Table T1 of the Normal distribution table which gives the probability of being outside the values of the mean −1.83 SD to mean +1.83 SD as 0.0672. Therefore the probability of having a birthweight of 4.5 kg or higher is 0.0672/2 = 0.0336 or 3.3%.

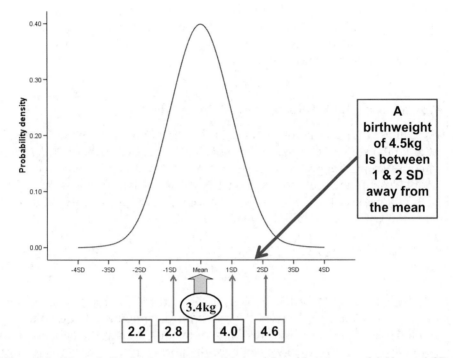

Figure 5.9 Normal distribution curve for birthweight with a mean of 3.4 kg and SD of 0.6 kg

The Normal distribution also has other uses in statistics and is often used as an approximation to the Binomial and Poisson distributions. Figure 5.2 shows that the Binomial distribution for any particular value of the parameter π approaches the shape of a Normal distribution as the other parameter n increases. The approach to Normality is more rapid for values of π near 0.5 than for values near to 0 or 1. Thus, provided n is large enough, a count may be regarded as approximately Normally distributed with mean $n\pi$ and SD $= \sqrt{[n\pi(1-\pi)]}$.

The Poisson distribution with mean λ approaches Normality as λ increases (see Figure 5.3). When λ is large a Poisson variable may be regarded as approximately Normally distributed with mean λ and SD $= \sqrt{\lambda}$.

5.6 Reference ranges

Diagnostic tests, as described in Chapter 4, use patient data to classify individuals as either normal or abnormal. A related statistical problem is the description of the variability in normal individuals, to provide a basis for assessing the test results of other individuals as we have seen in the previous chapter. The most common form of presenting such data is as a range of values or interval which contains the values obtained from the majority of a sample of normal subjects. The reference interval is often referred to as a normal range or reference range.

Worked example: Reference range – birthweight

We can use the fact that our sample birthweight data, from the O'Cathain et al (2002) study (see Figure 5.5); appear Normally distributed to calculate a reference range for birthweights. We have already mentioned that about 95% of the observations (from a Normal distribution) lie within 1.96 SDs either side of the mean. So a reference range for our sample of babies, from the O'Cathain et al (2002) study is:

$$3.391 - (1.96 \times 0.554) \text{ to } 3.391 + (1.96 \times 0.554)$$
$$\text{or } 2.31 \text{ to } 4.47 \text{ kg.}$$

A baby's weight at birth is strongly associated with mortality risk during the first year and, to a lesser degree, with developmental problems in childhood and the risk of various diseases in adulthood. If the data are not Normally distributed then we can base the normal reference range on the observed percentiles of the sample, that is, 95% of the observed data lie between the 2.5 and 97.5 percentiles. So a percentile-based reference range for our sample is: 2.19 kg to 4.43 kg.

Most reference ranges are based on samples larger than 3500 people. Over many years, and millions of births, the World Health Organization (WHO) has come up with a with a normal birthweight range for newborn babies. These ranges represent results than are acceptable in newborn babies and actually cover the middle 80% of the population distribution, that is, the 10th and 90th centiles. Low birthweight babies are usually defined (by the WHO) as weighing less than 2500 g (the 10th centile) regardless of gestational age, and large birth weight babies are defined as weighing above 4000 g (the 90th centile). Hence the normal birth weight range is around 2.5 kg to 4.0 kg. For our sample data, the 10 to 90th centile range was similar, at 2.75 to 4.03 kg.

Example from the literature: Reference or normal range – prolactin

Merza et al (2003) give the mean and standard deviation for prolactin concentration (prolactin is a hormone that is secreted by an endocrine gland) in 21 patients with chronic pain using opioid analgesia as 221 mIU/l and 91 mIU/l respectively. The prolactin concentration values in the sample ranged from a minimum of 103 mIU/l to a maximum of 369 mIU/l. If we assume the prolactin concentration has a Normal distribution in patients with chronic pain using opioid analgesia, then from this sample we would estimate a reference interval as 43 to 399 mIU/l. The paper states the normal reference range estimated from a large standard sample is actually 66 to 588 mIU/l. Here, none of the 21 chronic pain patients had a prolactin concentration value outside this normal reference range.

5.7 Points when reading the literature

1. What is the population from which the sample was taken? Are there any possible sources of bias that may affect the estimates of the population parameters?
2. Have reference ranges been calculated on a random sample of healthy volunteers? If not, how does this affect your interpretation? Is there any good reason why a random sample was not taken?
3. For any continuous variable, are the variables correctly assumed to have a Normal distribution? If not, how do the investigators take account of this?

5.8 Technical details

Binomial distribution

Data that can take only a 0 or 1 response, such as treatment failure or treatment success, follow the *Binomial distribution* provided the underlying population response rate π does not change. The Binomial probabilities are calculated from

$$\text{Prob}(r \text{ responses out of } n) = \frac{n!}{r!(n-r)!}\pi^r(1-\pi)^{n-r} \qquad 5.1$$

for successive values of r from 0 through to n. In the above $n!$ is read as n factorial and $r!$ as r factorial. For $r = 4$, $r! = 4 \times 3 \times 2 \times 1 = 24$. Both 0! and 1! are taken as equal to unity. It should be noted that the expected value for r, the number of successes yet to be observed if we treated n patients, is $n\pi$. The potential variation about this expectation is expressed by the corresponding standard deviation $SD(r) = \sqrt{[n\pi(1-\pi)]}$.

Poisson distribution

Suppose events happen randomly and independently in time at a constant rate. If the events happen with a rate of λ events per unit time, the probability of r events happening in unit time is

$$\text{Prob}(r \text{ events}) = \frac{\exp(-\lambda)\lambda^r}{r!} \qquad 5.2$$

where $exp(-\lambda)$ is a convenient way of writing the exponential constant e raised to the power $-\lambda$. (The constant e is the base of natural logarithms, which is 2.718281. . . .)

The mean of the Poisson distribution for the number of events per unit time is simply the rate, λ. The variance of the Poisson distribution is also equal to λ, and so the SD $= \sqrt{\lambda}$.

Normal distribution

The probability density, $f(x)$, or the height of the curve above the x axis (see Figures 5.5 and 5.6) of a Normally distributed random variable x, is given by the expression

$$f(x) = \frac{1}{\sigma\sqrt{2\pi}}\exp\left[-\frac{(x-\mu)^2}{2\sigma^2}\right], \qquad 5.3$$

where μ is the mean value of x and σ is the standard deviation of x. Note that for the Normal distribution π, is the mathematical constant 3.14159 . . . and not the parameter of a Binomial distribution.

The probability density simplifies for the Standard Normal distribution, since $\mu = 0$ and $\sigma = 1$, then the probability density, $f(x)$, of a Normally distributed random variable x, is

$$f(x) = \frac{1}{\sqrt{2\pi}}\exp\left[-\frac{x^2}{2}\right]. \qquad 5.4$$

5.9   Exercises

1. A GP estimates that about 50% of her patients have 'trivial' problems. What is the probability that four out of five patients in one evening's surgery have trivial problems?

2. Suppose a hospital Accident and Emergency department has an average of 10 new emergency cases per hour. Calculate the probability of observing exactly 10 new emergency cases in any given hour.

3. The systolic blood pressure of 16 middle age men before exercise has a Normal distribution with a mean of 141.1 mmHg and a standard deviation of 13.62 mmHg. What is the probability having a systolic blood pressure of 160 mmHg or higher?

4. The diastolic blood pressures (DBP) of a group of young men are Normally distributed with mean 70 mmHg and a standard deviation of 10 mmHg.

Decide whether the following statements are true or false.

   (i) About 95% of the men have a DBP between 60 and 80 mmHg.
   (ii) About 50% of the men have a DBP of above 70 mmHg.
   (iii) About 2.5% of the men have DBP below 50 mmHg.

5. Given the sample described in question 4.

   (i) What is the probability of a young man having a DBP of 95 mmHg or above?
   (ii) What is the probability of a young man having a DBP of 55 mmHg or less?
   (iii) What proportion of young men have a DBP between 55 mmHg and 95 mmHg?

6. A GP and partners have 6000 patients and refer 27 patients to neurology in one year. In the health authority region, there are 1400 neurology referrals from a population of 500 000. Is this GP's referral rate unusually high?

6 Populations, samples, standard errors and confidence intervals

Medical Statistics Fourth Edition, David Machin, Michael J Campbell, Stephen J Walters
© 2007 John Wiley & Sons, Ltd

Summary

In this chapter the concepts of a population and a population parameter are described. The sample from a population is used to provide the estimates of the population parameters. The standard error is introduced and methods for calculating confidence intervals for population means for continuous data having a Normal distribution and for discrete data which follow Binomial or Poisson distributions are given.

6.1   Populations

In the statistical sense a *population* is a theoretical concept used to describe an entire group of individuals in whom we are interested. Examples are the population of all patients with diabetes mellitus, or the population of all middle-aged men. Parameters are quantities used to describe characteristics of such populations. Thus the proportion of diabetic patients with nephropathy, or the mean blood pressure of middle-aged men, are characteristics describing the two populations. Generally, it is costly and labour intensive to study the entire population. Therefore we collect data on a *sample* of individuals from the population who we believe are *representative* of that population, that is, they have similar characteristics to the individuals in the population. We then use them to draw conclusions, technically make inferences, about the population as a whole. The process is represented schematically in Figure 6.1. So, samples are taken from populations to provide estimates

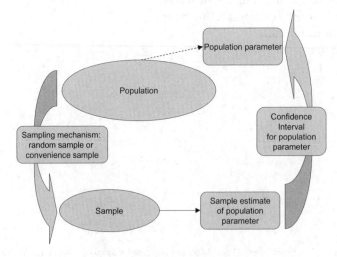

Figure 6.1   Population and sample

Table 6.1 Population parameters and sample statistics

	Population parameter	Sample statistic
Mean	μ	$\bar{x}$
Standard deviation	σ	s
Proportion	π	p
Rate	λ	r

of population parameters. Some common population parameters and their corresponding sample statistics or estimates are described in Table 6.1.

It is important to note that although the study populations are unique, samples are not as we could take more than one sample from the target population if we wished. Thus for middle-aged men there is only one normal range for blood pressure. However, one investigator taking a random sample from a population of middle-aged men and measuring their blood pressure may obtain a different normal range from another investigator who takes a different random sample from the same population of such men. By studying only some of the population we have introduced a sampling error. In this chapter we show how to use the theoretical probability distributions, outlined in Chapter 5 to quantify this error.

6.2 Samples

In some circumstances the sample may consist of all the members of a specifically defined population. For practical reasons, this is only likely to be the case if the population of interest is not too large. If all members of the population can be assessed, then the *estimate* of the parameter concerned is derived from information obtained on all members and so its value will be the population parameter itself. In this idealised situation we know all about the population as we have examined all its members and the parameter is estimated with no bias. The dotted arrow in Figure 6.1 connecting the population ellipse to population parameter box illustrates this. However, this situation will rarely be the case so, in practice, we take a sample which is often much smaller in size than the population under study.

Ideally we should aim for a *random sample*. A list of all individuals from the population is drawn up (the *sampling frame*), and individuals are selected randomly from this list, that is, every possible sample of a given size in the population has an equal chance of being chosen. Sometimes, there may be difficulty in constructing this list or we may have to 'make-do' with those subjects who happen to be available or what is termed a *convenience sample*. Essentially if we take a random sample then we obtain an unbiased estimate of the corresponding population parameter, whereas a convenience sample may provide a biased estimate but by how much we will not know. The different types of sampling are described more fully in Chapter 12.

6.3 The standard error

Standard error of the mean

So how good is the sample mean as an estimate of the true population mean? To answer this question we need to assess the uncertainty of our single sample mean. How can we do this? We shall use the birthweight data from the O'Cathain et al (2002) study. In Chapter 5 we showed that the birthweights of 3226 newborn babies are approximately Normally distributed with a mean of 3.39 kg and a standard deviation of 0.55 kg (Figure 5.5). Let us assume for expository purposes that this distribution of birthweights is the whole population. Obviously, the real population would be far larger than this and consist of the birthweights of millions of babies.

Suppose we take a random sample from this population and calculate the sample mean. This information then provides us with *our* estimate of the population mean. However, a different sample *may* give us a different estimate of the population mean. So if we take (say) 100 samples all of the same size, $n = 4$, we would get a spread of sample means which we can display visually in a dot plot or histogram like that in the top panel of Figure 6.2. These sample means range from as low as 2.4 to as high as 4.0 kg, whereas if we had taken samples of size $n = 16$ the range is less from 3.1 to 3.7 kg. This is because the mean from the larger sample absorbs or dilutes the effect of very small or very large observations in the sample more than does a sample of a smaller size that contains such observations.

The variability of these sample means gives us an indication of the uncertainty attached to the estimate of the population mean when taking only a single sample – very uncertain when the sample size is small to much less uncertainty when the sample size is large. Figure 6.2 clearly shows that the spread or variability of the sample means reduces as the sample size increases. In fact in turns out that sample means have the following properties.

Properties of the distribution of sample means

The mean of all the sample means will be the same as the population mean.

The standard deviation of all the sample means is known as the standard error (SE) of the mean or SEM.

Given a large enough sample size, the distribution of sample means, will be roughly Normal regardless of the distribution of the variable.

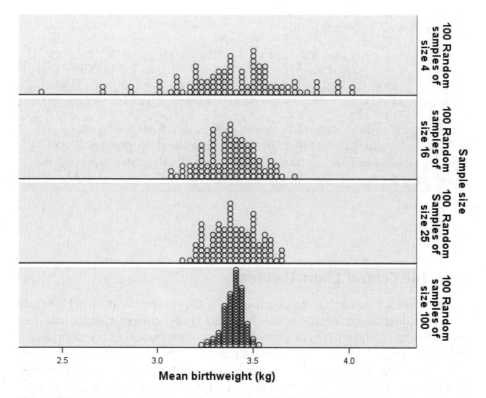

Figure 6.2   Dot plots showing mean birthweight (kg) for 100 random samples of size 4, 16, 25 and 100

The standard error or variability of the sampling distribution of the mean is measured by the standard deviation of the estimates. If we know the population standard deviation, σ, then the standard error of the mean is given by $\sigma/\sqrt{n}$. In reality, an investigator will only complete the study once (although it may be repeated for confirmatory purposes) so this single study provides a single sample mean, $\bar{x}$, and this is our best (and only) estimate of μ. The same sample also provides s, the standard deviation of the observations, as an estimate of σ. So with a *single* study, the investigator can then estimate the standard deviation of the distribution of the means by $s/\sqrt{n}$ without having to repeat the study at all.

Worked example: Standard error of a mean – birthweight of preterm infants

Simpson (2004) reported the birthweights of 98 infants who were born prematurely, for which $n = 98$, $\bar{x} = 1.31\,\text{kg}$, $s = 0.42\,\text{kg}$ and $SE(\bar{x}) = 0.42/\sqrt{98} = 0.04\,\text{kg}$.

The standard error provides a measure of the precision of our sample estimate of the population mean birthweight.

Properties of standard errors

The standard error is a measure of the precision of a sample estimate. It provides a measure of how far from the true value in the population the sample estimate is likely to be. All standard errors have the following interpretation:

- A large standard error indicates that the estimate is imprecise.
- A small standard error indicates that the estimate is precise.
- The standard error is reduced, that is, we obtain a more precise estimate, if the size of the sample is increased.

6.4   The Central Limit Theorem

It is important to note that the distribution of the sample means will be nearly Normally distributed, whatever the distribution of the measurement amongst the individuals, and will get closer to a Normal distribution as the sample size increases. Technically the fact that we can estimate the standard error from a single sample derives from what is known as the *Central Limit Theorem* and this important property enables us to apply the techniques we describe to a wide variety of situations.

To illustrate this, we will use the random number table Table T2 (p. 318). In this table each digit (0 to 9) is equally likely to appear and cannot be predicted from any combination of other digits. The first 15 digits (in sets of 5) read 94071, 63090, 23901. Assume that our population consists of all the 10 digits (0 to 9) in a random numbers table. Figure 6.3 shows the population distribution of these random digits, which is clearly not Normal, (in fact it is called a uniform distribution). Each digit has a frequency of 10%. The population mean value is 4.5.

Suppose we take a random sample of five digits from this distribution and calculate their mean and repeat this 500 times. So for example, reading across the first row of Table T4, the means would be 4.2, 3.6, 3.0, etc. Each of these is an estimate of the population value. How would these sample means (of size five) be distributed? One can imagine that mean values close to 0 or 9 are very unlikely, since one would need a run of five 0s or five 9s. However, values close to 4.5 are quite likely. Figure 6.4 shows the distribution of the means of these random numbers for different sized samples. The distribution for samples of size five is reasonably symmetric but well spread out. As we take means of size 50, the distributions become more symmetric and Normally distributed.

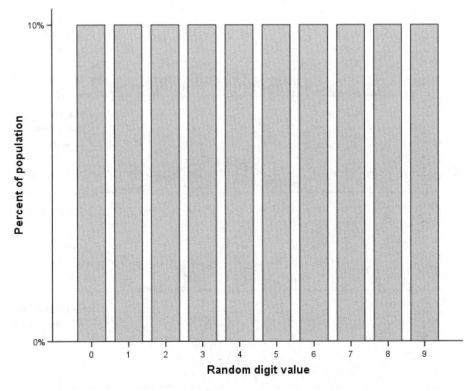

Figure 6.3 Distribution of a large number of random digits (0 to 9)

The important point is *whatever* the parent distribution of a variable, the distribution of the sample means will be nearly Normal, as long as the samples are large enough. Furthermore, as n gets larger the distribution of the sample means will become closer and closer to Normal. In practice the sample size restriction is not an issue when the parent distribution is unimodal and not particularly asymmetric (as in our example), as even for a sample size as small as ten, the distribution is close to Normal.

6.5 Standard errors for proportions and rates

Any estimate of a parameter obtained from data has a standard error and Table 6.3 (Section 6.10) gives formulae for means, proportions and rates. For example, we may be interested in the proportion of individuals in a population who possess some characteristic, such as having a disease. Having taken a sample of size n from the population, suppose r individuals have a particular characteristic. Our best estimate, p, of the population proportion, π, is given by $p = r/n$. If we were to take repeated samples of size n from our population and plot the estimates of the proportion as a histogram, then, provided $0.1 < \pi < 0.9$ and $n > 10$ resulting sampling distribution of the proportion

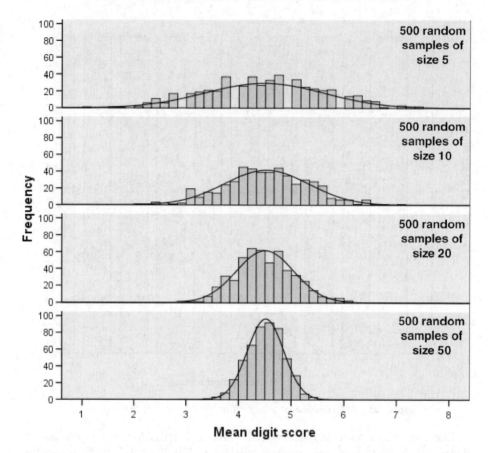

Figure 6.4 Observed distributions of the means of 500 random samples of size 5, 10, 20 and 50 taken from the distribution of random digits 0 to 9

would approximate a Normal distribution with mean value, π. The standard deviation of this distribution of estimated proportions is the *standard error of the proportion* or $SE(p)$. Similarly, if we counted the number of events over a given time we would get a rate.

Worked example: Standard error of a proportion – acupuncture and headache

Melchart et al (2005) give the proportion who responded to acupuncture treatment in 124 patients with tension type headache as $p = 0.46$. We assume the numbers who respond have a Binomial distribution and from Table 6.3 in Section 6.10 we find the standard error is

$$SE(p) = \sqrt{\frac{0.46(1-0.46)}{124}} = 0.04.$$

Worked example: Standard error of a rate – cadaveric heart donors

The study of Wight et al (2004) gave the number of organ donations calculated over a two-year period as $r = 1.82$ per day. We assume the number
of donations follows a Poisson distribution and from Table 6.3 in Section
6.10 we find the standard error is $SE(r) = \sqrt{(1.82/731)} = 0.05$.

Standard deviation or standard error?

There is often confusion about the distinction between the standard error
and standard deviation. The standard error always refers to an estimate of a
parameter. As such the estimate gets more precise as the number of observations gets larger, which is reflected by the standard error becoming smaller.
If the term standard deviation is used in the same way, then it is synonymous
with the standard error. However, if it refers to the observations then it is an
estimate of the population standard deviation and does not get smaller as the
sample size increases. The statistic, s, the calculation of which is described in
Section 3.1, is an estimator of the population parameter σ, that is, the population standard deviation.

In summary, the standard deviation, s, is a measure of the variability between
individuals with respect to the measurement under consideration, whereas the
standard error (SE), is a measure of the uncertainty in the sample statistic,
for example the mean, derived from the individual measurements.

6.6 Standard errors of differences

When two groups are to be compared, then it is the standard error of the
difference between groups that is important. The formulas for the standard
errors for the *difference* in means, proportions and rates are given in Table 6.4.

**Worked example: Difference in means – physiotherapy for
patients with lung disease**

Griffiths et al (2000) report the results of a randomised controlled trial to
compare a pulmonary rehabilitation programme (Intervention) with standard medical management (Control) for the treatment of chronic obstructive pulmonary disease. One outcome measure was the walking capacity
(distance walked in metres from a standardised test) of the patient assessed
6 weeks after randomisation. Further suppose such measurements can be
assumed to follow a Normal distribution. The results from the 184 patients
are expressed using the group means and standard deviations (SD) as
follows:

$$n_{Int} = 93, \bar{x}_{Int} = 211, SD(x_{Int}) = s_{Int} = 118$$
$$n_{Con} = 91, \bar{x}_{Con} = 123, SD(x_{Con}) = s_{Con} = 99.$$

From these data $\bar{d} = \bar{x}_{Int} - \bar{x}_{Con} = 211 - 123 = 88\,\text{m}$ and the correspond-

ing standard error from Table 6.4 is, $SE(\bar{d}) = \sqrt{\dfrac{118^2}{93} + \dfrac{99^2}{91}} = 16.04\,\text{m}.$

Worked example: Difference in proportions – post-natal urinary incontinence

The results of randomised controlled trial conducted by Glazener et al (2001) to assess the effect of nurse assessment with reinforcement of pelvic floor muscle training exercises and bladder training (Intervention) compared with standard management (Control) among women with persistent incontinence three months postnatally are summarised in Table 6.2. The primary outcome measure was urinary incontinence at 12 months postnatally.

The corresponding proportions of patients who improved (no urinary incontinence) is $p_{Int} = 111/279 = 0.40$ and $p_{Con} = 76/245 = 0.31$. The difference in the proportion of patients who improved on treatment is $p_{Int} - p_{Con} = 0.40 - 0.31 = 0.09$. Finally from Table 6.4 (Section 6.10) the standard error of this difference is:

$$SE(p_{Int} - p_{Con}) = \sqrt{\frac{0.40(1-0.40)}{279} + \frac{0.31(1-0.31)}{245}} = 0.042.$$

Table 6.2 Urinary incontinence rates at 12 months in women with persistent incontinence at three months postnatally (Glazener et al, 2001)

Urinary Incontinence	Intervention		Control	
	n		n	
Yes	167	(60%)	169	(69%)
No	112	(40%)	76	(31%)
Total	279		245	

From Glazener et al (2001). Conservative management of persistent postnatal urinary and faecal incontinence: randomised controlled trial. *British Medical Journal*, **323**, 1–5: reproduced by permission of the BMJ Publishing Group.

6.7 Confidence intervals for an estimate

Confidence interval for a mean

The sample mean, proportion or rate is the best estimate we have of the true population mean, proportion or rate. We know that the distribution of these parameter estimates from many samples of the same size will roughly be Normal. As a consequence, we can construct a confidence interval – a range of values in which we are confident the true population value of the parameter will lie. A confidence interval defines a range of values within which our population parameter is likely to lie. Such an interval for the population mean μ is defined by

$$\bar{x} - 1.96 \times SE(\bar{x}) \text{ to } \bar{x} + 1.96 \times SE(\bar{x})$$

and, in this case, is termed a 95% confidence interval as it includes the multiplier 1.96. Figure 6.5 illustrates that 95% of the distribution of sample means

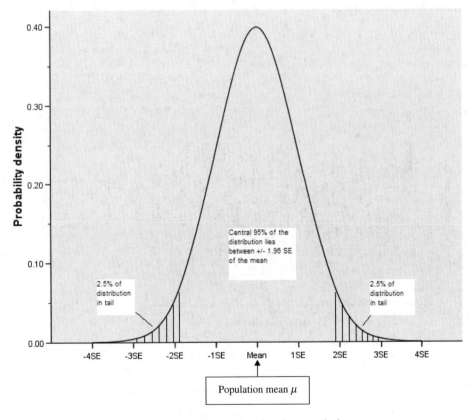

Figure 6.5 Sampling distribution for the population mean μ

lies within ±1.96 standard errors (the *standard deviation* of *this* distribution) of the population mean.

In strict terms the confidence interval is a range of values that is likely to cover the true but unknown population mean value, μ. The confidence interval is based on the concept of repetition of the study under consideration. Thus if the study were to be repeated 100 times, of the 100 resulting 95% confidence intervals, we would expect 95 of these to include the population parameter. Consequently a reported confidence interval from a particular study *may* or *may not* include the actual population parameter value of concern.

Figure 6.6 illustrates some of the possible 95% confidence intervals that could be obtained from different random samples of 25 babies from the 3226 babies whose birthweight data was recorded by O'Cathain et al (2002). Ninety-four (94%) of these 100 confidence intervals contain the population mean birthweight of 3.39 kg but 6 (6%) do not. This is close to what we would expect – that the 95% confidence interval will *not* include the true population mean 5% of the time.

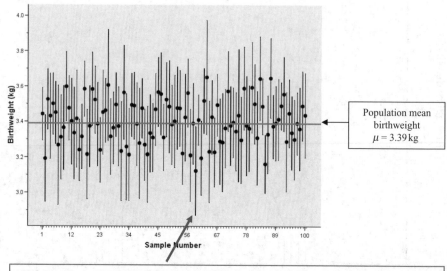

Unfortunately the CIs **ARE NOT** pre-labelled with 'I am a poor CI and do not include the population mean: do not choose me!'

Figure 6.6 One hundred different 95% confidence intervals for mean birthweight constructed from random samples of size 25. The arrow indicates one of the 6CIs which does not include $\mu = 3.39$ kg

In an actual study, only *one* 95% CI is obtained, and we would never know without detailed further study, whether it includes within it the true population mean's value.

Worked example: Confidence interval for a mean – birthweights of pre-term infants

Simpson (2004) reported the mean birthweight of 98 infants who were born prematurely as $\bar{x} = 1.31$ kg with $SE(\bar{x}) = 0.42/\sqrt{98} = 0.04$ kg. From these the 95% CI for the population mean is

$$1.31 - (1.96 \times 0.04) \text{ to } 1.31 + (1.96 \times 0.04)$$

or 1.23 to 1.39 kg.

Hence, loosely speaking, we are 95% confident that the true population mean birthweight for pre-term infants lies between 1.23 and 1.39 kg. Our best estimate is provided by the sample mean of 1.31 kg.

Strictly speaking, it is incorrect to say that there is a probability of 0.95 that the population mean birthweight lies between 1.23 and 1.39 kg as the population mean is a fixed number and not a random variable and therefore has no probability attached to it. However, most statisticians, including us, often describe confidence intervals in that way. The value of 0.95 is really the probability that the limits calculated from a random sample will include the population value. For 95% of the calculated confidence intervals it will be true to say that the population mean, μ, lies within this interval. The problem is, as Figure 6.6 shows, with a single study we just do not know which one of these 100 intervals we will obtain and hence we will not know if it includes μ. So we usually interpret a confidence interval as the range of values within which we are 95% confident that the true population mean lies.

Confidence interval for a proportion

Since a proportion, p, is a mean of a series of 0's and 1's, we can use a similar expression for a confidence interval for π as we did for μ with corresponding changes to the estimated parameter and the associated standard error. The Central Limit theorem will assure Normality. The standard error is given in Table 6.3 (Section 6.10) and so the confidence interval is just the *Estimate* $\pm$ $1.96 \times SE$ once more.

Example from the literature: Confidence interval for a proportion – acupuncture and headache

Melchart et al (2005) give the response rate to acupuncture treatment in 124 patients as $p = 0.46$, $SE(p) = 0.04$ giving a 95% confidence interval for π as $0.46 - 1.96 \times 0.04$ to $0.46 + 1.96 \times 0.04$ or 0.37 to 0.55, that is, from 37% to 55%.

We are 95% confident that the true population proportion of patients with migraine who response successfully with acupuncture treatment lies between 37% and 55% and our best estimate is 46%.

For technical reasons, this expression given for a confidence interval for π is an approximation and is referred to as the *traditional* approach. It is also only in situations in which reasonable agreement exists between the shape of the Binomial distribution and the Normal distribution (see Chapter 5) that we would use the confidence interval expression just given. The approximation will usually be quite good provided π is not too close to 0 or 1, situations in which either almost none or nearly all of the patients respond. The approximation improves with increasing sample size n.

If n is small, however, or π close to 0 or 1, the disparity between the Normal and Binomial distributions with the same mean and standard deviation, similar to those illustrated in Figure 5.2, increases and the Normal distribution can no longer be used to approximate the Binomial distribution.

The preferred or *recommended* method for calculating a confidence interval for a single proportion described by Altman et al (2000) and given in Section 6.10, has better statistical properties than the traditional method just given.

Confidence interval for a rate

Provided the sample size is reasonably large we can use the general formula, *Estimate* $\pm 1.96 \times SE$, for the confidence interval of a rate.

Worked example: Confidence interval for a rate – cadaveric heart donors

In the example from Wight et al (2004) the estimated heart donor rate was $r = 1.82$ with $SE(r) = 0.05$.

Therefore the 95% confidence interval for the population rate λ is $1.82 - 1.96 \times 0.05$ to $1.82 + 1.96 \times 0.05$ or 1.72 to 1.92 organ donations per day. This confidence interval is quite narrow suggesting that the true value of (strictly range for) λ is well established.

6.8 Confidence intervals for differences

To calculate a confidence interval for a difference in means, for example $\delta = \mu_A - \mu_B$, the same structure for the confidence interval of a single mean is used but with $\bar{x}$ replaced by $\bar{x}_1 - \bar{x}_2$ and $SE(\bar{x})$ replaced by $SE(\bar{x}_1 - \bar{x}_2)$. Algebraic expressions for these standard errors are given in Table 6.4 (Section 6.10). Thus the 95% CI is given by

$$(\bar{x}_1 - \bar{x}_2) - 1.96 \times SE(\bar{x}_1 - \bar{x}_2) \text{ to } (\bar{x}_1 - \bar{x}_2) + 1.96 \times SE(\bar{x}_1 - \bar{x}_2).$$

Example from the literature: CI for the difference between two means – physiotherapy for patients with lung disease

In the study by Griffiths et al (2000) described earlier there was a difference in walking capacity between intervention and control of 88 m, with standard error 16 m.

Thus a 95% CI is

$$88 - 1.96 \times 16 \text{ to } 88 + 1.96 \times 16,$$

which is 56.6 to 119.4 m.

It is therefore plausible that the intervention could improve walking capacity by as little as 57 m or by as much as 119 m.

Provided the sample sizes in the two groups are large, this method of calculating a confidence interval can be adapted for the comparison of two proportions or the comparison of two rates with appropriate changes.

Worked example: CI for difference between two proportions – post-natal urinary incontinence

In the study by Glazener et al (2001) described in Table 6.2 the difference in proportions was 0.09, with $SE = 0.042$. Thus the 95% CI for the true difference in proportions is given by $0.09 - (1.96 \times 0.042)$ to $0.09 + (1.96 \times 0.042)$ or 0.008 to 0.172.

Therefore we are 95% confident that the true population estimate of the effect of this intervention lies somewhere between 0.008 (0.8%) and 0.172 (17.2%), but our best estimate is 0.09 (9%). These data are therefore consistent with the Intervention improving continence over control by between 1% and 17%.

6.9 Points when reading the literature

1. When authors give the background information to a study they often quote figures of the form $a \pm b$. Although it is usual that a represents the value of the sample mean, it is not always clear what b is. When the intent is to describe the variability found in the sample then b should be the *SD*. When the intent is to describe the precision of the mean then b should be the *SE*. This ± method of presentation tends to cause confusion and should be avoided.

2. A useful mnemonic to decide which measure of variability to use is: 'If the purpose is **D**escriptive use Standard **D**eviation, if the purpose is **E**stimation, use the Standard **E**rror'.

3. What is the population from which the sample was taken? Are there any possible sources of bias that may affect the estimates of the population parameters?

4. Have reference ranges been calculated on a random sample of healthy volunteers? If not, how does this affect your interpretation? Is there any good reason why a random sample was not taken?

5. Have confidence intervals been presented? Has the confidence level been specified (e.g. 95%)?

6. Has a Normal approximation been used to calculate confidence intervals for a Binomial proportion or Poisson rate? If so, is this justified?

6.10 Technical details

Standard errors

Table 6.3 Population parameters of the Normal, Binomial and Poisson distributions, their estimates and the associated standard errors (*SE*) for a single group

Distribution	Parameters	Population values	Sample estimate	Standard error (SE)
Normal	Mean	μ	$\bar{x}$	$\dfrac{s}{\sqrt{n}}$
Binomial	Proportion	π	p	$\sqrt{\dfrac{p(1-p)}{n}}$
Poisson	Rate	λ	r	$\sqrt{\dfrac{r}{n}}$

Table 6.4 Population parameters of the Normal, binomial and Poisson distributions, their estimates and the associated standard errors (SE) for comparing two groups

Distribution	Parameter	Population value	Estimated difference	SE (difference)
Normal	Mean	$\mu_1 - \mu_2$	$\bar{x}_1 - \bar{x}_2$	$\sqrt{\dfrac{s_1^2}{n_1} + \dfrac{s_2^2}{n_2}}$
Binomial	Proportion	$\pi_1 - \pi_2$	$p_1 - p_2$	$\sqrt{\dfrac{p_1(1-p_1)}{n_1} + \dfrac{p_2(1-p_2)}{n_2}}$
Poisson	Rate	$\lambda_1 - \lambda_2$	$r_1 - r_2$	$\sqrt{\dfrac{r_1}{n_1} + \dfrac{r_2}{n_2}}$

More accurate confidence intervals for a proportion, p = r/n

To use this method we first need to calculate three quantities:

$$A = 2r + z^2; B = z\sqrt{z^2 + 4r(1-p)}; \text{ and, } C = 2(n + z^2)$$

where z is as before the appropriate value, $z_{1-\alpha/2}$, from the standard Normal distribution of Table T1. Then the recommended confidence interval for the population proportion is given by:

$$\frac{(A-B)}{C} \text{ to } \frac{(A+B)}{C}.$$

When there are no observed events, $r = 0$ and hence $p = 0/n = 0$ (0%), the recommended confidence interval simplifies to 0 to $\dfrac{z^2}{(n+z^2)}$, while when $r = n$ so that $p = 1$ (100%), the interval becomes $\dfrac{n}{(n+z^2)}$ to 1.

Worked example: CI for a proportion – prolactin concentration

Of 15 patients with chronic pain using non-opioid analgesia, Merza et al (2003) found, one to have a prolactin hormone concentration outside the normal range. Here $p = 1/15 = 0.07$. To calculate the recommended 95% confidence interval:

$$A = 2 \times 1 + 1.96^2 = 5.84;$$
$$B = 1.96 \times \sqrt{(1.96^2 + 4 \times 1 \times 0.93)} = 5.39;$$
$$C = 2 \times (15 + 1.96^2) = 37.68.$$

Then the 95% confidence interval for the prevalence of abnormal prolactin hormone concentrations in the population of such chronic pain patients is

$$\frac{(5.84-5.39)}{37.68}=0.01 \text{ to } \frac{(5.84+5.39)}{37.68}=0.30,$$

that is, from 1% to 30%.

In the same study, there were 21 chronic pain patients using opioid analgesia, none of whom had prolactin hormone concentrations outside the normal range. The estimated prevalence of abnormal prolactin hormone concentrations for this group is 0 (0%), with 95% confidence interval from 0 to $\frac{1.96^2}{(21+1.96^2)}=0.15$, that is 0 to 15%.

6.11 Exercises

Decide whether the following are true or false:

1. As the size of a random sample increases:

    (a) The standard deviation decreases.
    (b) The standard error of the mean decreases.
    (c) The mean decreases.
    (d) The range is likely to increase.
    (e) The accuracy of the parameter estimates increases.

2. A 95% confidence interval for a mean

    (a) Is wider than a 99% confidence interval.
    (b) In repeated samples will include the population mean 95% of the time.
    (c) Will include the sample mean with a probability of 1.
    (d) Is a useful way of describing the accuracy of a study.
    (e) Will include 95% of the observations of a sample.

3. Assume that the mid-upper arm circumference in a population of rural Indian children aged 12 to 60 months follows a Normal distribution with unknown mean, μ. Ten samples each of four children are drawn from this population by a formal process of random sampling with replacement. The results are shown in Table 6.5.

    (a) Calculate the sample mean and standard deviation for random sample number 10.
    (b) Display the sample means on a dot plot.
    (c) Calculate the standard error of the mean using the standard deviation, s, of random sample number 10 in Table 6.5.

Table 6.5 Mid-upper arm circumference (mm) in a rural Indian population aged 12 to 60 months (10 random samples of size 4)

Sample	Observations, X				Sample mean, $\bar{x}$	Standard deviation, s
1	128	162	158	156	151.00	15.53
2	148	148	146	136	144.50	5.74
3	164	150	148	158	155.00	7.39
4	154	172	128	136	147.50	19.62
5	144	158	154	168	156.00	9.93
6	136	140	128	138	135.50	5.26
7	144	158	140	142	146.00	8.16
8	154	148	148	138	147.00	6.63
9	154	140	154	152	150.00	6.73
10	156	154	140	158		

4. Table 6.6 shows ten random samples of size 16 drawn from the same population of Indian children.

   (a) Display as a dot plot alongside the previous one, the means of the ten random samples of size 16 shown in Table 6.6.
   (b) Calculate the standard error of the mean using the standard deviation of random sample number 4 in Table 6.6.
   (c) Compare the standard error (of the mean) for $n = 4$ with the standard error (of the mean) for $n = 16$.

Table 6.6 Mid-upper arm circumference (mm) in a rural Indian population aged 12 to 60 months: random samples of size 16

Sample	Observations, x	Sample mean	Standard deviation
1	146 160 144 140 162 162 128 176 148 146 144 176 146 138 146 138	150.00	13.54
2	142 158 156 190 164 148 138 130 142 152 150 148 146 154 142 148	150.50	13.36
3	130 142 138 144 144 150 174 138 154 150 154 136 162 152 156 138	147.63	11.15
4	146 160 158 140 128 150 172 154 140 162 162 136 150 152 156 154	151.25	11.19
5	142 148 154 152 140 140 156 122 164 130 148 140 162 162 136 142	146.13	11.88
6	148 142 134 158 130 156 144 154 148 138 168 140 146 154 146 152	147.38	9.63
7	140 140 146 146 138 154 156 136 146 146 152 142 138 156 156 154	146.63	7.18
8	156 140 152 158 164 148 140 128 132 156 148 162 164 142 156 134	148.75	11.61
9	146 160 138 134 162 148 156 154 148 172 154 154 162 152 150 156	153.00	9.27
10	152 142 148 150 154 136 148 144 158 144 134 140 144 176 144 148	147.62	9.80

5. (a) Estimate the 95% confidence interval for one selected sample of size 4 (sample number 10 in Table 6.5) and display this on the dot plot for $n = 4$.

   (b) Estimate the 95% confidence interval for one selected sample of size 16 (sample number 4 in Table 6.5) and display this on the dot plot for $n = 16$.

6. A surgeon in a large hospital is investigating acute appendicitis in people aged 65 and over. As a preliminary study he examines the hospital case notes over the previous 10 years and finds that of 120 patients in this age group with a diagnosis confirmed at operation 73 were women and 47 were men. Calculate a 95% confidence interval for the proportion of females with acute appendicitis.

7 *p*-values and statistical inference

Medical Statistics Fourth Edition, David Machin, Michael J Campbell, Stephen J Walters
© 2007 John Wiley & Sons, Ltd

Summary

The main aim of statistical analysis is to use the information gained from a sample of individuals to make inferences about the population of interest. There are two basic approaches to statistical analysis: Estimation (with Confidence intervals) and Hypothesis Testing (with *p*-values). The concepts of the null hypothesis, statistical significance, the use of statistical tests, *p*-values and their relationship to confidence intervals are introduced.

7.1   Introduction

We have seen that in sampling from a population which can be assumed to have a Normal distribution the sample mean can be regarded as estimating the corresponding population mean μ. Similarly, s estimates the population standard deviation, σ. We therefore describe the distribution of the population with the information given by the sample statistics $\bar{x}$ and s. More generally, in comparing two populations, perhaps the population of subjects exposed to a particular hazard and the population of those who were not, two samples are taken, and their respective summary statistics calculated. We might wish to compare the two samples and ask: 'Could they both come from the same population?' That is, does the fact that some subjects have been exposed, and others not, influence the characteristic or variable we are observing? If it does not, then we regard the two populations as if they were one with respect to the particular variable under consideration.

7.2   The null hypothesis

Statistical analysis is concerned not only with summarising data but also with investigating relationships. An investigator conducting a study usually has a theory in mind; for example, patients with diabetes have raised blood pressure, or oral contraceptives may cause breast cancer. This theory is known as the *study* or *research hypothesis*. However, it is impossible to prove most hypotheses; one can always think of circumstances which have not yet arisen under which a particular hypothesis may or may not hold. Thus one might hold a theory that all Chinese children have black hair. Unfortunately, having observed 1000 or even 1 000 000 Chinese children and checked that they all have black hair would not have proved the hypothesis. On the other hand, if only one fair-haired Chinese child is seen, the theory is disproved. Thus there is a simpler logical setting for disproving hypotheses than for proving them. The converse of the study hypothesis is the *null hypothesis*. Examples are: diabetic patients do not have raised blood pressure, or oral contraceptives do not cause breast cancer. Such a hypothesis is usually phrased in the negative and that is why it is termed *null*.

In Section 6.5 we described the results of a randomised trial conducted by Griffiths et al (2000) of 184 patients with chronic obstructive pulmonary disease to compare a pulmonary rehabilitation programme (Intervention) with standard medical management (Control). One outcome measure was the walking capacity (distance walked in metres using a standardised test) of the patient assessed 6 weeks after randomisation. The sample means $\bar{x}_{Int} = 211$ m and $\bar{x}_{Con} = 123$ m estimate the two population mean distances walked μ_{Int} and μ_{Con} respectively. In the context of a clinical trial the population usually refers to those patients, present and future, who have the disease and for whom it would be appropriate to treat with either the Intervention or Control. Now if both approaches are equally effective, μ_{Int} equals μ_{Con} and the difference between $\bar{x}_{Int}$ and $\bar{x}_{Con}$ is only a chance difference. After all, subjects will differ between themselves, so we would not be surprised if differences between $\bar{x}_{Int}$ and $\bar{x}_{Con}$ are observed, even if the approaches are identical in their effectiveness. The statistical problem is: when can it be concluded that the difference between $\bar{x}_{Int}$ and $\bar{x}_{Con}$ is of sufficient magnitude to suspect that μ_{Int} is not equal to μ_{Con}?

The null hypothesis states that $\mu_{Int} = \mu_{Con}$ and this can be alternatively expressed as $\mu_{Int} - \mu_{Con} = 0$. The problem is to decide if the observations, as expressed by the sample means and corresponding standard deviations, appear consistent with this hypothesis. Clearly, if $\bar{x}_{Int} = \bar{x}_{Cont}$ exactly, we would be reasonably convinced that $\mu_{Int} = \mu_{Cont}$ but what of the actual results given above? To help decide it is necessary to first calculate $\bar{d} = \bar{x}_{Int} - \bar{x}_{Con} = 211 - 123 = 88$ m and also calculate the corresponding standard deviation of the difference, $SD(\bar{d})$ termed $SE(\bar{d})$. The formula for the standard error is given in Table 7.4 in Section 7.9.

The formula given here differs from that given in Table 6.4, which was used when calculating a confidence interval for the true difference between means, δ. The change arises as the standard error is now calculated under the assumption that the two groups have the same population standard deviation, σ. This implies that both s_1 and s_2 are estimating the same quantity and so these are combined into the so-called pooled estimate, s_{Pooled}, of Table 7.4. However in this example there is very little difference numerically in the estimates and so $SE_{Pooled}(\bar{d}) = 16.1$ m also.

Now, if indeed the two populations of distances walked can be assumed each to have approximately Normal distributions, then $\bar{d}$ will also have a Normal distribution. This distribution will have its own mean $\mu_{Int-Con}$ and standard deviation $\sigma_{Int-Con}$, which are estimated by $\bar{d}$ and $SE_{Pooled}(\bar{d})$, respectively. One can even go one step further, if samples are large enough, and state that the ratio $\bar{d}/SE_{Pooled}(\bar{d})$ will have a Normal distribution with mean $\mu_{Int-Con}$ and a standard deviation of unity. If the null hypothesis were true, this distribution would have mean $\delta = 0$.

However, the observed values are $\bar{d} = 88\,\mathrm{m}$ with $SE_{\text{Pooled}}(\bar{d}) = 16.1\,\mathrm{m}$ and therefore a ratio of mean to standard error equal to $z = 88/16.1$ or more than five standard deviations for this distribution from the null hypothesis mean of zero. This is a very extreme observation and very unlikely to arise by chance since 95% of observations sampled from a Normal distribution with specified mean and standard deviation will be within 1.96 standard deviations of its centre. A value of δ greater than zero seems very plausible. It therefore seems very unlikely that the measurements come from a Normal distribution whose mean is in fact $\delta = \mu_{\text{Int}} - \mu_{\text{Con}} = 0$. There is strong evidence that μ_{Int} and μ_{Con} differ perhaps by a substantial amount. As a consequence the notion of equality of effect of the two treatments suggested by the null hypothesis is rejected. The conclusion is that the Intervention results in further distances walked in patients with chronic obstructive pulmonary disease than Control management.

Provided the sample sizes in the two groups are large, the method of analysis used for comparing the mean distances walked in two groups can be utilised for the comparison of two proportions with minor changes. Thus the population proportions of success, π_{Int} and π_{Con}, replace the population means μ_{Int} and μ_{Con}. Similarly the sample statistics p_{Int} and p_{Con} replace $\bar{x}_{Int}$ and $\bar{x}_{Con}$. However, the standard error is now given by the expression of Table 7.4, which is calculated under the null hypothesis that the two proportions are the same, so that p_1 and p_2 both estimate a common value, π, and so these are combined into the so-called pooled estimate, p_{Pooled} or more briefly p.

Example from the literature: Post-natal urinary incontinence

One of the outcomes from the randomised trial conducted by Glazener et al (2001) to assess the effect of nurse assessment with reinforcement of pelvic floor muscle training exercises and bladder training (Intervention) compared with standard management (Control) among women with persistent incontinence three months postnatally included urinary incontinence rates at 12 months postnatally and are summarised in Table 6.2. From these data, $\bar{d} = 0.40 - 0.31 = 0.09$ and $p = \dfrac{(279 \times 0.40) + (245 \times 0.31)}{279 + 245} = 0.357$, or more simply the total number of mothers with no urinary incontinence, $r = 188$ divided by the total number of patients in the trial, $N = 524$. This leads to

$$SE_{\text{Pooled}}(\bar{d}) = \sqrt{[0.357 \times (1 - 0.357)]\left(\frac{1}{279} + \frac{1}{245}\right)} = 0.042.$$ (Compare this with

Chapter 6 with $SE(\bar{d}) = 0.042$). Finally, $z = \bar{d} / SE_{\text{Pooled}}(\bar{d}) = 0.09/0.042 = 2.14$.

7.3 The p-value

All the examples so far have used 95% when calculating a confidence interval, but other percentages could have been chosen. In fact the choice of 95% is quite arbitrary although it has now become conventional in the medical literature. A general $100(1 - \alpha)\%$ confidence interval can be calculated using

$$\bar{d} - z_\alpha \times SE(\bar{d}) \text{ to } \bar{d} + z_\alpha \times SE(\bar{d}).$$

In this expression z_α is the value, along the axis of a Normal distribution (Table T1), which leaves a total probability of α equally divided in the two tails. In particular, if $\alpha = 0.05$, then $100(1 - \alpha)\% = 95\%$, $z_\alpha = 1.96$ and the 95% confidence interval is given as before by

$$\bar{d} - 1.96 \times SE(\bar{d}) \text{ to } \bar{d} + 1.96 \times SE(\bar{d}).$$

In the comparison of the 12-month post-natal urinary incontinence rates between the Intervention and Control groups in the Glazener et al (2001) study, the expression for the more general confidence interval for δ is

$$0.09 - (z_\alpha \times 0.042) \text{ to } 0.09 + (z_\alpha \times 0.042).$$

Suppose that z_α is now chosen in this expression, in such a way that the left-hand or lower limit of the above confidence interval equals zero. That is, it just includes the null hypothesis value of $\delta = (\pi_A - \pi_B) = 0$. Then the resulting equation is

$$0.09 - (z_\alpha \times 0.042) = 0.$$

This equation can be rewritten to become

$$z_\alpha = 0.09/0.042 = 2.14,$$

and this is termed the z-test. It is in fact the estimate of the difference between treatments divided by the standard error of that difference.

We can now examine Table T1 to find an α such that $z_\alpha = 2.14$. This determines α to be 0.0324 and $100(1 - \alpha)\%$ to be 97%. Thus a 97% confidence interval for δ is

$$0.09 - (2.14 \times 0.042) \text{ to } 0.09 + (2.14 \times 0.042)$$

or 0 to 0.18. This interval just includes the null hypothesis value of zero difference as we have required. The value of α so calculated is termed the p-value. The p-value can be interpreted as the probability of obtaining the observed difference, or one more extreme, if the null hypothesis is true.

Example: p-value – change in blood pressure

The systolic blood pressure in 16 middle-aged men before and after a standard exercise programme are shown in Table 7.1.

If the change in blood pressure, d, was calculated for each patient and if the null hypothesis is true that there is no effect of exercise on blood pressure, then the mean of the $n = 16$ d's should be close to zero. The d's are termed the paired differences and are the basic observations of interest. Thus $\bar{d} = \Sigma d/n = 6.63$ and $SD(d) = \sqrt{\dfrac{\Sigma(d - \bar{d})^2}{(n-1)}} = 5.97\,\text{mmHg}$.

This gives $SE(\bar{d}) = SD(d)/\sqrt{n} = 1.49\,\text{mmHg}$ and $z = 6.63/1.49 = 4.44$.
Using Table T1 with $z = 4.44$, a p-value <0.001 is obtained.

A statistical significance test considers the p-value obtained from the study. If it is small, conventionally less than 0.05, the null hypothesis is rejected as implausible. While if $p > 0.05$ this is often taken as suggesting that insufficient information is available to discount the null hypothesis.

Table 7.1   Systolic blood pressure levels (mmHg) in 16 men before and after exercise (data from Altman et al, 2000) sorted by before exercise levels for convenience

Subject	Before exercise	After exercise	Difference
16	116	126	10
15	126	132	6
9	128	146	18
7	132	144	12
4	134	148	14
3	136	134	−2
5	138	144	6
13	138	146	8
6	140	136	−4
2	142	152	10
8	144	150	6
1	148	152	4
12	150	162	12
14	154	156	2
11	162	162	0
10	170	174	4
		Mean, $\bar{d}$	6.63
		SD	5.97
		SE $(\bar{d})$	1.49

Example: z-test – difference in fatigue severity scores

Stulemeijer et al (2005) report the mean and standard deviation of the fatigue severity score in a randomised controlled trial to compare immediate Cognitive Behaviour Therapy (CBT) with Waiting Listing for Therapy (WLT) in 69 adolescents with chronic fatigue patients. The 35 patients in the CBT group had a mean fatigue severity score of 30.2 (SD = 16.8) and 34 patients in the WLT control group had a mean score of 44.0 (SD = 13.4).

An appropriate null hypothesis is that there is no difference in fatigue severity score at 5 months between the two groups. From the above summary, $\bar{d}$ = 30.2 – 44.0 = –13.8 and from Table 7.4, SE($\bar{d}$) = 3.67.

A z-test gives z = 13.8/3.67 = 3.76 and use of Table T1 gives p = 0.0002. This is much smaller than 0.05 and so we would reject the null hypothesis of equal mean fatigue severity scores for the two 'populations' of adolescent patients and so conclude that the two patient groups do have different mean of levels of fatigue.

7.4 Statistical inference

Hypothesis testing is a method of deciding whether the data are consistent with the null hypothesis. The calculation of the p-value is an important part of the procedure. Given a study with a single outcome measure and a statistical test, hypothesis testing can be summarised in four steps.

Hypothesis testing: main steps

- State your null hypothesis (H_0) (*Statement you are looking for evidence to disprove*)
- State your alternative hypothesis (H_A)
- Choose a *significance level*, α, of the test
- Conduct the study, observe the outcome and compute the probability of observing your results, or results more extreme, if the null hypothesis is true (p-value)
- Use your p-value to make a decision about whether to reject, or not reject, your null hypothesis.

That is: If the p-value is less than or equal to α conclude that the data are not consistent with the null hypothesis. Whereas if the p-value is greater than α, do not reject the null hypothesis, and view it as 'not yet disproven'.

Step 1 *State your null hypothesis (H$_0$) and alternative hypothesis (H$_A$)*

It is easier to disprove things than to prove them. In a court of law the defendant is assumed innocent until proven guilty. Often statistical analyses involve comparisons between different treatments, such as between standard and new – here we assume that the treatment effects are equal until proven different. Therefore the null hypothesis is often the negation of the research hypothesis which is that the new treatment will be more effective than the standard.

Step 2 *Choose a significance level, α, for your test*

For consistency we have to specify at the planning stage a value, α, so that once the study is completed and analysed, a *p*-value below this would lead to the null hypothesis (which is specified in step 1) being rejected. Thus if the *p*-value obtained from a trial is $\leq \alpha$, then one rejects the null hypothesis and concludes that there is a statistically significant difference between treatments. On the other hand, if the *p*-value is $> \alpha$ then one does not reject the null hypothesis. Although the value of α is arbitrary, it is often taken as 0.05 or 5%.

p-value	
Small $< \alpha$	Large $\geq \alpha$
Your results are *unlikely* when the null hypothesis is true	Your results are *likely* when the null hypothesis is true

Step 3 *Obtain the probability of observing your results, or results more extreme, if the null hypothesis is true (p-value)*

First calculate a test statistic using your data (reduce your data down to a single value). The general formula for a test statistics is:

$$\text{Test statistic} = \frac{\text{Observed value} - \text{Hypothesised value}}{\text{Standard error of the observed value}}$$

This test statistic is then compared to a distribution that we expect if the null hypothesis is true (such as the Normal distribution with mean zero and standard deviation unity) to obtain a *p*-value.

Step 4 *Use your p-value to make a decision about whether to reject, or not reject, your null hypothesis*

We say that our results are statistically significant if the *p*-value is less than the significance level α, usually set at 5% or 0.05.

Result is	p-value ≤ 0.05	p-value > 0.05
	Statistically significant	Not statistically significant
Decide	That there is sufficient evidence to reject the null hypothesis and accept the alternative	That there is insufficient evidence to reject the null hypothesis ↑ We cannot say the null hypothesis is true, only that there is not enough evidence to reject it.

It is important to distinguish between the (preset) significance level and the p-value obtained after the study is completed. If one rejects the null hypothesis when it is in fact true, then one makes what is known as a *Type I error*. The significance level α is the probability of making a Type I error. This is set before the test is carried out. The p-value is the result observed after the study is completed and is based on the observed result.

The term *statistically significant* is spread throughout the published medical literature. It is a common mistake to state that it is the probability that the null hypothesis is true as the null hypothesis is *either* true *or* it is false. The null hypothesis is not, therefore, 'true' or 'false' with a certain probability. However, it is common practice to assign probabilities to events, such as 'the chance of rain tomorrow is 30%'. So in some ways, the p-value can be thought of as a measure of the strength of the belief in the null hypothesis.

How to interpret p-values (*adapted from Bland, 2000*)

We can think of the p-values as indicating the strength of evidence but always keep in mind the size of the study being considered

p-value	Interpretation
Greater than 0.10	Little or no evidence of a difference or a relationship*
Between 0.05 and 0.10	Evidence of a difference or relationship
Between 0.01 and 0.05	Weak evidence of a difference or a relationship
Less than 0.01:	Strong evidence of a difference or relationship
Less than 0.001:	Very strong evidence of a difference or relationship.

*Although we have talked in terms of detecting differences in this chapter, the same principles arise when testing relationships as in Chapter 9 for example.

In Chapter 4 we discussed different concepts of probability. The p-value is a probability, and the concept in this instance is closest to the idea of a repeated sample. If we conducted a large number of similar studies and repeated the test each time, when the null hypothesis is true, then in the long run, the proportion of times the test statistic equals, or is greater than the observed value is the *p*-value.

In terms of the notation of Chapter 4 the *p*-value is equivalent to the probability of the data (*D*), given the hypothesis (*H*), that is, $P(D|H)$ (strictly the probability of the observed data, or data more extreme). It is not $P(H|D)$, the probability of the hypothesis given the data, which is what most people want. Unfortunately, unlike diagnostic tests we cannot go from $P(D|H)$ to $P(H|D)$ using Bayes' theorem, because we do not know the *a priori* probability (that is before collecting any data) of the null hypothesis being true $P(H)$, which would be analogous to the prevalence of the disease. Some people try to quantify their *subjective* belief in the null hypothesis, but this is *not objective* as different investigators will have different levels of belief and so different interpretations from the same data will arise.

Whenever a significance test is used, the corresponding report should quote the exact *p*-value to a sensible number of significant figures together with the value of the corresponding test statistic. Merely reporting whichever appropriate, $p < 0.05$ or worse, $p > 0.05$, or $p =$ 'NS' meaning 'Not statistically significant', is not acceptable.

Example: Interpreting a *p*-value – blood pressure before and after exercise

In the example of examining change in blood pressure before and after exercise in 16 men the *p*-value was less than 0.001.

What does p < 0.001 *mean?*

Your results are unlikely when the null hypothesis is true.

Is this result statistically significant?

The result is statistically significant because the *p*-value is less than the significance level α set at 5% or 0.05.

You decide?

That there is sufficient evidence to reject the null hypothesis and accept the alternative hypothesis that there is a difference (a rise) in the mean blood pressure of middle-aged men before and after exercise.

7.5 Statistical power

Type I error, test size and significance level

We said that the first step in hypothesis testing is to choose a value α, so that once the study is completed and analysed, a *p*-value below this would lead to the null hypothesis being rejected. Thus if the *p*-value obtained from

Table 7.2 Possible errors arising when performing a hypothesis test

You decide to	The null hypothesis is actually	
	True	False
Reject the null hypothesis (test is statistically significant)	Incorrect	Correct
Not reject the null hypothesis (test is not statistically significant)	Correct	Incorrect

a trial is $\leq \alpha$, then one rejects the null hypothesis and concludes that there is a statistically significant difference between treatments. On the other hand, if the p-value is $> \alpha$ then one does not reject the null hypothesis. This seems a clear-cut decision with no chance of making a wrong decision. However, as Table 7.2 shows there are two possible errors when using a p-value to make a decision.

Even when the null hypothesis is in fact true there is still a risk of rejecting it. To reject the null hypothesis when it is true is to make a type I error. Plainly the associated probability of rejecting the null hypothesis when it is true is equal to α. The quantity α is interchangeably termed the test size, significance level or probability of a type I (or false-positive) error.

Type II error and power

The clinical trial could yield an observed difference $\bar{d}$ that would lead to a p-value $> \alpha$ even though the null hypothesis is really not true, that is, μ_{Int} is indeed not equal to μ_{Con}. In such a situation, we then accept (more correctly phrased as 'fail to reject') the null hypothesis although it is truly false. This is called a Type II (false-negative) error and the probability of this is denoted by β.

The probability of a Type II error is based on the assumption that the null hypothesis is not true, that is, $\delta = \mu_{\text{Int}} - \mu_{\text{Con}} \neq 0$. There are clearly many possible values of δ in this instance and each would imply a different alternative hypothesis, H_A, and a different value for the probability β.

The power is defined as one minus the probability of a Type II error, thus the power equals $1 - \beta$. That is, the *power* is the probability of obtaining a 'statistically significant' p-value when the null hypothesis is truly false.

The relationship between Type I and II errors and significance tests is given in Table 7.3.

These concepts of Type I error and Type II error parallel the concepts of sensitivity and specificity that we discussed in Section 4.2. The Type I error is equivalent to the false positive rate (1 – specificity) and the Type II error is equivalent to the false negative rate (1 – sensitivity).

Table 7.3 Relationship between Type I and Type II errors and significance tests

Test statistically significant	Difference exists (H_A true)	Difference does not exist (H_0 true)
Yes	Power $(1 - \beta)$	Type I error (α)
No	Type II error (β)	

Example from the literature: Aspirin for non-fatal myocardial infarction

In a randomised trial of 1239 patients, Elwood and Sweetnam (1979) discovered the mortality after a non-fatal myocardial infarction to be 8.0% in a group given aspirin and 10.7% in a group given placebo. The difference, 2.7%, has 95% confidence interval −0.5% to 6.0%.

Based on this result, a reader might conclude that there was little evidence for an effect of aspirin on mortality after myocardial infarction. However, shortly after this another study was published by the Persantine-Aspirin Reinfarction Research Study Group (1980). This showed 9.2% mortality in the aspirin group, and 11.5% in the placebo, a difference of 2.3%, which is less than that of Elwood and Sweetnam. However, the sample size was 6292 and the 95% *CI* 0.8% to 3.8%.

The larger study had greater power, and so achieved a narrower confidence interval whose lower limit was further from the null hypothesis value of zero than in the first study.

7.6 Confidence intervals rather than *p*-values

All that we know from a hypothesis test is, for example, that there is a difference in the mean blood pressure of middle aged men before and after exercise. It does not tell us what the difference is or how large the difference is. To answer this we need to supplement the hypothesis test with a confidence interval which will give us a range of values in which we are confident the true population mean difference will lie.

Simple statements in a study report such as '$p < 0.05$' or '$p = $ NS' do not describe the results of a study well, and create an artificial dichotomy between significant and non-significant results. Statistical significance does not necessarily mean the result is clinically significant. The *p*-value does not relate to the clinical importance of a finding, as it depends to a large extent on the size of the study. Thus a large study may find small, unimportant, differences that are highly significant and a small study may fail to find important differences.

Supplementing the hypothesis test with a confidence interval will indicate the magnitude of the result and this will aid the investigators to decide whether the difference is of interest clinically (see Figure 7.1). The confidence interval gives an estimate of the precision with which a statistic estimates a population value, which is useful information for the reader. This does not mean that one should not carry out statistical tests and quote *p*-values, rather that these results should supplement an estimate of an effect and a confidence interval. Many medical journals now require papers to contain confidence intervals where appropriate and not just *p*-values.

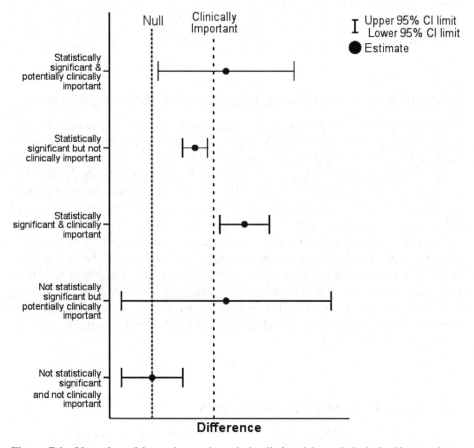

Figure 7.1 Use of confidence intervals to help distinguish statistical significance from clinical importance

> ### Example: Clinical importance – blood pressure before and after exercise
>
> The mean difference in systolic blood pressure following exercise was 6.63 mmHg with a <u>SD</u> of 5.97 mmHg. The standard error (of the mean difference) is $5.97/\sqrt{16} = 1.49$ mmHg and so the 95% CI is
>
> $$6.63 - (1.96 \times 1.49) \text{ to } 6.63 + (1.96 \times 1.49) \text{ or } 3.71 \text{ to } 9.55 \text{ mmHg}.$$
>
> Therefore we are 95% confident that the true population mean difference in systolic blood pressure lies somewhere between 3.7 and 9.6 mmHg, but the best estimate we have is 6.6 mmHg.
>
> Suppose the difference is clinically important if a mean blood pressure change of 10 mmHg or more is observed, then the above result is not clinically important although it is statistically significant. Hence this situation corresponds to the second confidence interval down in Figure 7.1.

Relationship between confidence intervals and statistical significance

Different though hypothesis testing and confidence intervals may appear there is in fact a close relationship between them. If the 95% CI does not include zero (or, more generally the value specified in the null hypothesis) then a hypothesis test will return a statistically significant result. If the 95% CI does include zero then the hypothesis test will return a non-significant result. The confidence interval shows the magnitude of the difference and the uncertainty or lack of precision in the estimate of interest. Thus the confidence interval conveys more useful information than *p*-values. For example, whether a clinician will use a new treatment that reduces blood pressure or not will depend on the amount of that reduction and how consistent the effect is across patients. So, the presentation of both the *p*-value and the confidence interval is desirable – but if only one is to be presented the *p*-value would be omitted. Presenting a 95% CI indicates whether the result is statistically significant at the 5% level.

7.7 One-sided and two-sided tests

The *p*-value is the probability of obtaining a result at least as extreme as the observed result when the null hypothesis is true, and such extreme results can occur by chance equally often in either direction. We allow for this by calculating a two-sided *p*-value. In the vast majority of cases this is the correct procedure. In rare cases it is reasonable to consider that a real difference can occur in only one direction, so that an observed difference in the opposite direction must be due to chance. Here, the alternative hypothesis is restricted to an effect in one direction only, and it is reasonable to calculate a one-sided p-value by considering only one tail of the distribution of the test statistic. For a test statistic with a Normal distribution, the usual two-sided 5% cut-off point is 1.96, whereas the corresponding one-sided 5% cut-off value is 1.64.

One-sided tests are rarely appropriate. Even when we have strong prior expectations, for example that a new treatment cannot be worse than an old one, we cannot be sure that we are right. If we could be sure we would not need to conduct the study! If it is felt that a one-sided test really is appropriate, then this decision must be made *before* the data are collected; it must not depend on the observed outcome data from the study itself. In practice, what is often done is that a two-sided p-value is quoted, but the result is given more weight, in an informal manner, if the result goes in the direction that was anticipated.

Key points

- Research questions need to be turned into a statement for which we can find evidence to disprove – the null hypothesis.
- The study data is reduced down to a single probability – the probability of observing our result, or one more extreme, if the null hypothesis is true (p-value).
- We use this p-value to decide whether to reject or not reject the null hypothesis.
- But we need to remember that 'statistical significance' does not necessarily mean 'clinical significance'.
- Confidence intervals should always be quoted with a hypothesis test to give the magnitude and precision of the difference.

7.8 Points when reading the literature

1. Have clinical importance and statistical significance been confused?
2. Is it reasonable to assume that the continuous variables have a Normal distribution?
3. Have confidence intervals of the main results been quoted?
4. Is the result medically or biologically plausible and has the statistical significance of the result been considered in isolation, or have other studies of the same effect been taken into account?

7.9 Technical details

Table 7.4 Population parameters of the Normal and binomial distributions, their estimates and the associated standard errors (SE) for comparing two groups under the null hypothesis of no difference between groups

Distribution	Parameters	SE (Difference)	
Normal	Mean difference $\delta = \mu_1 - \mu_2$	$s_{Pooled}\sqrt{\dfrac{1}{n_1}+\dfrac{1}{n_2}}$	$s_{Pooled} = \sqrt{\dfrac{(n_1-1)s_1^2 + (n_2-1)s_2^2}{(n_1-1)+(n_2-1)}}$
Binomial	Difference in proportions $\delta = \pi_1 - \pi_2$	$\sqrt{p(1-p)\left(\dfrac{1}{n_1}+\dfrac{1}{n_2}\right)}$	$p = \dfrac{n_1 p_1 + n_2 p_2}{n_1 + n_2}$

7.10 Exercises

1. Gaffney et al (1994) compared 141 babies who developed cerebral palsy to a control group of (control) babies made up from the babies who appeared immediately after each cerebral palsy case in the hospital delivery book. The corresponding hospital notes were reviewed by a researcher, who was blind to the baby's outcome, with respect to medical staff response to signs of fetal stress. Failure to respond to signs of fetal distress by the medical staff was noted in 25.8% of the cerebral palsy babies and in 7.1% of the next delivery controls: a difference of 18.7%. This difference had standard error 4.2% and the 95% CI was 10.5 to 26.9%.

    (a) What is the statistical null hypothesis for this study? What is the alternative hypothesis?
    (b) What is meant by 'the difference was 18.7%'?
    (c) What can we conclude from the 95% CI?

2. A randomised controlled trial was conducted to investigate the cost-effectiveness of community leg ulcer clinics (Morrell et al 1998). A total of 233 patients were randomly allocated to either intervention (120 patients, treatment at a leg ulcer clinic) or control (113, usual care at home by district nursing service). At the end of 12 months the mean time (in weeks) that each patient was free from ulcers during follow up was 20.1 and 14.2 in the clinic and control groups, respectively. On average, patients in the clinic group had 5.9 more ulcer-free weeks (95% CI 1.2 to 10.6 weeks) than the control patients. Mean total costs were £878 per year for the clinic group and £863 for the control group ($p = 0.89$).

(a) Is there a statistically significant difference between the two groups with respect to the number of ulcer-free weeks?
(b) What is the standard error of the difference in mean ulcer free weeks?
(c) Is there a statistically significant difference between the two groups with respect to the cost of treating the patients over the 12 month period? Would you expect the confidence interval for this difference to include the value for 'no difference'?
(d) What would you conclude from the information above?

3. A study by Taylor et al (2002) investigated whether the measles, mumps and rubella (MMR) vaccination was associated with bowel problems and developmental regression in children with autism. The authors reviewed the case notes for 278 children with core autism and 195 with atypical autism from five health districts in north-east London, England born between 1979 and 1998. This time frame was chosen as it included the date when the MMR vaccination was introduced in October 1988. The authors examined whether the proportions with developmental regression and those with bowel problems changed during the 20 years. The p-values associated with the change over time were 0.50 and 0.47 respectively.

In addition the authors examined whether there was any association between bowel problems and developmental regression. Of the 118 children with developmental regression, 26% reported bowel problems, whilst of the 351 without developmental regression 14% reported bowel symptoms. The difference was 12.3% (95% CI 4.2% to 21.5%).

(a) Write suitable statistical null hypotheses for this study. What are the alternative hypotheses to these?
(b) Was there a statistically significant difference in the proportions with developmental regression during the 20-year study period?
(c) Was there a statistically significant difference in the proportions with bowel problems during the 20-year study period?
(d) What does the confidence interval for the difference in with bowel problems for the children with and without developmental regression tell you? Would you expect the p-value for this difference to be greater than or less than 0.05?

4. A UK study by Peacock et al (1995) of factors affecting the outcome of pregnancy among 1513 women reported that the overall incidence of pre-term births was 7.5%, SE 0.68% and 95% CI 6.1 to 8.8%.

(a) What is meant by $SE = 0.68\%$?
(b) What is meant by 95% CI 6.1 to 8.8%?
(c) How would the confidence interval change if 90% limits were used?
(d) How would the confidence interval change if 99% limits were used?

Another study conducted at about the same time in Denmark (Kristensen et al, 1995) and including 51 851 women, reported that the overall incidence of pre-term birth was 4.5% (95% CI 4.3 to 4.7%).

(e) Explain why this 95% CI is narrower than that reported in the UK study. Do you think that there is a real difference in pre-term birth rates between the two populations being studied?

8 Tests for comparing two groups of categorical or continuous data

Medical Statistics Fourth Edition, David Machin, Michael J Campbell, Stephen J Walters
© 2007 John Wiley & Sons, Ltd

Summary

In this chapter we will now be putting some of the theory into practice and looking at some of the more basic statistical tests that you will come across in the literature and in your own research. The choice of method of analysis for a problem depends on the comparison to be made and the data to be used. We explain some of the basic methods appropriate for comparing two groups. We consider the comparison of two independent groups such as groups of patients given different treatments and the comparison of paired data, for example, the response of one group under different conditions as in a cross-over trial, or of matched pairs of subjects.

8.1   Introduction

There are often several different approaches to even a simple problem. The methods described here and recommended for particular types of question may not be the only methods, and may not be universally agreed as the best method. However, these would usually be considered as valid and satisfactory methods for the purposes for which they are suggested here.

What type of statistical test? Five key questions to ask

1. What are the aims and objectives of the study?
2. What is the hypothesis to be tested?
3. What type of data is the outcome data?
4. How is the outcome data distributed?
5. What is the summary measure for the outcome data?

   Given the answers to these five key questions, an appropriate approach to the statistical analysis of the data collected can be decided upon. The type of statistical analysis depends fundamentally on what the main purpose of the study is. In particular, what is the main question to be answered? The data type for the outcome variable will also govern how it is to be analysed, as an analysis appropriate to continuous data would be completely inappropriate for binary categorical data. In addition to what type of data the outcome variable is, its distribution is also important, as is the summary measure to be used. Highly skewed data require a different analysis compared to data that are Normally distributed.

   The choice of method of analysis for a problem depends on the comparison to be made and the data to be used. This chapter outlines the methods appropriate for two common problems in statistical inference as outlined below.

Two common problems in statistical inference

1. Comparison of independent groups, for example, groups of patients given different treatments.
2. Comparison of the response for paired observations, for example, in a cross-over trial, or for matched pairs of subjects.

Before beginning any analysis it is important to examine the data, using the techniques described in Chapters 2 and 3; adequate description of the data should precede and complement the formal statistical analysis. For most studies and for randomised controlled trials in particular, it is good practice to produce a table that describes the initial or baseline characteristics of the sample.

Example dataset

We shall illustrate some of various statistical tests by using data from a randomised controlled trial which aimed to compare a new treatment regime for patients with leg ulcers with usual care (Morrell et al 1998). In this trial, 233 patients with venous leg ulcers were randomly allocated to the Intervention (120) or the Control (113) group. The intervention consisted of weekly treatment with four layer bandaging in a leg ulcer clinic (Intervention group) or usual care at home by the district nursing service (Control group). Patients were treated and followed up for 12 months. The trial used a variety of outcomes which included: time to complete ulcer healing (in weeks); ulcer status (healed or not healed) at 3 and 12 months; ulcer free weeks (amount of time that patient was ulcer free during the 12 month follow-up period) and patient health-related quality of life (HRQoL) at baseline, 3 months and 12 months. HRQoL was measured using the general health dimension of the SF-36. This outcome is scored on a 0 (poor health) to 100 (good health) scale.

8.2 Comparison of two groups of paired observations – continuous outcomes

One common problem is the comparison of paired data, for example, the response of one group under different conditions as in a cross-over trial, or of matched pairs of subjects. When there is more than one group of observations it is vital to distinguish the case where the data are paired from that where the groups are independent. Paired data may arise when the same individuals are studied more than once, usually in different circumstances, or when individuals are paired as in a case-control study. For example, as part of the leg ulcer trial, data were collected on health related quality of life (HRQoL) at baseline, 3 months and 12 months follow-up. We may be interested in seeing if there is change in HRQoL between baseline and three months follow-up in those patients whose leg-ulcer had healed at 3 months? Methods of analysis for paired samples are summarised in Figure 8.1.

HRQoL at baseline and 3 months are both continuous variables and the data are paired as measurements are made on the same individuals at baseline and 3 months; therefore interest is in the mean of the differences not the difference between the two means. If we assume that the paired differences are Normally distributed, then the most appropriate summary measure for the data is the sample mean, at each time point, and the best comparative summary measure is the mean of the paired difference in HRQoL between baseline and 3 months. In this example a suitable null hypothesis (H_0) is that

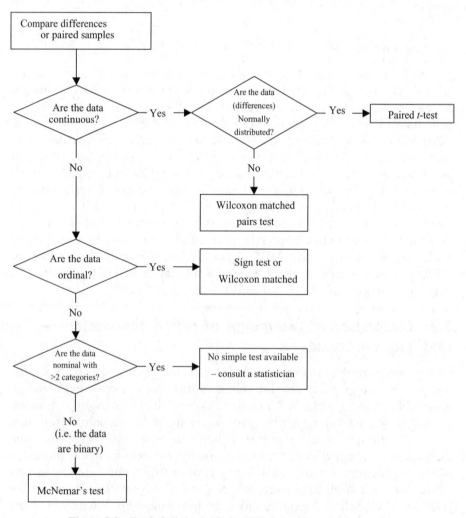

Figure 8.1   Statistical methods for differences or paired samples

there is no difference (or change) in mean HRQoL at baseline and 3 months follow-up in patients whose leg ulcer had healed by 3 months, that is, $\mu_{3\text{Month}} - \mu_{\text{Baseline}} = 0$. The alternative hypothesis (H_A) is that there is a difference (or change) in mean HRQoL at baseline and 3 months follow-up in patients whose leg ulcer had healed by 3 months, that is $\mu_{3\text{Month}} - \mu_{\text{Baseline}} \neq 0$. Using the flow diagram of Figure 8.1, the most appropriate hypothesis test appears to be the paired t-test.

Paired t-test

Two groups of paired observations, $x_{11}, x_{12}, \ldots, x_{1n}$ in Group 1 and $x_{21}, x_{22}, \ldots, x_{2n}$ in Group 2 such that x_{1i} is paired with x_{2i} and the difference between them, $d_i = x_{1i} - x_{2i}$. The null hypothesis is that the mean difference in the population is zero.

Assumptions

- The d_i's are plausibly Normally distributed. It is not essential for the original observations to be Normally distributed.
- The d_i's are independent of each other.

Steps

- Calculate the differences $d_i = x_{1i} - x_{2i}$, $i = 1$ to n.
- Calculate the mean $\bar{d}$ and standard deviation, s_d of the differences d_i.
- Calculate the standard error of the mean difference $SE(\bar{d}) = s_d / \sqrt{n}$
- Calculate the test statistic $t = \dfrac{\bar{d}}{SE(\bar{d})}$

Under the null hypothesis, the test statistic, t is distributed as Student's t, with degrees of freedom (df), $df = n - 1$.

It is a common mistake to assume in such cases that because the basic observations appear not to have Normal distributions, then the methods described here do not apply. However, it is the differences, that is, the 3-month minus baseline HRQoL, that have to be checked for the assumption of a Normal distribution, and not the basic observations. In fact the differences appear to have an approximately symmetrical distribution, as shown by the histogram in Figure 8.2.

There were 36 patients with a healed leg ulcer at 3 months and the summary statistics for the HRQoL of these subjects are shown in the top half of the computer output in Table 8.1. We have a mean difference $\bar{d} = 7.3$ and the $SD(d) = 16.5$, and hence $SD(\bar{d}) = SE(\bar{d}) = 16.5/\sqrt{36} = 2.8$. In this example the data are paired and the degrees of freedom are therefore one less than the number of patients in the study, that is, $df = n - 1 = 36 - 1 = 35$. The test or t-statistic is $t = 7.3/2.8 = 2.66$. This value is then compared to values of

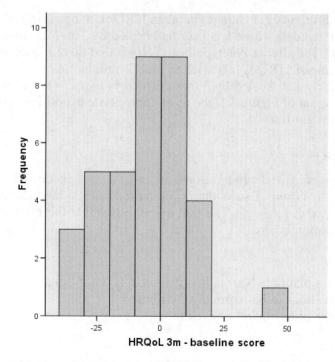

Figure 8.2   Histogram of differences in HRQoL between baseline and 3 months ($n = 36$)

the t-distribution with $df = 35$ df. Table T3 (p. 319), which only goes up to df = 30, suggests a p-value of somewhere between 0.02 and 0.01. The computer output in Table 8.1 gives a precise p-value = 0.012.

The 100 $(1 - \alpha)$% confidence interval for the mean difference in the population is:

$$\bar{d} - \left[t_{df,\alpha} \times SE\left(\bar{d}\right)\right] \text{ to } \bar{d} + \left[t_{df,\alpha} \times SE\left(\bar{d}\right)\right],$$

where $t_{df,\alpha}$ is taken from the t distribution with $df = n - 1$ degrees of freedom.

From Table T1 with $df = 35$, $t_{35,.05} \approx 2.03$, giving the 95% CI for the mean difference as

$$7.3 - (2.03 \times 2.8) \text{ to } 7.3 + (2.03 \times 2.8)$$

or 1.7 to 12.9.

The computer output for the comparison of HRQoL for these 36 patients at baseline and 3 months shows that the result is statistically significant (Table 8.1). The confidence interval of the difference suggests that we are 95% confident that HRQoL has changed by between 1.7 and 12.9

Table 8.1 Computer output for paired t-test

Paired samples statistics

	Mean	n	SD	SE
Health related quality of life: baseline	66.3	36	18.8	3.1
Health related quality of life: 3 months	58.9	36	22.0	3.7

Paired samples t-test

	Paired differences							
				95% CI of the Difference				
HRQoL	Mean	SD	SE	Lower	Upper	t	df	p-value
Baseline – 3-month	7.3	16.5	2.8	1.7	12.9	2.661	35	0.012*

*The p-value or probability of observing the test statistic of 2.661 or more extreme under the null hypothesis is 0.012. This means that this result is unlikely when the null hypothesis is true (of no difference in HRQoL). The result is said to be *statistically significant* because the p-value is less than the significance level (α) set at 5% and there is sufficient evidence to reject the null hypothesis. The alternative hypothesis that there is a difference or change in mean HRQoL between baseline and 3 months in patients whose leg ulcer had healed by 3 months, is accepted.

points over the period and the best estimate is a mean change of 7.3 points. In actual fact HRQoL has declined over time from a mean of 66.3 at baseline to 58.9 at 3 months.

The assumptions underlying the use of the paired t-test are outlined above. If these are not met, Figure 8.1 shows that a non-parametric alternative, the Wilcoxon signed rank sum test, can be used, to assess whether the differences are centred around zero.

Wilcoxon (matched pairs) signed rank test

This is used when the assumptions underlying the paired t-test are not valid. It is a test of the null hypothesis that there is no tendency for the outcome under one set of conditions (in this current example – at the start of the study) to be higher or lower than under the comparison set of conditions (in this current example – after 3 months). The computer output for the comparison of HRQoL for these 36 patients at baseline and 3 months shows that the result is statistically significant (Table 8.2) with a p-value = 0.012.

Table 8.2   Example computer output for Wilcoxon signed rank sum test

	Ranks	n	Mean rank	Sum of ranks
HRQoL: 3 months – Baseline	Negative	22[a]	16.11	354.50
	Positive	8[b]	13.81	110.50[d]
	Ties	6[c]		
	Total	36		

[a]HRQoL: 3 months < Baseline.
[b]HRQoL: 3 months > Baseline.
[c]HRQoL: 3 months = Baseline.
[d]T^+, the sum of the positive ranks.

Test statistics

	HRQoL: 3 month – Baseline
z	−2.511[a]
p-value	0.012

[a]Based on positive ranks.
The p-value or probability of observing the test statistic of −2.511 or more extreme under the null hypothesis is 0.012. This means that this result is unlikely when the null hypothesis is true (of no difference in HRQoL). The result is said to be *statistically significant* because the p-value is less than the significance level (α) set at 5% or 0.05 and there is sufficient evidence to reject the null hypothesis. The alternative hypothesis that there is a difference or change in HRQoL between baseline and 3 months in patients whose leg ulcer had healed, is accepted.

Wilcoxon (matched pairs) signed rank test

Two groups of paired observations, $x_{11}, x_{12}, \ldots, x_{1n}$ in Group 1 and $x_{21}, x_{22}, \ldots, x_{2n}$ in Group 2 such that x_{1i} is paired with x_{2i} and the difference between them, $d_i = x_{1i} - x_{2i}$. The null hypothesis is that the *median* difference in the population is zero.

Assumptions

• The d_i's come from a population with a symmetric distribution.
• The d_i's are independent of each other.

Steps

• Calculate the differences $d_i = x_{1i} - x_{2i}$, $i = 1$ to n.
• Ignoring the signs of the differences, rank them in order of increasing magnitude from 1 to n', with zero values being ignored (so n' is the number of non-zero differences, and so may be less than the original sample size n). If some of the observations are numerically equal, they are given tied ranks equal to the mean of the ranks which would otherwise have been used.

- Calculate, T^+, the sum of the ranks of the positive values.

- Calculate the test statistic $z = \dfrac{T^+ - \left(\dfrac{n'(n'+1)}{4}\right)}{\sqrt{\dfrac{[n'(n'+1)(2n'+1)]}{24}}}$

Under the null hypothesis, z has an approximately Normal distribution, with mean $n'(n'+1)/4$ and variance $n'(n'+1)(2n'+1)/24$.

8.3 Comparison of two independent groups – continuous outcomes

Before comparing two independent groups it is important to decide what type of data the outcome is and how it is distributed, as this will determine the most appropriate analysis. This section describes the statistical methods available for comparing two independent groups, when we have a continuous outcome.

For example, one of the main questions of interest in the leg ulcer trial was whether there was a difference in the number of ulcer-free weeks between the Intervention and the Control groups. As the number of ulcer-free weeks is continuous data and there are two independent groups, assuming the data are Normally distributed in each of the two groups, then the most appropriate summary measure for the data is the sample mean and the best comparative summary measure is the difference in the mean number of ulcer free weeks between the two groups. Under these assumptions, the flow diagram of Figure 8.3 suggests that the two independent samples t-test should be used. The independent samples t-test is used to test for a difference in the mean value of a continuous variable between two groups.

When conducting any statistical analysis one should check that the assumptions which underpin the chosen method are valid. The assumptions underlying the two independent samples t-test are outlined below.

Independent two-sample t-test for comparing means

Suppose we wish to test the null hypothesis that the means from two populations, estimated from two independent samples, are equal.

- Sample 1: number of subjects n_1, mean $\bar{x}_1$, standard deviation s_1,
- Sample 2: number of subjects n_2, mean $\bar{x}_2$, standard deviation s_2.

Assumptions

1. The groups are independent.
2. The variables of interest are continuous.
3. The data in both groups have similar standard deviations.
4. The data is Normally distributed in both groups.

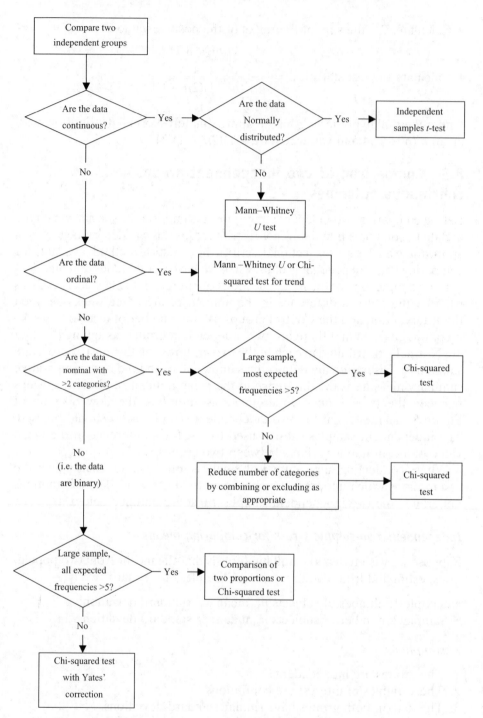

Figure 8.3   Statistical methods for comparing two independent groups or samples

Steps

1. First calculate the mean difference between groups $\bar{x}_1 - \bar{x}_2$.

2. Calculate the pooled standard deviation $SD_{pooled} = \sqrt{\dfrac{(n_1-1)s_1^2 + (n_2-1)s_2^2}{n_1+n_2-2}}$.

3. Then calculate the standard error of the difference between two means

$$SE(\bar{x}_1 - \bar{x}_2) = SD_{pooled} \times \sqrt{\dfrac{1}{n_1} + \dfrac{1}{n_2}}.$$

4. Calculate the test statistic $t = \dfrac{\bar{x}_1 - \bar{x}_2}{SE(\bar{x}_1 - \bar{x}_2)}$.

5. Compare the test statistic with the t distribution with $n_1 + n_2 - 2$ degrees of freedom. This gives us the probability of the observing the test statistic t or more extreme under the null hypothesis.

The assumption of Normality can be checked by plotting two histograms, one for each sample; these do not need to be perfect, just roughly symmetrical. The two standard deviations should also be calculated and as a rule of thumb, one should be no more than twice the other. At this stage, we shall assume the outcome, ulcer free weeks, is Normally distributed in both groups, but we will check this assumption later on. In this example a suitable null hypothesis (H_0) is that there is no difference in mean ulcer free weeks between Intervention and Control groups, that is, $\mu_{Intervention} - \mu_{Control} = 0$ weeks. The alternative hypothesis (H_A) is that there is a difference in mean ulcer free weeks between Intervention and Control groups i.e. $\mu_{Intervention} - \mu_{Control} \neq 0$ weeks.

The summary statistics for the ulcer free weeks for the Intervention and Control groups are shown in the top half of the computer output in Table 8.3. We have a mean difference between the groups, $\bar{x}_1 - \bar{x}_2 = 20.1 - 14.2 = 5.9$ weeks and the standard error of this mean difference $SE(\bar{x}_1 - \bar{x}_2) = 2.4$ weeks. In this example the degrees of freedom are, $df = n_1 + n_2 - 2$ or $120 + 113 - 2 = 231$. The test or t-statistic is $t = 5.9/2.4 = 2.485$. This value is then compared to values of the t-distribution with $df = 231$. From Table T3, the closest tabulated value is with $df = 30$ but with such large df we can use the final row of the table which has infinite degrees of freedom suggesting a p-value of somewhere between 0.02 and 0.01. This is clearly less than 0.05. The computer output in Table 8.3 shows that the exact p-value = 0.014.

The $100\,(1 - \alpha)\%$ confidence interval for the mean difference in the population is:

$$(\bar{x}_1 - \bar{x}_2) - [t_{df,\alpha} \times SE(\bar{x}_1 - \bar{x}_2)] \text{ to } (\bar{x}_1 - \bar{x}_2) + [t_{df,\alpha} \times SE(\bar{x}_1 - \bar{x}_2)],$$

where $t_{df,\alpha}$ is taken from the t distribution with $df = n_1 + n_2 - 2$. For a 95% CI $t_{231,0.05} = 1.970$. Thus giving the 95% CI for the mean difference as: $5.9 - (1.970 \times 2.4)$ to $5.9 + (1.970 \times 2.4)$ or 1.2 to 10.5 weeks.

Table 8.3 Computer output from the two independent samples t-test

Group statistics

	Group	n	Mean	SD	SE
Leg ulcer-free time (weeks)	Intervention	120	20.1	18.5	1.7
	Control	113	14.2	17.6	1.7

The standard deviations for the two groups are similar.

Independent samples t-test

				t-test for equality of means			
	t	df	p-value	Mean difference	SE difference	95% CI of the difference	
						Lower	Upper
Leg ulcer-free time (weeks)	2.485	231	0.014*	5.9	2.4	1.2	10.5

*The p-value is 0.014. Thus the results are unlikely when the null hypothesis (that there is no difference between the groups is true). The result is said to be statistically significant because the p-value is less than the significance level (α) set at 5% or 0.05 and there is sufficient evidence to reject the null hypothesis and accept the alternative hypothesis, that there is a difference in mean ulcer free weeks between the Intervention and Control groups.

Table 8.3 shows the computer output for comparing ulcer-free weeks between the two groups using the two independent samples t-test. It can be seen that there is a significant difference between the groups; the 95% CI for the difference suggests that patients in the clinic group have between 1.2 and 10.5 more ulcer-free weeks than patients in the control group and the best estimate is a mean difference of 5.9 more ulcer-free weeks.

When conducting any statistical analysis it is important to check that the assumptions which underpin the chosen method are valid. For the two independent samples t-test, the assumption that the outcome is Normally distributed in each group can be checked by plotting two histograms, one for each sample. Figure 8.4 shows two histograms for the ulcer-free weeks outcome. The outcome in both groups is clearly not Normally distributed and both distributed appear positively skewed. Hence in these circumstances it looks like the two-independent samples t-test is not the most appropriate test. The flow diagram of Figure 8.3, suggests that the Mann–Whitney U test may be a more suitable alternative. An alternative would be to use the log rank test, suitable for survival data and described in Chapter 10.

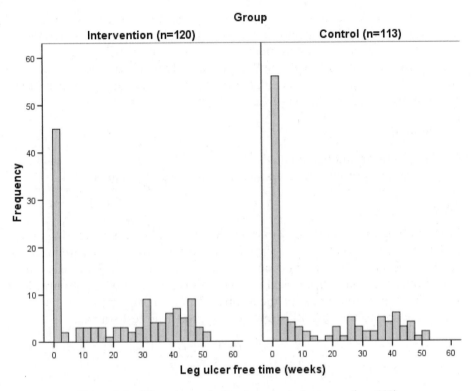

Figure 8.4   Histograms of ulcer free weeks by group (n = 233)

Mann–Whitney U test

When the assumptions underlying the t-test are not met, then the non-parametric equivalent, the Mann–Whitney U test, may be used. There are two derivations of the test, one due to Wilcoxon and the other to Mann and Whitney. It is better to call the method the Mann–Whitney U test to avoid confusion with the paired test due to Wilcoxon.

The Mann–Whitney test requires all the observations to be ranked as if they were from a single sample. We can now use two alternative test statistics, U and W. The statistic W (due to Wilcoxon) is simply the sum of the ranks in the smaller group and is easier to calculate by hand. The statistic U (due to Mann and Whitney) is more complicated. U is the number of all possible pairs of observations comprising one from each sample for which the value in the first group precedes a value in the second group. Whilst the independent samples t-test is specifically a test of the null hypothesis that the groups have the same mean value, the Mann–Whitney U test is a more general test of the null hypothesis that the distribution of the outcome variable in the two groups is the same; it is possible for the outcome data in the two groups to have similar measures of central tendency or location, such as mean and medians, but different distributions.

Suppose we wish to test the null hypothesis that two samples come from the same from populations. The data are at least ordinal and from two independent groups of size n_1 and n_2 respectively.

Assumptions

1. The groups are independent.
2. The variables of interest are at least ordinal (can be ranked).

Steps

First combine the two groups and rank the entire data set in increasing order (smallest observation to the largest). If some of the observations are numerically equal, they are given tied ranks equal to the mean of the ranks which would otherwise have been used. Sum the ranks for one of the groups. Let W be the sum of the ranks for the n_1 observations in this group.

If there are no ties or only a few ties, calculate the test statistic

$$z = \frac{W - \left(\dfrac{n_1 (n_1 + n_2 + 1)}{2} \right)}{\sqrt{\dfrac{n_1 n_2 (n_1 + n_2 + 1)}{12}}}.$$

Under the null hypothesis that the two samples come from the same population, the test statistic, z, is approximately Normally distributed with mean zero, and standard deviation of 1, and can be referred to Table T1 to calculate a p-value.

Many text books give special tables for the Mann–Whitney U test, when sample sizes are small, that is when n_1 and n_2 are less than 20. However, the above expression is usually sufficient. The formula is not very accurate if there any many ties in the data. The reader is referred to Armitage et al (2002) in such situations.

Examining the output from the Mann–Whitney U test in Table 8.4 we see there is sufficient evidence to reject the null hypothesis and accept the alternative hypothesis that there is a difference in ulcer free weeks between the Intervention and Control groups.

However, this example illustrates that the t-test is very robust to violations of the assumptions of Normality and equal variances, particularly for moderate to large sample sizes, as the p-values and conclusions, from both the t-test and Mann–Whitney test are the same, despite the non-Normal distribution of the data.

Table 8.4 Computer output for Mann–Whitney U test

Ranks

	Group	n	Mean rank	Sum of ranks
Leg ulcer-free time (weeks)	Intervention	120	126.87	15 224.0
	Control	113	106.52	12 037.0
	Total	233		

Test statistics

	Leg ulcer-free time (weeks)
Mann–Whitney U	5 596.0
Wilcoxon W	12 037.0
z	–2.388
p-value	0.017*

*p-value: probability of observing the statistic, W or U, under the null hypothesis. As the value of 0.017 is less than the significance level (α) set at 0.05 or 5% this means that the result obtained is unlikely when the null hypothesis is true. Thus there is sufficient evidence to reject the null hypothesis and accept the alternative hypothesis that there is a difference in ulcer free weeks between the Intervention and Control groups.

Discrete count data

In the majority of cases it is reasonable to treat discrete count data, such as number of children in a family or number of visits to a general practice clinic in a year, as if they were continuous, at least as far as the statistical analysis goes. Ideally, there should be a large number of different possible values, but in practice this is not always necessary. However, where ordered categories are numbered such as stage of disease or social class, the temptation to treat these numbers as statistically meaningful must be resisted. For example, it is not sensible to calculate the average social class or stage of cancer, and in such cases the data should be treated in statistical analyses as if they are ordered categories.

Comparing more than two groups

The methods outlined above can be extended to more than two groups. For the independent samples t-test, the analogous method for more than two groups is called the Analysis of Variance (ANOVA) and the assumptions underlying it are similar. The non-parametric equivalent for the method of ANOVA when there are more than two groups is called the Kruskall–Wallis test. A fuller explanation of these methods is beyond the scope of this chapter and the interested reader is referred to Altman (1991) or Armitage et al (2002).

8.4   Comparison of two independent groups – categorical outcomes

When comparing two independent groups where the outcome is categorical rather than continuous, for example in the leg ulcer trial, we may wish to know whether there was a difference between the groups in the proportions with healed ulcers at 3 months follow-up. With two independent groups (Intervention and Control) and a binary (ulcer healed versus not healed) rather than a continuous outcome, the data can be cross-tabulated as in the top part of the computer output in Table 8.5. This is an example of a 2×2 contingency table with two rows (for treatment) and two columns (for outcome), that is, four cells in total. The most appropriate summary measure is simply the proportion in the sample whose leg ulcer has healed at 3 months and the best comparative summary measure is the difference in proportions healed between the two groups.

Table 8.5   Computer output for the chi-squared test

Leg ulcer healed at 3 months – group crosstabulation

			Group		
			Intervention	Control	Total
Leg ulcer healed at 3 months	Not healed	Count	98	96	194
		% within Group	(81.7%)	(85.0%)	(83.3%)
	Healed	Count	22	17	39
		% within Group	(18.3%)	(15.0%)	(16.7%)
Total		Count	120	113	233
		% within Group	(100.0%)	(100.0%)	(100.0%)

Chi-square tests

	Value	df	p-value	Exact p-value
Pearson chi-square	0.452[b]	1	0.502[c]	
Continuity correction[a]	0.247	1	0.620	
Fisher's exact test				0.599
n of valid cases	233			

[a]Computed only for a 2×2 table. To improve the approximation for a 2×2 table, Yates' correction for continuity is sometimes applied.
[b]0 cells (0%) have expected count less than 5.
The minimum expected count is 18.91. This suggests that the chi-squared test is valid as all the counts are greater than 5.
[c]The p-value of 0.502 indicates that the results obtained are likely if the null hypothesis (of no association between the rows and columns of the contingency table above) is true. Thus there is insufficient evidence to reject the null hypothesis and the results are said to be not statistically significant.
In a 2×2 table when expected cell counts are less than 5, or any are less than 1 even Yates' correction does not work and Fisher's exact test is used.

Figure 8.3 shows that there are several different approaches to analysing these data. One approach which we outlined in Chapter 7 would be to compare the proportions of ulcers healed at 3 months follow-up in the two groups. In this example a suitable null hypothesis (H_0) is that there is no difference in outcomes, the proportion of patients with healed leg ulcers, at 3 months between Intervention and Control groups, that is, $\pi_{Int} - \pi_{Con} = 0$. The alternative hypothesis (H_A) is that there is a difference in outcomes, proportion of patients with healed leg ulcers, at 3 months, between Intervention and Control groups, that is, $\pi_{Int} - \pi_{Con} \neq 0$.

The hypothesis test assumes that there is a common proportion, π, estimated by $p = \dfrac{(n_1 p_1 + n_2 p_2)}{(n_1 + n_2)}$ and standard error for the difference in proportions is estimated by $SE(p_1 - p_2) = \sqrt{p(1-p)\left(\dfrac{1}{n_1} + \dfrac{1}{n_2}\right)}$ (see Table 7.4).

From this we can compute the test statistic: $z = (p_1 - p_2)/SE(p_1 - p_2)$.

We can then compare this value to what would be expected under the null hypothesis of no difference, in order to get a p-value. The computer output in the top half of Table 8.5 gives: $n_1 = 120$, $p_1 = 22/120 = 0.18$; $n_2 = 113$, $p_2 = 17/113 = 0.15$ and $p_1 - p_2 = 0.033$.

$$p = \frac{(n_1 p_1 + n_2 p_2)}{(n_1 + n_2)} = \frac{[(120 \times 0.183) + (113 \times 0.150)]}{(120 + 113)} = \frac{(38.91)}{233} = 0.167$$

$$and\ SE(p_1 - p_2) = \sqrt{p(1-p)\left(\frac{1}{n_1} + \frac{1}{n_2}\right)} = \sqrt{0.167(1 - 0.167)\left(\frac{1}{120} + \frac{1}{113}\right)} = 0.049$$

The test statistics is: $z = (p_1 - p_2)/SE(p_1 - p_2) = 0.033/0.049 = 0.673$ and the probability of observing the test statistic $z = 0.67$ or more extreme under the null hypothesis, using Table T1, is 0.502.

The 95% CI for the difference in proportions is:

$$(p_1 - p_2) \pm [1.96 \times SE(p_1 - p_2)]$$

For the calculation of the confidence interval, we do not need to make any assumptions about there being a common proportion π and use the formula in Table 6.7 for the $SE(p_1 + p_2)$:

$$SE(p_1 - p_2) = \sqrt{\frac{p_1(1 - p_1)}{n_1} + \frac{p_2(1 - p_2)}{n_2}} = \sqrt{\frac{0.18 \times 0.82}{120} + \frac{0.15 \times 0.85}{113}} = 0.049$$

The 95% CI for the difference in proportions is:

$(0.033)-[1.96 \times 0.049]$ to $(0.033)+[1.96 \times 0.049]$ which is -0.063 to 0.129.

Therefore we are 95% confident that the true population difference in the proportion of leg ulcers healed, at 12 weeks, between the Clinic and Home treated patients lies somewhere between –6.3% to 12.9%, but our best estimate is 3.3%.

Figure 8.3 also shows that an alternative approach to the comparisons of two proportions, assuming a large sample and all expected frequencies >5, is the chi-squared test. The null hypothesis is that the two classifications (group and ulcer-healed status at 3 months) are unrelated in the relevant population (leg ulcer patients). More generally the null hypothesis, H_0, for a contingency table is that there is no association between the row and column variables in the table, that is, they are independent. The general alternative hypothesis, H_A, is that there is an association between the row and column variables in the contingency table and so they are *not* independent or unrelated. For the chi-squared test to be valid two key assumptions need to be met, as outlined below. If these are not met, Figure 8.3 suggests that Fisher's exact test can be used for 2 × 2 tables.

Chi-squared test for association in r × c contingency tables

Suppose we wish to test the null hypothesis, for an $r \times c$ contingency table, that there is no association between the row and column variables in the table, i.e. they are independent.

Assumptions

- Two independent unordered categorical variables that form an $r \times c$ contingency table.
- At least 80% of expected cell counts >5.
- All expected cell counts >1.

Steps

1. Calculate the expected frequency (E_{ij}) for the observation in row i and column j of the $r \times c$ contingency table:

$$E_{ij} = \frac{Row\ total\,(R_i) \times Column\ total\,(C_j)}{N}, \text{ where } N \text{ is the total sample size.}$$

2. For each cell in the table calculate the difference between the observed value and the expected value ($O_{ij} - E_{ij}$).
3. Square each difference and divide the resultant quantity by the expected value $(O_{ij} - E_{ij})^2/E_{ij}$.
4. Sum all of these to get a single number, the χ^2 statistic.

$$\chi^2 = \sum_{i=1}^{r} \sum_{j=1}^{c} \frac{(O_{ij} - E_{ij})^2}{E_{ij}} = \sum \frac{(O-E)^2}{E}$$

5. Compare this number with tables of the chi-squared distribution with the following degrees of freedom: $df = $ (no. of rows $- 1) \times$ (no. of columns $- 1$).

Table 8.6 shows more details of the calculations and how we compare what we have observed (O) with what we would have expected (E) under the null hypothesis of no association. If what we have observed is very different from what we would have expected, then we reject the null hypothesis.

The value of $\sum \frac{(O-E)^2}{E}$ is 0.45; this is given in Table 8.5 as 'Pearson chi-square'. This value can be compared with tables for the chi-squared distribution with $df = $ (no. of rows $- 1) \times$ (no. of columns $- 1) = (2-1) \times (2-1) = 1$. Under the null hypothesis of no association the probability of observing this value of the test statistic χ^2 or more, is p-value $= 0.502$.

If more than 20% of expected cell counts are less than 5 then the test statistic does not approximate a chi-squared distribution. If any expected cell counts are <1 then we cannot use the chi-squared distribution. In large tables we may have to combine categories to make bigger numbers (providing it's meaningful). The bottom half of Table 8.5 shows the typical computer output for a chi-squared test. In this example it appears that the chi-squared test is valid as all the expected counts are greater than 5.

In 2×2 tables, even when expected cell counts are bigger than 5, the observed value of χ^2 (calculated from count data) can be made closer to the true χ^2 value (calculated on a continuous scale) using *Yates' continuity correction*, χ^2_{CC}. This simply involves subtracting 0.5 from the absolute value for the difference between the observed and expected cell values,

$$\chi^2_{CC} = \sum \frac{(|O-E|-0.5)^2}{E}.$$

Table 8.6 Observed and expected cell counts for leg ulcer data

	O	E	$O - E$	$(O - E)^2/E$
Intervention/healed	22	20.1	1.9	0.18
Intervention/not healed	98	99.9	1.9	0.04
Control/healed	17	18.9	−1.9	0.19
Control/not healed	96	94.1	−1.9	0.04
Total	233	233	0	0.45

$$\chi_{CC}^2 = \frac{(|98 - 99.9| - 0.5)^2}{99.9} + \frac{(|22 - 20.1| - 0.5)^2}{20.1} + \frac{(|96 - 94.1| - 0.5)^2}{94.1} +$$

$$\frac{(|17 - 18.9| - 0.5)^2}{18.9}$$

$$= \frac{(1.4)^2}{20.1} + \frac{(1.4)^2}{94.1} + \frac{(1.4)^2}{18.9} = 0.247$$

Again this value can be compared with Table T4 for the chi-squared distribution with $df = 1$. Under the null hypothesis of no association, the probability of observing this value of the test statistic or more, is about 0.620.

Fisher's exact test

In a 2×2 table, when all the expected cell counts are smaller than 5, or any <1 even Yates' correction does not work. There is also a special method known as Fisher's exact test for 2×2 tables with very small expected frequencies. We need to go back to definitions of basic probability and estimate the probability of falsely rejecting the null hypothesis directly, based on all the possible tables, or more extreme than we could have observed. This is very time-consuming by hand! Fortunately, most computer packages will calculate Fisher's exact test for all 2×2 tables, as the output in Table 8.5 shows. A fuller explanation of how to derive Fisher's exact test is given in Section 8.9.

Chi-squared test for trend in a 2 × c table

An important class of tables are $2 \times c$ tables, where the multi-level factor has c ordered levels. For example patients might score their pain on an integer scale from 1 to 5 on one of two treatments. In this case the chi-squared test is very inefficient, because it fails to take account of the ordering and one should use the chi-squared test for trend. A fuller explanation of the chi-squared test for trend in a $2 \times c$ table is given in Section 8.9.

8.5 Comparison of two groups of paired observations – categorical outcomes

Just as for continuous data, a special analysis is required if paired or matched data are involved. As we said before, these can arise from cross-over clinical trials and matched-pair case–control studies.

Example from the literature: Matched case–control study – testicular cancer

Brown et al (1987) studied all cases of testicular cancer in a defined area from 1 January 1976 to 30 June 1986. The controls were men in the same hospital as the cases, who were within two years of age and belonged to the same ethnic group as the cases but suffering from a malignancy other than testicular cancer. They conducted a matched case-control study, and one of the questions asked of both cases and controls was whether or not their testes were descended at birth. Part of the results of their study is given in Table 8.7.

Consider the following four case–control pairs:

- Pair 1 Both with undescended testes
- Pair 2 Both with descended testes
- Pair 3 Case with undescended testes, control with descended testes
- Pair 4 Case with descended testes, control with undescended testes.

If all matched pairs were like pairs 1 and 2 we would be unable to answer the question: 'Do undescended testes result in a greater risk of testicular cancer?' It is only the discordant pairs 3 and 4 that provide relevant information in that cases and controls differ in their response. If there were many more matched pairs like pair 3 than pair 4, we would have evidence against the null hypothesis, and answer the above question in the affirmative. If there were about the same number of matched pairs like pair 3 and pair 4, we would answer the above question in the negative. If there were many more matched pairs like pair 4 than pair 3, we would have evidence that undescended testes exert a protective effect.

In this example the appropriate null hypothesis is that the expected values of f and g are equal. Given that we have $f + g$ discordant pairs, we would expect half to be pair 3 (cases exposed, controls not) and half to be pair 4 (controls exposed, cases not). Thus $O_1 = f$ while

Table 8.7 Results of a matched case–control study (Brown et al, 1987)

			Controls without testicular cancer		Total
			Undescended testes		
			Yes	No	
Cases with	Undescended	Yes	4 (e)	11 (f)	15
testicular	testes	No	3 (g)	241 (h)	244
cancer		Total	7	252	259

$E_1 = (f + g)/2$ and $O_2 = g$ while $E_2 = (f + g)/2$. A chi-squared test using the general expression for χ^2 given in Section 8.4 leads to the *McNemar's* test.

$$\chi^2_{\text{McNemar}} = \frac{(f - g)^2}{f + g}.$$

For the data of Brown et al (1987) we have $\chi^2_{\text{McNemar}} = \frac{(11 - 3)^2}{11 + 3} = 4.57$. We compare this with the χ^2 distribution with $df = 1$ (Table T4) and find that p is approximately 0.0325.

McNemar's test may be adjusted for small values of either f or g, to $\chi^2_C = \frac{(|f - g| - 1)^2}{f + g}$. The correction of -1 makes little difference to the calculations in large samples. For the data of Brown et al (1987) we have $\chi^2_C = \frac{(|11 - 3| - 1)^2}{11 + 3} = 3.5$. We compare this with the tabulated values of χ^2 with $df = 1$ and find that p-value ≈ 0.05. In fact, more exact calculations may be obtained by using the fact that the square root of a χ^2 distribution with $df = 1$ is a standard Normal distribution. The square root of 3.5 is $z = 1.87$, and referring to Table T1 (p. 316) gives $p = 0.06$ so we do not have enough evidence to reject the null hypothesis. An exact test for paired data, equivalent to Fisher's exact test for unpaired data, is described in Section 8.10.

8.6 Non-Normal distributions

Non-parametric tests

Non-parametric methods such as the Wilcoxon signed rank test and the Mann–Whitney U test described here provide alternative data analysis techniques without assuming anything about the shape of the data i.e. they do not assume an underlying distribution for the data. Hence, non-parametric methods often referred to as 'distribution free' methods. Non-parametric techniques are usually based on the ordered or ranked values of the observations in the sample and not the actual data. Non-parametric methods are used when:

- Data does not seem to follow any particular shape or distribution (for example, the Normal distribution);
- Assumptions underlying parametric tests are not met;
- A plot of the data appears to be very skewed;
- There are potential outliers in the dataset.

It is important to note that it is the test that is non-parametric, *not* the data. Non-parametric methods should not be considered as an alternative way to find significant p-values!

Why not always use non-parametric tests?

It can be argued that since non-parametric tests can always be used-why not use them always! The argument has much appeal but can be answered albeit in somewhat technical terms. It turns out that if a non-parametric test is used when the data follow a Normal distribution, then the calculated p-value will always exceed that that would be obtained using the t-test. Thus one is less likely to declare a result significant using a non-parametric test than using a parametric test with the same data. In these circumstances the non-parametric test is termed less powerful, although the loss of power is often not very great. This is because the more assumptions one is prepared to make about the data the more precisely one can investigate hypotheses. The corresponding non-parametric confidence intervals will also be wider and more difficult to calculate, although help with this is provided by Gardner et al (2000, Chapter 5).

However, the overwhelming argument against the routine use of non-parametric procedures is that they are not flexible enough. For example, they do not easily allow for analyses such as multiple regression, which take into account other characteristics of the groups being compared.

There is also some misunderstanding about the flexibility of parametric tests. For example, for the data summarised in Figure 8.4, it is clearly indicated that a Normal distribution for the outcome, ulcer-free weeks, does not seem reasonable for either of the Intervention or Control groups. However, this does not in itself invalidate the use of the t-test. We are interested in comparing the sample means of the two groups and the Central Limit Theorem, which we described in Chapter 6, ensures that the sample means will be approximately Normally distributed, when the sample size is sufficiently large (over 100 subjects per group in this example).

8.7 Degrees of freedom

The number of degrees of freedom has been discussed in two situations: the first with respect to t-tests and the second with respect to χ^2 tests. In fact, the number of degrees of freedom depends on two factors: first, the number of groups we wish to compare; and second, the number of parameters we need to estimate to calculate the standard deviation of the contrast of interest. Thus for the χ^2 test for the comparison of two proportions, which is equivalent to a z-test in large samples (see Section 8.4), there are two groups to compare; hence we have $df = 1$ for the between-groups comparison. Once the proportion is estimated in each group, a direct estimate of the standard error is $\sqrt{(pq/n)}$, without estimation of an additional parameter. This is because the binomial distribution, for a particular n, is completely determined by p.

In contrast, when comparing two means, whereas there are degrees of freedom for between-groups, there are also degrees of freedom for estimating σ. How the degrees of freedom are calculated depends on the particular problem. For a paired situation df = (number of subjects minus one); for an unpaired situation df = (total number of subjects minus two), in the case of equal group sizes this is $n - 1$ for each group. Thus the t-test has implicitly two sets of degrees of freedom attached to it. The first, a degree of freedom for between-groups, the second one for within-groups. However, the first of these degrees of freedom is not usually explicitly referred to as it is always unity. The z-test is similar to the t-test, but since in this case σ is assumed known effectively the within-groups degrees of freedom are infinite and so these also are seldom explicitly referred to.

8.8 Points when reading the literature

1. Have clinical importance and statistical significance been confused?
2. Has the sample size been taken into account when determining the choice of statistical tests; that is, are small-sample tests used when appropriate?
3. Is it reasonable to assume that the continuous variables have a Normal distribution?
4. Have paired tests been utilised in the appropriate places?
5. Have confidence intervals of the main results been quoted?
6. Is the result medically or biologically plausible and has the statistical significance of the result been considered in isolation, or have other studies of the same effect been taken into account?

8.9 Technical details

Student's t-distribution

In discussing the z-test in Chapter 7 two assumptions were made. The first is that the variable under consideration follows an approximately Normal distribution, and second, that samples from the respective population have always been relatively large. However, it is intuitively obvious that with small samples one can make less precise statements about population parameters than one can with large samples. Thus it is necessary to recognise that if samples are small $\bar{x}$ and s will not always be necessarily close to μ and σ respectively. How does the sample size influence the calculations? In one way sample size is already taken into account through the calculation of the standard deviation of the mean, $SE(\bar{x})$, when dividing by $\sqrt{n}$, the square-root of the sample size. In small samples, however, values of s very far from σ will not be uncommon, and one consequence is that although $\bar{x}$ will still have a Normal distribution, it can no longer be assumed that the ratio, $z = \bar{x}/SE(\bar{x})$, will. The previous discussion effectively assumed that s was close in value to the (unknown) population parameter σ.

As a consequence it is necessary to modify the calculation of both the p-value and a confidence interval. For the confidence interval z_α is replaced by $t_{df,\alpha}$, in the expression given for a confidence interval for the difference between two means in Section 6.2, to obtain

$$\bar{d} - t_{df,\alpha} \times SE(\bar{d}) \text{ to } \bar{d} + t_{df,\alpha} \times SE(\bar{d}),$$

while the expression for z is relabelled, $t = \dfrac{\bar{d}}{SE(\bar{d})}$. This then known as Student's t-statistic. Under the null hypothesis of no difference in the means t is assumed to be distributed as Student's t-distribution rather than as a Normal distribution.

In the expression for the confidence interval the particular value for t_α, depends not only on α but also on the number of degrees of freedom, df, on which σ is estimated. We explain how to calculate degrees of freedom in Section 8.8. Table T3 gives some values of t_α for different values of df and α. Examination of the bottom row of Table T3 shows that with $df = \infty$, that is with very large degrees of freedom, the same value for t_α is obtained as for z_α in Table T1 for each value of α. However, the values of t_α get larger as the df get smaller. This reflects the increasing uncertainty concerning the estimate of σ as sample sizes get smaller.

Fisher's exact test

If any expected value in a 2×2 table is less than about 5, the p-value given by the chi-squared test is not strictly valid.

Given the notation of Table 8.8, the probability of observing the particular table is $\dfrac{m!n!r!s!}{N!a!b!c!d!}$, where $n!$ means $1 \times 2 \times 3 \times \ldots \times (n-1) \times n$ and 0! and 1! are both taken to be unity. We next calculate the probability of other tables that can be identified that have the same marginal totals, m, n, r, s and also give as much or more evidence for an association between the factors. These probabilities are then summed and for a two-sided test we double the probability so obtained.

Worked example: calculation of Fisher's exact test

The probability of observing this table, is

$$P(i) = \frac{8!32!20!20!}{40!2!6!18!14!} = 0.095760.$$

There are two rearrangements of the table (Table 8.10), which give as much or more evidence for the association between mortality and type of orthopaedic ward; that is, greater odds ratios. These are:

The probabilities associated with these tables are $P(ii) = 0.020160$ and $P(iii) = 0.001638$. Thus the total probability is $0.095760 + 0.020160 + 0.001638 = 0.117558$. For a two-sided test we double this to get p-value = 0.24.

Table 8.8 Notation for unmatched 2×2 table. Number of subjects classified by factors A and B

		Factor A		Total
		Present	Absent	
Factor B	Present	a	c	m
	Absent	b	d	n
Total		r	s	N

Table 8.9 Deaths in 6 months after fractured neck of femur in a specialised orthopaedic ward (A) and general ward (B)

Deaths	Ward		Total
	A	B	
Yes	2	6	8
No	18	14	32
Total	20	20	40

Table 8.10 (ii) Odds ratio = 10.2 and (iii) Odds ratio = ∞

Deaths	Ward		Total	Ward		Total
	A	B		A	B	
Yes	1	7	8	0	8	8
No	19	13	32	20	12	32
Total	20	20	40	20	20	40

Chi-squared test for trend (2 × c table)

An important class of tables are $2 \times c$ tables, where the multi-level factor has ordered levels. For example patients might score their pain on an integer scale from 1 to 5 on one of two treatments. In this case the chi-squared test is very inefficient, because it fails to take account of the ordering and one should use the chi-squared test for trend. In this test one must assign scores to the ordered outcome. So long as the scores reflect the ordering, the actual values affect the result little.

Example Consider the notation in Table 8.11, which gives the results of a parallel group clinical trial with ordered outcomes.
   With the notation given in Table 8.11, calculate

$$T_{xp} = \sum_{i=1}^{c} n_i (p_i - \bar{p})(x_i - \bar{x}) = \sum_{i=1}^{c} a_i x_i - \frac{\sum_{i=1}^{c} a_i \sum_{i=1}^{c} n_i x_i}{N} \quad \text{and}$$

$$T_{xx} = \sum_{i=1}^{c} n_i x_i^2 - \frac{\left(\sum n_i x_i\right)^2}{N}.$$

Finally calculate $X_{\text{trend}}^2 = \dfrac{T_{xp}^2}{\left(T_{xx}\,\bar{p}\bar{q}\right)}$ where $\bar{q} = 1 - \bar{p}$. This chi-squared test for

trend has $df = 1$.
   Thus from Table 8.11, $T_{xp} = -26 - 144 \times (-12)/196 = -17.18$, $T_{xx} = 228 - (-12)^2/196 = 227.27$ and $\chi_{\text{trend}}^2 = (-17.18)^2/(227.27 \times 0.2653 \times 0.7347) = 6.66$. From Table T4, we find $p = 0.01$.

Table 8.11   Results of a parallel group clinical trial of two treatments

	Outcome of trial					
	Worse	Same	Slightly better	Moderately better	Much better	Total
Treatment A (a_i)	11	53	42	27	11	144
Treatment B	1	13	16	15	7	52
Total (n_i)	12	66	58	42	18	196 (N)
$p_i = a_i/n_i$	0.0833	0.1970	0.2759	0.3571	0.3889	0.2653 ($\bar{p}$)
Score (x_i)	−2	−1	0	1	2	

Exact test for small samples with paired binary outcomes

The exact test requires the calculation of $P = \dfrac{(f+g)!}{f!g!}\left(\dfrac{1}{2}\right)^{f+g}$ for the table observed and those indicating a stronger association with the same total $f + g$ of discordant pairs. These probabilities are then summed and for a two-sided test we double the probability so obtained.

Example   In the case–control study of Brown et al (1987) the four tables for calculation are:

(i)		(ii)		(ii)		(iv)	
4	11	4	12	4	13	4	14
3	241	2	241	1	241	0	241

Giving

$$P(i) = \frac{14!}{11!3!}\left(\frac{1}{2}\right)^{14} = 0.022217,\ P(ii) = \frac{14!}{12!2!}\left(\frac{1}{2}\right)^{14} = 0.005554$$

$$P(iii) = \frac{14!}{13!1!}\left(\frac{1}{2}\right)^{14} = 0.000854,\ P(iv) = \frac{14!}{14!0!}\left(\frac{1}{2}\right)^{14} = 0.000061.$$

Thus the total probability is 0.028686. For a two-sided test $p = 0.057$. This is very close to the value $p = 0.06$ calculated in Section 8.5 using a McNemar's test with Yates's correction.

An approximate 95% CI for the true difference in proportions can be calculated as follows. First calculate $p_1 = (e + f)/N$ and $p_2 = (e + g)/N$ and the difference between them is $p_1 - p_2 = \dfrac{(f-g)}{N}$. The standard error for the difference $p_1 - p_2$ is given by $SE(p_1 - p_2) = \dfrac{\sqrt{f + g - \{(f-g)^2/N\}}}{N}$. Hence, the 95% confidence interval for the true difference in proportion is $(p_1 - p_2) - \{1.96 \times SE(p_1 - p_2)\}$ to $(p_1 - p_2) + \{1.96 \times SE(p_1 - p_2)\}$.

8.10   Exercises

1. Table 8.12 shows the 24 hour total energy expenditure of groups of lean and obese women. The aim of this study was to compare total energy expenditure between the lean and obese women.

Table 8.12 24 hour total energy expenditure (MJ/day) in groups of lean and obese women (Prentice et al, 1986)

	Lean ($n = 13$)	Obese ($n = 9$)
	6.13	8.79
	7.05	9.19
	7.48	9.21
	7.48	9.68
	7.53	9.69
	7.58	9.97
	7.90	11.51
	8.08	11.85
	8.09	12.79
	8.11	
	8.40	
	10.15	
	10.88	
Mean	**8.066**	**10.298**
SD	**1.238**	**1.398**

From Prentice et al (1986). High levels of energy expenditure in obese women. *British Medical Journal*, **292**, 983–987: reproduced by permission of the BMJ Publishing Group.

(a) Write out a suitable null and alternative hypothesis for this problem and data.

(b) Do these data suggest that women in the lean group have a different total energy expenditure to women in the obese group? *Stating any assumptions you make,* perform an appropriate hypothesis test to compare mean 24 hour total energy expenditure (MJ/day) between the groups of lean and obese women. Comment on the results of this hypothesis test.

(c) Calculate a 95% CI for the difference in mean 24 hour total energy expenditure (MJ/day) between the groups of lean and obese women. Discuss whether the confidence interval suggests that women in the obese group might have higher total energy expenditure than women in the lean group.

2. Table 8.13 shows the results of a randomised, double-blind, placebo-controlled trial examining whether patients with chronic fatigue syndrome

Table 8.13 Outcomes from the RCT (Cox et al, 1991)

Treatment	Outcome		
	Felt better	Did not feel better	Total
Magnesium	12	3	15
Placebo	3	14	17

(CFS) improved 6 weeks after treatment with intramuscular magnesium. The group who received the magnesium were compared to a group who received a placebo and outcome was feeling better (Cox et al, 1991).

(a) Do these data suggest that the magnesium-treated CFS patients have different outcomes to placebo treated patients after 6 weeks of treatment? Stating any assumptions you make, perform an appropriate hypothesis test to compare the difference in proportions feeling better between the Magnesium and Placebo treated groups. Comment on the results of this hypothesis test.

(b) Calculate a 95% CI for the difference in the proportion of patients feeling better between the Magnesium and Placebo groups. Does the CI estimate from this data suggest that patients in the Magnesium group have a better outcome at six weeks than patients in the Placebo group?

3. A prospective double-blind clinical trial was conducted in 11 young, health, normally menstruating female subjects to detect any differences in energy intake in the pre and post phases of the menstrual cycle. The data is shown in Table 8.14.

(a) Write out a suitable null and alternative hypothesis for this problem and data.

Table 8.14 Mean daily dietary intake (kJ) over 10 pre-menstrual and 10 post-menstrual days

Subject	Dietary intake (kJ)		
	Pre-menstrual	Post-menstrual	Difference
1	5260	3910	1350
2	5470	4220	1250
3	5640	3885	1755
4	6180	5160	1020
5	6390	5645	745
6	6515	4680	1835
7	6805	5265	1540
8	7515	5975	1540
9	7515	6790	725
10	8230	6900	1330
11	8770	7335	1435
Mean	**6753.6**	**5433.2**	**1320.5**
SD	**1142.1**	**1216.8**	**366.7**

From Manocha et al (1986). A study of dietary intake in pre- and post-menstrual period. *Human Nutrition – Applied Nutrition*, **40**, 213–216.

(b) Do these data suggest that the mean daily dietary intake over the 10 pre and 10 post-menstrual days is different? *Stating any assumptions you make,* perform an appropriate hypothesis test to compare mean daily dietary intake (kJ/day) between the pre and post-menstrual phases in this sample of 11 women. Comment on the results of this hypothesis test.

(c) Calculate a 95% CI for the difference in mean daily dietary intake (kJ/day) between the pre and post-menstrual phases in this sample of 11 women. Discuss whether the confidence interval suggests that women might have a lower dietary intake in the post-menstrual phase than women in the pre-menstrual phase.

9 Correlation, linear and logistic regression

Medical Statistics Fourth Edition, David Machin, Michael J Campbell, Stephen J Walters
© 2007 John Wiley & Sons, Ltd

Summary

Correlation and linear regression are techniques for dealing with the relationship between two or more continuous variables. In correlation we are looking for a linear association between two variables, and the strength of the association is summarised by the correlation coefficient. In regression we are looking for a dependence of one variable, the dependent variable, on another, the independent variable. In linear regression the dependent variable is continuous whereas in logistic regression it is binary. The relationship is summarised by a regression equation consisting of a slope and an intercept. In linear regression the slope represents the amount the dependent variable increases with unit increase in the independent variable, and the intercept represents the value of the dependent variable when the independent variable takes the value zero. In logistic regression the slope represents the change in log odds for a unit increase in the independent variable and the intercept the log odds when the independent variable is zero. In multiple regression we are interested in the simultaneous relationship between one dependent variable and a number of independent variables.

9.1   Introduction

Given two continuous variables measured on a group of subjects, possibly the simplest question to ask in this situation is: 'Are the variables associated?'. The first task would then be to plot the data. If the association appears linear then it is reasonable to ask: 'How strongly are they associated?'. This is the question answered by correlation.

On the other hand, where it is believed that one variable is a direct cause of the other, or that if the values of one variable is changed, then as a direct consequence the other variable also changes, or if the main purpose of the analysis is prediction of one variable from the other, then the associations between them are better explored using regression rather than by simple correlation. The simplest possible method of describing a relationship between two continuous variables is by a straight line. In this case one variable changes in proportion to the other, and this type of relationship has proved very useful in medical research.

Example: Correlation or regression – anaemia in women

Consider a survey of anaemia in women, from a pre-defined geographical area. They had a blood sample taken and their haemoglobin (Hb) level and packed cell volume (PCV) measured. They were also asked their age, and whether or not they had experienced the menopause. Results from a random sample of 20 women from the group are given in Table 9.1, which we will use to illustrate the ideas underlying correlation and linear regression.

It is not clear whether Hb affects PCV or the other way around. Here one is interested in the association between these two variables and would use correlation techniques.

On the other hand, if there is a relationship between Hb and age then it is clear that it is growing old that affects Hb, and not the other way around. Thus one might wish to predict a value of Hb given a patient's age, and so one would use regression for this purpose.

9.2 Correlation

Some facts about the correlation coefficient

In Chapter 3 we described methods of plotting data when associations between two variables are to be explored. In such cases we would like a statistic that summarises the strength of the relationship, in much the same way that the mean and standard deviation summarise the location and variability of the data.

Example: Correlation – Hb and PCV

The scatter diagram of Figure 9.1 illustrates the relationship between Hb and PCV in the 20 women of Table 9.1. In this situation we are not really interested in causation, that is whether a high PCV causes a high Hb; but rather, is a high packed cell volume associated with a high Hb? The sample correlation coefficient, r, enables us not only to summarise the strength of the relationship but also to test the null hypothesis that the population correlation coefficient ρ is zero; that is, whether an apparent association between the variables would have arisen by chance.

The correlation coefficient is a dimensionless quantity ranging from −1 to +1. A positive correlation is one in which both variables increase together. A negative correlation is one in which one variable increases as the other decreases. When variables are exactly linearly related, then the correlation coefficient equals either +1 or −1. Values for different strengths of association are shown in Figure 9.2.

The correlation coefficient is unaffected by the units of measurement. Thus, if assessing the strength of association between, say, blood pressure

Table 9.1 Haemoglobin level (Hb), packed cell volume (PCV), age and menopausal status in a group of 20 women

Subject number	Hb (g/dl)	PCV (%)	Age (years)	Menopause 0 = No, 1 = Yes
1	11.1	35	20	0
2	10.7	45	22	0
3	12.4	47	25	0
4	14.0	50	28	0
5	13.1	31	28	0
6	10.5	30	31	0
7	9.6	25	32	0
8	12.5	33	35	0
9	13.5	35	38	0
10	13.9	40	40	1
11	15.1	45	45	0
12	13.9	47	49	1
13	16.2	49	54	1
14	16.3	42	55	1
15	16.8	40	57	1
16	17.1	50	60	1
17	16.6	46	62	1
18	16.9	55	63	1
19	15.7	42	65	1
20	16.5	46	67	1

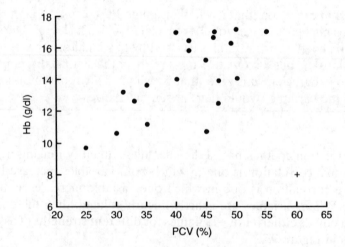

Figure 9.1 Scatter diagram of haemoglobin (Hb) and packed cell volume (PCV) in 20 women (+ marks an additional and hypothetical data point to illustrate an outlier)

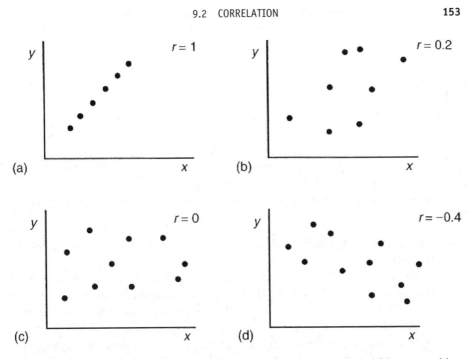

Figure 9.2   Scatter plots showing data sets with different correlations: (a) strong positive, (b) weak positive, (c) uncorrelated and (d) weak negative

and age it does not matter whether blood pressure is measured in mmHg, lb per square inch or kPa per square cm, or PCV expressed as a percentage or a proportion, as the correlation coefficient remains unaffected.

The square of the correlation coefficient gives the proportion of the variation of one variable 'explained' by the other.

Example: Correlation – Hb and PCV

For the data from Figure 9.1, the correlation between Hb and PCV is found to be $r = 0.6734$ which we would quote as 0.67. Thus $0.6734^2 = 0.4535$ or 45% (only about half) of the variability of Hb can be explained by PCV, or vice versa.

When not to use the correlation coefficient

To determine whether the correlation coefficient is an appropriate measure of association, a first step should always be to look at a plot of the raw data. The situations where it might be not be appropriate to use the correlation coefficient are:

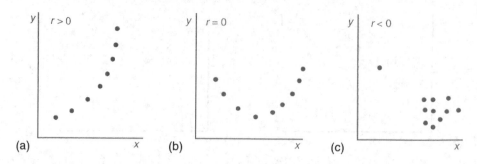

Figure 9.3   Examples where the use of the correlation coefficient is not appropriate

(i) The correlation coefficient should not be used if the relationship is non-linear.

Figure 9.3(a) shows a situation in which y is related to x by means of the equation $y = a + bx + cx^2$. In this case it is possible to predict y exactly for each value of x. There is therefore a perfect association between x and y. However, it turns out that r is not equal to one. This is because the expression for y involves an x^2 term, or what is known as a quadratic term, and so the relationship is non-linear as is clear from the figure. Figure 9.3(b) shows a situation in which y is also clearly strongly associated with x and yet the correlation coefficient is zero. Such an example may arise if y represented overall mortality of a population and x some measure of obesity. Very thin and obese people both have higher mortality than people with average weight for their height.

In the situations depicted by both Figure 9.3(a) and (b) there is clearly a close relationship between y and x, but it is not linear. In situations such as these, one should abandon trying to find a single summary statistic of the relationship.

(ii) The correlation coefficient should be used with caution in the presence of outliers.

For example, Figure 9.3(c) shows a situation in which one observation is well outside the main body of the data. This observation has a great deal of influence on the estimated value of the correlation coefficient. Since it is so extreme it is possible that this observation in fact comes from a different population from the others. Such an observation may arise in a study of blood loss and its relation to Hb level following insertion of an IUD. The outlier might be one woman who happens to have a disease that causes heavy blood loss and also renders her anaemic. If she is excluded from the data set, the correlation coefficient becomes close to zero for the remainder.

(iii) The correlation coefficient should be used with caution when the variables are measured over more than one distinct group.

One situation where this may occur is if observations, say PCV and Hb, are made on a group of patients, and also in a group of healthy controls. Such studies may result in two distinct clusters of points with zero correlation within each cluster but when combined produce the same effect as the outlier in Figure 9.3(c).

(iv) The correlation coefficient should not be used in situations where one of the variables is determined in advance.

For example, if one were measuring responses to different doses of a drug, one would not summarise the relationship with a correlation coefficient. It can be shown that the choice of the particular drug dose levels used by the experimenter will result in different correlation coefficients, even though the underlying dose-response relationship is fixed. Thus if the dose range chosen to investigate is narrow estimates of the correlation will tend to be small while if the doses are very disparate the estimates will tend to be large.

Tests of significance

Having plotted the data, and established that it is plausible the two variables are associated linearly, we have to decide whether the observed correlation could have arisen by chance, since even if there were no association between the variables, the calculated correlation coefficient is extremely unlikely to be exactly zero. The associated statistical test of the null hypothesis $\rho = 0$ is $t = r/\text{SE}(r)$, where r is the estimated correlation coefficient calculated as described in Section 9.6 and $\text{SE}(r) = \sqrt{\dfrac{1 - r^2}{n - 2}}$. This follows a Students' t-distribution with $df = n - 2$.

Example: Significance test of a correlation – Hb and PCV

For the data from Figure 9.1, with the number of observations $n = 20$, $r = 0.6734$, $\text{SE}(r) = \sqrt{\dfrac{1 - 0.6734^2}{20 - 2}} = 0.1742$. The test is $t = r/\text{SE}(r) = 0.6734/0.1742 = 3.86$ with $df = 18$. From Table T3, $t_{18, 0.001} = 3.922$, hence the p-value is a little larger than 0.001.

Thus the relationship can be summarised by saying there is a correlation of 0.67, and the probability of such a correlation, or one more extreme, arising by chance when there is in fact no relation is approximately 1 in 1000. Thus we reject the null hypothesis and accept that Hb and PCV are associated.

Assumptions underlying the test of significance

The assumption underlying the test of significance of a correlation coefficient is that the observations are random samples, and at least one of the two variables has a Normal distribution. Outlying points, away from the main body of the data, suggest a variable may not have a Normal distribution and hence invalidate the test of significance. In this case, it may be better to replace the recorded value of each variable by their ranks. That is replace the continuous variable, say the x_i of individual i, by its' corresponding rank position amongst the n individuals in the study. The rank having a value of between 1, if the observation was the smallest of the group, to n if it was the largest. The correlation coefficient is then calculated in the same manner but with the ranks for each variable replacing the original observation pair for each subject.

When the correlation coefficient is based on the original observations it is known as the *Pearson* correlation coefficient. When it is calculated from the ranks of the data it is known as the *Spearman rank* correlation coefficient – the assumption of Normality is no longer required for this.

Example: Spearman and Pearson correlation coefficients – Hb and PCV

Consider an additional subject for Table 9.1, with a Hb level of 8 g/dl and a PCV of 60%, shown by a '+' in Figure 9.1. As one can see, such a woman is well outside the main body of the data. Including her, the estimated Pearson correlation coefficient is now reduced from 0.67 to 0.29, and the test of significance becomes $t = 1.32$, $df = 19$. Use of Table T3 gives $p = 0.20$, which is no longer statistically significant.

For the 20 women of Table 9.1 the corresponding Spearman rank correlation coefficient is $r_{Spearman} = 0.63$, $df = 18$ and $p = 0.003$ while including the outlying (extra) point reduces $r_{Spearman}$ to 0.41, with $df = 19$ and $p = 0.067$. Thus, the reduction is not as great for the Spearman as the Pearson correlation coefficient.

However, in both cases the overall effect of including the additional subject is to reduce the correlation, and to render the statistical test less significant.

9.3   Linear regression

The regression line

In regression, we assume that a change in x will lead directly to a change in y – hence, as opposed to when considering correlation, x and y have a different status. Often we are interested in predicting y for a given value of x and it would not be logical in these circumstances to believe that y caused x. It is conventional to plot the dependent variable on the vertical or y-axis and the independent variable on the horizontal or x-axis.

Example: Linear regression – Hb and age

The data from Table 9.1 of Hb level and age are plotted in Figure 9.4. It is logical to believe that increasing age may affect Hb level, and not the other way around.

The equation $y = \alpha + \beta x$ is defined as the linear regression equation, where α is the *intercept*, and β is the *regression coefficient*. As we have done earlier, the Greek letters are used to show that these are *population parameters*. The regression equation is an example of what is often termed a *model* with which one attempts to model or describe the relationship between y and x. On a graph, α is the value of the equation when $x = 0$ and β is the *slope* of the line. When x increases by one unit, y will change by β units.

Given a series of n pairs of observations $(x_1, y_1), (x_2, y_2) \ldots (x_n, y_n)$, in which we believe that y is linearly related to x, what is the best method of estimating α and β? We think of the parameters α and β as characteristics of a population and we require estimates of these parameters calculated from a sample taken from the population. We label these estimates a and b respectively. If

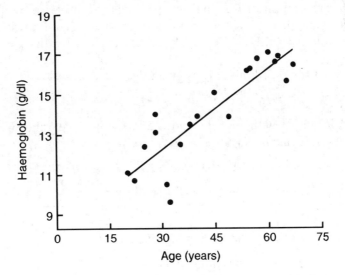

Figure 9.4 A scatter plot of haemoglobin and age in 20 women with the corresponding fitted regression line

we had estimates for a and b then, for any subject i with value x_i, we could predict their y_i by $Y_i = a + bx_i$. Clearly, we would like to choose a and b so that y_i and Y_i are close and hence make our prediction error as small as possible. This can be done by choosing a and b to minimise the sum $\Sigma(y_i - Y_i)^2$. This leads us to call a and b the *least-squares estimates* of the *population parameters* α and β. The model now becomes $y_i = \alpha + \beta x_i + \varepsilon_i$. The ε_i are the error terms and are usually assumed to be Normal and to have an average value of zero. They are the amount that the observed value differs from that predicted by the model, and represent the variation not explained by fitting the straight line to the data.

All sample estimates like b have an inherent variability, estimated by the $SE(b)$. To calculate the degrees of freedom associated with the standard error, given n independent pairs of observations, two degrees of freedom are removed for the two parameters α and β that have been estimated; thus $df = n - 2$.

Tests of significance and confidence intervals

To test the hypothesis that there is no association between Hb and age, we compare $t = b/SE(b)$ with a t-statistic with $df = n - 2$.

Example: Linear regression – Hb and age

From Table 9.1, we obtained the following result for the relationship between Hb and age: $b = 0.134\,\text{g/dl/year}$, $SE(b) = 0.017$ and $df = 18$.

The interpretation of b is that we expect Hb to increase by $0.134\,\text{g/dl}$ for every year of age. The corresponding test for significance is given by calculating $t = 0.134/0.017 = 7.84$. Use of Table T3 with $df = 18$ gives $p < 0.001$.

A 95% CI for β with $n - 2$ df is given by

$$b - t_{n-2,0.05} \times SE(b) \text{ to } b + t_{n-2,0.05} \times SE(b).$$

From Table T3 with $df = 18$ and a 5% significance value we obtain $t_{18,0.05} = 2.101$. Thus the 95% CI for β is given by

$$0.134 - 2.101 \times 0.017 \text{ to } 0.134 + 2.101 \times 0.017,$$

$$\text{or } 0.10 \text{ to } 0.17\,\text{g/dl/year}.$$

Assumptions underlying the test of significance

(i) *The relationship is approximately linear.*

This is most easily verified by plotting y_i against x_i as shown in Figure 9.4. A further plot that can be useful is to plot the residuals $e_i = y_i - Y_i$, that is the observed y minus the predicted y, denoted Y_i against x_i. These are the sample estimates of the error terms ε_i defined earlier. If there is any discernible relationship between the residuals e_i and x_i, then it is likely that the relationship between y_i and x_i is not linear.

Example: Residuals – Hb and age

The residuals remaining, after fitting age to Hb, are plotted against age, the independent variable, in Figure 9.5. There is no discernible correlation remaining, so we conclude that the linear regression provides an adequate model with which to describe the data. If the graph had indicated a correlation it would suggest that perhaps some other variable may also be influencing Hb levels in addition to age, or perhaps that the relationship is not linear.

(ii) *The prediction error is unrelated to the predicted value.*

It sometimes happens that if a small x is predicting a small y the residual is much smaller than when a large x is predicting a large y. To examine if this is the case, plot the residuals e_i against the fitted values Y_i. If the residuals appear to get larger with increasing values of Y_i, then the assumption that the prediction error is unrelated to the predicted value clearly cannot hold. If this is the case, then one may attempt to remedy the situation by using a transformation of the y variable, perhaps the logarithm of y, and then repeat both the calculation of the regression line and the plots.

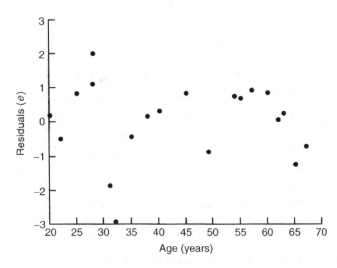

Figure 9.5   A scatter plot of residuals from linear regression against age

Example: Residuals – Hb and age

The plot of the Hb residuals against the fitted values is shown in Figure 9.6. There is some evidence in this plot that the scatter of the residuals is actually decreasing with increasing Hb. This would suggest that age is not the only variable to determine Hb levels. Note that in the case of only one independent variable x (we discuss the case of several independent variables later), Figures 9.5 and 9.6 are essentially the same.

(iii) *The residuals about the fitted line are Normally distributed.*

This does not imply that the y_i's themselves must be Normally distributed, or even that they must be continuous variables. Thus a simple rating scale variable may take only values such as 0, 1, 2, 3, but when related to some x variable by means of linear regression may give residuals about that line that are Normally distributed. One method of verifying Normality is to plot the histogram of the residuals, with the best-fit Normal distribution superimposed on it. An example of a best-fit Normal curve is given in Figure 5.4. A more efficient way of examining the results is to plot the residuals against their ordered Normal scores or Normal ordinates, as described in Section 9.9, in which deviations from linearity indicate lack of Normality.

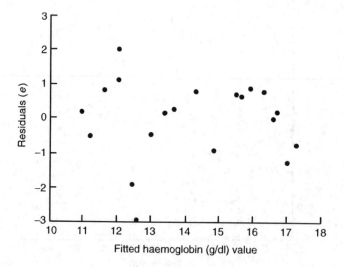

Figure 9.6 A scatter plot of residuals from linear regression against fitted values

Example: Normal scores – Hb and age

A scatter plot of the ordered Normal scores obtained after a linear regression of Hb on age is shown in Figure 9.7. It can be seen that the data plausibly lie along a straight line and are therefore approximately Normally distributed. However, there is a possibility that the residual corresponding to subject 7 is rather too low to be considered part of the same sample. Perhaps this point should be investigated further, but its presence does not affect the test of significance unduly.

(iv) *The residuals are independent of each other.*

In the case where we have single measurements on separate individuals, then there is no problem with independence as there is no reason to suppose that measurements made on one individual are likely to affect a different individual. There are two situations in which the assumption of independence might be violated: (1) if the observations are ordered in time, or (2) if different numbers of observations are made on some individuals, but all the observations are treated equally. In this latter case the study size is regarded (incorrectly) as the number of data points within the regression rather than the number of individuals providing data.

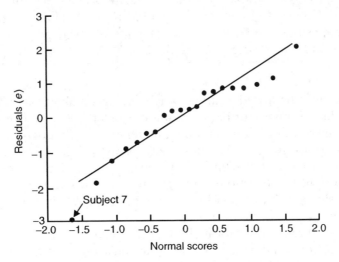

Figure 9.7 A scatter plot of residuals from the linear regression of Hb on age against their ordered Normal scores

Example from the literature: Non-random residuals – patients with AIDS

Figure 9.8(a) shows the monthly number of acquired immune deficiency syndrome (AIDS) cases identified in the UK from January 1983 to December 1986, with the best-fit straight line of cases on time (Tillett et al, 1988). The number of cases clearly increased substantially over the period. Figure 9.8(b) is a plot of the residuals from this best-fit line against time and it can be seen that one positive residual tends to be followed by another positive one and a negative residual tends to be followed by another negative one (in contrast with Figure 9.5 where the points appear to be randomly scattered). The residuals are not random and this suggests the model is not appropriate for the data. In fact, Figure 9.8(a) shows this to be the case in the first months and also towards the close of the study period. The non-random residuals also lead to an underestimate of the standard error of the slope, and so tests of significance are not valid.

Example from the literature: Non-independent observations – white-matter water content and longitudinal relaxation time

Figure 9.9 shows the relationship between the percentage white-matter water content and longitudinal relaxation time, T_1, from a study by Bell et al (1987). The authors refer to 19 patients in the study, and yet there are 30 points on the graph, so some of the patients must have had at least two observations. The regression equation is not estimated correctly in these circumstances, if all 30 observation pairs are included in the calculations of a and b in the manner described in Section 9.7.

Suppose one conducted a survey of Hb and age, making one observation per individual. Suppose further there was one elderly woman with a high Hb level, but the rest of the data showed little relationship between Hb and age. On the spurious grounds that this relationship is 'interesting', a clinician could recall this woman five times for blood tests, to produce five extra points in the top right-hand section of the graph. These would then generate an artificially strong relationship which would then appear to be (falsely) statistically significant.

One procedure to adopt for multiple measurements is to take an average for each individual and treat each average as single observation. This, at least, ensures that the observations are independent. The variances of the observations may vary, but this is usually less of a problem than lack of independence and can be allowed using a *weighted* analysis.

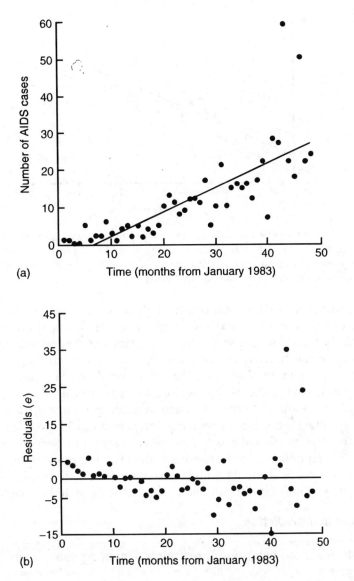

Figure 9.8 (a) A scatter plot of monthly number of AIDS cases in the UK from January 1983 to December 1986 against time, and (b) the residuals from linear regression against time (Tillett et al, 1988)

Do the assumptions matter?

The art in statistics occurs when deciding how far the assumptions can be stretched without providing a seriously misleading summary and when the procedure should be abandoned altogether and other methods tried. In general,

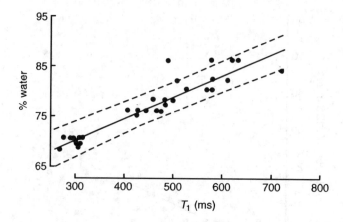

Figure 9.9 Percentage of water in the cortex and longitudinal relaxation time T_1 (reprinted from *The Lancet* Vol **i**, Bell et al, Brain water measured by magnetic resonance imaging. Correlation with direct estimation and changes after mannitol and dexamethasone, pp. 66–69, copyright © 1987, by permission of Elsevier)

lack of Normality of the residuals is unlikely to affect seriously the estimates of a regression equation, although it may affect the standard errors and the size of the *p*-value. Similarly, a lack of constant variance of the residuals is unlikely to seriously affect the estimates, but again will have some influence on the final *p*-value. In either case the advice would be to proceed, but with caution, particularly if the *p*-value is close to some critical value such as 0.05.

The lack of linearity is more serious, and would suggest either a transformation of *y* before fitting the regression equation on *x*, or a model involving quadratic (squared) or higher terms of *x* using multiple regression (see Section 9.5).

Lack of independence of the residuals can also be serious. If the data form a time sequence, or if the data involve repeated measures on individuals, a correct analysis may be difficult and expert advice should be sought.

Regression and prediction

> **Example from the literature: Prediction – running speed and pulse rate**
>
> In a study of 98 half-marathon runners, Campbell (1985) showed that one was able to predict the running speed of an athlete from his resting pulse rate (RPR) measured in beats/min by means of the regression model
>
> $$\text{Finishing time} = 71 + 0.35 \times \text{RPR}$$
>
> Here $a = 71$ and $b = 0.35$, that is, for every 1 beat/min increase in RPR the finishing time in the half marathon increased by 0.35 min. This predicts a runner with RPR = 60 beat/min will have a finishing time of 92 min.

In these situations it is important to be aware that the prediction equation is valid only within the range of the independent variable from which it was derived. In the above example, the range of resting pulse rates in the sample was 40 to 94 beats/min. It would be unwise to use the derived equation to predict a running speed of a runner whose resting pulse was 110 beats/min.

9.4 Comparison of assumptions between correlation and regression

The tests of significance for a correlation coefficient and a regression coefficient yield identical t-statistics and p-values for a particular data set.

It is one of the nice coincidences in statistics that two completely different sets of assumptions lead to the same test of significance. This would seem logical since one would not expect to have a significant correlation in the absence of a significant regression effect. Unfortunately this has often led to confusion between correlation and regression. The major difference in assumptions is that in regression there is no stipulation about the distribution of the independent variable x. It is often the case that the x's are determined by the experimenter. In an anaemia survey one might choose fixed numbers of women in specified age groups; in a laboratory survey one might be interested in the responses of patients to fixed levels of a drug chosen by the experimenter. Moreover, choosing fixed values for the x's violates the assumption underlying the correlation coefficient, namely that the x's (as well as the y's) have a Normal distribution.

Example: Selecting extreme observations – Hb and PCV

Selecting only the six women with a PCV of 35% and less, and the three women with 50% and more, in Table 9.1, the correlation coefficient between Hb and PCV becomes $r = 0.91$ as compared with 0.67 for the full data set. Thus selecting only women whose values are at the extreme of the x range can increase the apparent correlation coefficient.

In contrast it is perfectly valid in regression problems to have x variables that can take only two values (say) 0 and 1. These are clearly very far from being Normally distributed. It is worth noting that the test of significance of a regression coefficient when x is a binary 0/1 variable is equivalent to the t-test for the difference between two means. One mean is the mean value of y for those subjects with $x = 0$ and the other the mean value of y for those with $x = 1$. This result is useful because computer packages that can carry out regression can also be used to do t-tests.

9.5   Multiple regression

The multiple regression equation

Life is rarely simple, and outcome variables in medical research are usually affected by a multitude of factors. Fortunately the simple linear regression situation with one independent variable is easily extended to multiple regression. In that case the corresponding model is

$$y = \alpha + \beta_1 x_1 + \ldots + \beta_k x_k + \varepsilon$$

where x_1 is the first independent variable, x_2 is the second, and so on up to the kth independent variable x_k.

The term α is the intercept or constant term. It is the value of y when all the independent variables are zero. The regression coefficients $\beta_1, \ldots, \beta_k$ are again estimated by minimising the sum of the squares of the differences from the observed and predicted outcome variables, y and Y. Although the variables $x_1, \ldots, x_k$ are termed the independent variables, it should be noted that this is a misnomer since they need not be independent of one another. Although it is not essential that investigators understand the computational details of multiple regression, it is such a commonly used technique that they will need to be able to understand both computer output from a multiple regression calculation and read papers which use the results of multiple regression.

Uses of multiple regression

(i) *To look for relationships between continuous variables, allowing for a third variable.*

In the examples above we found a significant correlation between Hb and PCV, and a significant regression between Hb and age. This stimulates us to ask: Is the relationship between Hb and PCV only apparent because they both increase with age? In other words: Does age act as a *confounding variable* or covariate?

Example: Multiple regression – influence of age on the relation between Hb and PCV

Suppose the variable of major interest is in Hb (our y), then edited output from a multiple regression program of two independent variables PCV and age is given in Table 9.2.

The constant 5.24 is the estimated value of α, the intercept, of the equation. It is the Hb level estimated for someone with PCV and age of zero and, as is often the case, has no real interpretation since such patients are rare! However, it is usually produced by multiple regression programs and is needed in the prediction equation. PCV and Age are the two independent variables and the regression coefficients are the estimates of the β's in the regression equation. We therefore write

$$\text{Predicted Hb} = 5.24 + 0.097 \,(\text{PCV}) + 0.110 \,(\text{Age}).$$

The interpretation of the regression coefficient associated with PCV is that for a *given* age, Hb increases by 0.097 g/dl for every unit increase in PCV. Note that this is less than the value 0.134 calculated earlier when age was *not* taken into account in the relationship. For a *given* value of PCV, Hb increases by 0.110 g/dl for every year of age.

Every parameter estimate has associated with it a standard error. The corresponding t-value is the regression coefficient estimate, b, divided by its SE and the df are given by the number of observations minus the number of estimated parameters – here α, β_{PCV} and β_{Age}. In this case, $df = 20 - 3 = 17$. From these we can derive the p-value by use of Table T3. These are given in Table 9.2. The p-values correspond to the probability of observing that particular regression coefficient, or one more extreme, on the null hypothesis assumption that the true regression coefficient is in fact zero. Since the regression coefficient associated with PCV is still highly significant, the conclusion is that Hb and PCV are related even when age is taken into account.

Table 9.2 Output obtained from a multiple regression of the dependent variable Hb on PCV and age

Variable	Regression coefficient	Estimate	SE	t	p-value
Constant	α	5.24	1.21		
PCV	β_{PCV}	0.097	0.033	2.98	0.0085
Age	β_{Age}	0.110	0.016	6.74	0.0001

(ii) *To adjust for differences in confounding factors between groups.*

Example: Haemoglobin and menopausal status

Suppose an investigator wished to test whether, on average, women of Table 9.1 who have experienced the menopause, have a different Hb level than women who have not. The mean and standard deviation of Hb for pre-menopausal women are 12.29 and 1.57 g/dl, whereas those for post-menopausal women are 16.36 and 0.63 respectively.

A two independent groups t-test (as described in Chapter 8) yields a difference between the pre- and post-menopausal women of -4.07 g/dl ($t = 7.3$, $df = 18$, $p < 0.001$), which is very highly significant. However, women who have experienced the menopause clearly will be older than women who have not. If there were a steady rise in Hb with age this might account for the difference observed and not the menopausal status itself.

However, menopausal status can be added to a multiple regression, which includes age, by use of a dummy variable. Such a variable takes the value 1 if the woman is post-menopausal and 0 if she is not. The output from a multiple regression program is given in Table 9.3.

Note that the size of the coefficient associated with age has reduced from the 0.110 of Table 9.2. This is because the probability of being menopausal is age related, and age and menopausal status are being fitted simultaneously. The interpretation of the coefficient associated with the variable menopause is that, allowing for age, women who are post-menopausal have a Hb level 1.88 g/dl higher than women who are not.

However, the corresponding 95% confidence interval for $\beta_{\text{Menopause}}$ with $df = 17$ is

$$1.884 - t_{17,0.05} \times 1.032 \text{ to } 1.884 + t_{17,0.05} \times 1.032$$

or -0.29 to 4.06. This interval includes zero, and so the conclusion made previously that there was a difference between pre- and post-menopausal women is largely discounted. It is the relative ages of the women in the two groups that accounts for most of the difference in Hb levels.

Nevertheless with a larger study an effect of the menopause, independent of age, might have been demonstrated. In which case the scatter plot of Hb against age although linear within each menopausal group will 'jump' to a higher level around the usual age of menopause – say 45 to 55 years.

Note that these are not the best data to answer the question: 'Do post-menopausal women have a higher Hb level than pre-menopausal women?'. For a cross-sectional study it would be better to collect data from women who are immediately pre- or post-menopausal. Better still would be a longitudinal study which measured Hb levels in women before and after their menopause.

Table 9.3 Output obtained from a multiple regression of Hb on age and menopausal status

Variable	Regression coefficient	Estimate	SE	t	p-value
Constant	α	9.74			
Age	β_{Age}	0.081	0.033	2.41	0.028
Menopause	$\beta_{\text{Menopause}}$	1.884	1.032	1.82	0.086

9.6 Logistic regression

One independent variable

In linear regression the dependent variable is continuous, but in logistic regression (sometimes known as binary logistic regression) the dependent variable is binary; that is it can only take a value of one of two categories and these are coded 0 and 1. Logistic regression is used to predict binary outcomes such as whether a patient has (code 1) or does not have (code 0) a disease in the presence of a particular diagnostic feature. Another application is to examine whether the chance of cure (success) in patients with, for example, a particular type of cancer depends on the stage of their disease (risk factor). The model needs to be described with care. It is written in terms of the expected value of a positive result (success) for the outcome variable and assumes that the expected (or population) probability of a positive result for a subject with risk factor x is π. Then the logistic model is

$$\log\left(\frac{\pi}{1-\pi}\right) = \alpha + \beta x.$$

The values of the regression coefficients α and β are chosen as the ones that give expected proportions that are closest (in a particular mathematical sense) to the observed proportions, usually using a technique known as maximum likelihood.

The above equation may be compared with that for linear regression in Section 9.3. The right-hand side of the logistic equation has the same form, but y on the left-hand side is replaced not by π, but by the so-called logit of π. The essential reason for this is that π itself can take only values between 0 and 1, whereas the logit which is $\log[\pi/(1-\pi)]$ may range from $-\infty$ to $+\infty$, as can the continuous variable y. Essentially this transformation ensures that the probabilities, which we want to estimate, lie between 0 and 1.

The logit transform has the useful property that if an independent variable, x, in the model is binary with values 0 or 1, and has associated regression coefficient β, then $\exp(\beta)$ is the odds ratio, OR, of someone with $x = 1$ having a positive result.

Example: Logistic regression – anaemia in women

If in Table 9.1 we classified women into 'anaemic' or 'non-anaemic' groups by defining those with Hb less than 12.0 g/dl as anaemic, then this implies that subjects 1, 2, 6 and 7 are categorised as anaemic using this definition. Suppose we were interested in whether women aged less than 30 were at particular risk of anaemia. We define a new (independent) variable 'age-30' to take the value of 1 if a woman is less than 30, and 0 otherwise.

A logistic regression with 'anaemia' as the outcome variable gives the output summarised in Table 9.4, from which the OR is estimated by $\exp(1.4663) = 4.33$. We can relate this to the 2×2 table of Table 9.5 from which the $OR = (2 \times 13)/(2 \times 3) = 4.33$.

The p-values obtained are approximately equal to those from the conventional χ^2 test for 2×2 tables, especially when the numbers in the table are large. An estimated 95% CI for the OR is

$$\exp(b - 1.96 \times SE) \text{ to } \exp(b + 1.96 \times SE).$$

For example, from Table 9.4, the OR for 'anaemia' for a woman aged under 30 years is 4.3, with 95% CI of 0.4 to 44.4. This CI is very wide, reflecting the paucity of data and hence the lack of statistical significance.

The multiple logistic regression equation

In the same way that multiple regression is an extension of linear regression, we can extend logistic regression to multiple logistic regression with more than one independent variable. We can also extend it to the case where some independent variables are categorical and some are continuous. Thus if there are k risk variables $x_1, x_2, \ldots, x_k$, then the model is:

$$\log\left(\frac{\pi}{1 - \pi}\right) = \alpha + \beta_1 x_1 + \ldots + \beta_k x_k.$$

If the independent variables are categorical, as is 'Age < 30' in the example above, we can tabulate the data by all levels of the covariables. Thus we tabulate the women by whether or not they are younger than 30 years. The model then implies that all women in a particular 'age' cell of the table will have the same probability of being anaemic, say π_i, and this probability may differ from cell to cell. The π_i can be estimated by p_i which is the proportion of women who are anaemic in that cell.

Table 9.4 Output obtained from a logistic regression analysis with dependent variable 'Anaemia', independent binary variable 'Age < 30' (date of Table 9.1)

Variable	Regression coefficient	Estimate	SE	Wald*	df	p-value	$OR = \exp(\beta_{30})$
Constant	α	−1.8718	0.7596				
Age < 30	β_{30}	1.4663	1.1875	1.5246	1	0.2169	4.333

*'Wald' refers to a statistical test based on the ratio of the estimate (for example, b the estimate of β) to its standard error.

Table 9.5 Relationship between anaemia and age in 20 women (data of Table 9.1)

Age < 30	x	'Anaemic'	'Non-anaemic'	Total	Proportion anaemic
Yes	1	2	3	5	0.40
No	0	2	13	15	0.13
Total		4	16	20	

Table 9.6 Output obtained from a logistic regression analysis with dependent variable 'Anaemia', independent continuous variable 'Age' (date of Table 9.1)

Variable	Regression coefficient	Estimate	SE	Wald	df	p-value	$OR = \exp(\beta_{30})$
Constant	α	5.6219	3.6223				
Age	β_{Age}	−0.2077	0.1223	2.8837	1	0.0895	0.8125

If the independent variables are continuous, then such a table cannot be sensibly drawn up. However, if one were to do so, there would be very many cells. In fact possibly many more cells than there are women! In which case, many cells would be likely to be empty and many contain only a single individual. Thus the resulting proportions responding in each cell, would almost all be zero or one.

Nevertheless, it is perfectly possible to get valid estimates of the parameters of a logistic model in this extreme(the continuous variable) case. In which case, if an independent variable x is continuous and β is the associated regression coefficient, then $\exp(\beta)$ is the increase in odds associated with a unit increase in x.

Example: Logistic regression – anaemia and age

For example, if we use age as a continuous variable in the above example we obtain Table 9.6.

We can rewrite the fitted multiple logistic regression equation as:

$$p = \frac{\exp(a + b_1 x_1 + \ldots + b_k x_k)}{1 + \exp(a + b_1 x_1 + \ldots + b_k x_k)}.$$

Here p is the estimated probability of anaemia for a woman with covariates or risk factors $x_1, \ldots, x_k$; $a, b_1, \ldots, b_k$ are the estimates of $\alpha, \beta_1, \ldots, \beta_k$.

Example: Logistic regression – anaemia and age

For the single continuous covariate 'Age' the above model for p_{Age}, the corresponding proportion with 'Anaemia', is

$$p_{Age} = \frac{\exp(5.6219 - 0.2077 \times Age)}{[1 + \exp(5.6219 - 0.2077 \times Age)]}$$

For example, a woman aged 30 has an estimated probability p_{30} = exp(5.6219 − 0.2077 × 30)/[1 + exp(5.6219 − 0.2077 × 30)] = 0.35 of being anaemic. For a woman age 31 the corresponding OR = exp(−0.2077) = 0.81 times less likely to be 'anaemic' than a woman age 30. This in turn implies that she is 0.81 times 0.81 = 0.81^2 = 0.66 times less likely to be 'anaemic' than a woman two years younger. Thus $\exp(\beta_{Age})$ is the change (decrease) in the odds ratio of becoming anaemic for every increase of one year of age.

Use of logistic regression in case–control studies

Logistic regression is particularly useful in the analysis of case–control studies. It can be shown that if the case or control status (1 or 0) is made the dependent variable in a logistic regression then the model will provide valid estimates of the odds ratios associated with risk factors. These odds ratios will give estimates of relative risks (RR) provided the incidence of the disease is reasonably low, say below 20% (see also Section 12.7).

Example from the literature: Logistic regression – risk factors for chlamydial infection

Oakeshott et al (1998) describe a cross-sectional study in patients attending a general practice of the risk factors associated with *Chlamydia trachomatis* infection detected following a cervical smear. The outcome variable was binary (infection, no infection) and the potential risk factors investigated were age under 25, race and number of sexual partners. Each of these potential associations with chlamydial infection was tested separately using a χ^2 test and found to be statistically significant.

A logistic regression analysis showed, for example, that being aged under 25 carried a risk of infection three times that of the over-25s and that for a particular racial group the risk increased by a factor of 2. As a consequence, someone in a particular racial group who is also aged under 25 is then expected to have a risk which is 2 × 3 = 6 times that of someone without those risk factors.

The overall prevalence of chlamydial infection was quite low, so the estimated OR can be interpreted as the *Relative Risk*.

Consequences of the logistic model

A question that remains is: Is there any interaction between the input variables? For example, if a patient tested has more than one risk factor, such as being 'Age < 25' *and* in the 'Racial group' of highest risk then added together these may give more risk than would be predicted from each risk factor separately?

However, since the logistic model is described in terms of logarithms, what is additive on a logarithmic scale is multiplicative on the linear scale. To quantify the potential interaction between two binary covariates, say x_1 and x_2, the multiple logistic regression model is extended by adding a third covariate $x_3 = x_1 \times x_2$. The magnitude of the associated regression coefficient then indicates whether the two factors interact together in a synergistic (either more or less than multiplicative) way or are essentially independent of each other, in which case the associated estimated regression coefficient will be close to zero.

Example: Interaction – chlamydial infection by young age and ethnic group

For the study of Oakeshott et al (1998) someone in a particular racial group who is also aged under 25 is expected to have a risk which 6 times that of someone without either of these risk factors. Thus if 'Race' takes the value 1 for someone who is of a particular race and 0 otherwise, and 'Age < 25' takes the value 1 for someone aged under 25 and 0 otherwise, then to investigate interaction between these variables, a new variable 'Age/Race', equal to 'Race' multiplied by 'Age < 25', must be included in the logistic model.

Model checking

An important question is whether the logistic model describes the data well. If the logistic model is obtained from grouped data, then there is no problem comparing the observed proportions in the groups and those predicted by the model.

There are a number of ways the model may fail to describe the data well and these include:

1. lack of an important covariate
2. outlying observations
3. 'extra-binomial' variation.

The first problem can be investigated by trying all available covariates, and the possible interactions between them. Provided the absent covariate is not a confounder, then inference about the particular covariate of interest is usually not affected by its absence. Suppose the proportion of people aged under 25 in the study by Oakeshott et al (1998) was the same in each racial group. For example the proportion of (say) Welsh people aged under 25 was the same as the proportion of (say) English people aged under 25. Then the estimated risk of chlamydial infection for people aged under 25 will not be affected by whether race is or is not included in the model.

Outlying observations can be difficult to check when the outcome variable is binary. However, some statistical packages do provide standardised residuals; that is, residuals divided by their estimated standard errors. These values can be plotted against values of independent variables to examine patterns in the data. It is important also to look for influential observations, perhaps a subgroup of subjects that if deleted from the analysis would result in a substantial change to the values of regression coefficient estimates.

Extra-binomial variation can occur when the data are not strictly independent; for example, if the data comprise repeated outcome measures from the same individuals rather than a single outcome from each individual, or if patients are grouped for treatment which may be the case in an intervention trial randomised by clusters rather than for each individual (see Section 13.5). In such cases, although the estimates of the regression coefficients are not unduly affected, the corresponding standard errors are usually underestimated. This then leads to a Type I error rate higher than the expected (say 5%).

9.7   Correlation is not causation

One of the most common errors in the medical literature is to assume that simply because two variables are correlated, therefore one causes the other. Amusing examples include the positive correlation between the mortality rate in Victorian England and the number of Church of England marriages, and the negative correlation between monthly deaths from ischaemic heart disease and monthly ice-cream sales. In each case here, the fallacy is obvious because all the variables are time-related. In the former example, both the mortality rate and the number of Church of England marriages went down during the 19th century, in the latter example, deaths from ischaemic heart disease are higher in winter when ice-cream sales are at their lowest. However, it is always worth trying to think of other variables, confounding factors, which may be related to both of the variables under study. Further details on assessing causation are given in Section 12.9.

9.8 Points when reading the literature

1. When a correlation coefficient is calculated, is the relationship likely to be linear?
2. Are the variables likely to be Normally distributed?
3. Is a plot of the data in the paper? (This is a common omission.)
4. If a significant correlation is obtained and the causation inferred, could there be a third factor, not measured, which is jointly correlated with the other two, and so accounts for their association?
5. Remember correlation does not necessarily imply causation.
6. If a scatter plot is given to support a linear regression, is the variability of the points about the line roughly the same over the range of the independent variable? If not, then perhaps some transformation of the variables is necessary before computing the regression line.
7. If predictions are given, are any made outside the range of the observed values of the independent variable?
8. Sometimes logistic regression is carried out when a dependent variable is dichotomised, such as the example of Tables 9.4 and 9.5 when Hb level was dichotomised to 'Anaemic' or 'Non-anaemic'. It is important that the cut point is not derived by direct examination of the data for example to find a 'gap' in the data which maximises the discrimination between the selected groups as this can lead to biased results. It is best if there are *a priori* grounds for choosing a particular cut point.

9.9 Technical details

Correlation coefficient

Given a set of pairs of observations $(x_1, y_1), (x_2, y_2), \ldots, (x_n, y_n)$ the Pearson correlation coefficient is given by

$$r = \frac{\sum_{i=1}^{n}(y_i - \bar{y})(x_i - \bar{x})}{\sqrt{\sum_{i=1}^{n}(y_i - \bar{y})^2 \sum_{i=1}^{n}(x_i - \bar{x})^2}}.$$

To test whether this is significantly different from zero, calculate

$$t = \frac{r}{\sqrt{(1 - r^2)/(n - 2)}}.$$

This is compared with the *t*-distribution of Table T3 with $df = n - 2$.

Worked example: Correlation coefficient

The results of forced expiratory volume (FEV_1) measurements and height in 5 patients with asthma are given in Table 9.7.

Thus, $n = 5$, $\bar{y} = 1.86$, $\bar{x} = 168.6$, $\Sigma(y - \bar{y})^2 = \Sigma y^2 - n\bar{y}^2 = 0.572$, $\Sigma(x - \bar{x})^2 = \Sigma x^2 - n\bar{x}^2 = 149.2$, $\Sigma(x - \bar{x})(y - \bar{y}) = \Sigma xy - n\bar{x}\bar{y} = 8.32$ and so

$$r = \frac{8.32}{\sqrt{149.2 \times 0.572}} = \frac{8.32}{9.2381} = 0.9006.$$

Thus $SE(r) = \sqrt{(1 - 0.9006^2)/3} = 0.2509$ and $t = 0.9006/0.2509 = 3.59$.

From Table T3, with $df = 5 - 2 = 3$, $t_{3,0.03} = 3.896$, $t_{3,0.04} = 3.482$, hence $0.03 < p < 0.04$; computer output gives a p value of 0.037.

Spearman's rank correlation is calculated from Pearson's correlation coefficient on the ranks of the data. An alternative, and easier to calculate, formula is

$$r_{Spearman} = 1 - \frac{6\sum d_i^2}{n^3 - n},$$

where d_i is the difference in ranks for the ith individual. In the above example, the estimated $r_{Spearman} = 1$ precisely, as the ranks for FEV_1 and height for each patient are the same and so all $d_i = 0$.

Linear regression

Given a set of pairs of observations $(x_1, y_1), (x_2, y_2), \ldots, (x_n, y_n)$ the regression coefficient of y given x is

$$b = \frac{\sum_{i=1}^{n}(x_i - \bar{x})(y_i - \bar{y})}{\sum_{i=1}^{n}(x_i - \bar{x})^2}.$$

The intercept is estimated by $a = \bar{y} - b\bar{x}$.

Table 9.7 Relationship beween FEV_1 and height in five patients with asthma

	FEV_1 (litres) y	Height (cm) x	xy	y^2	x^2
	1.5	160	240.0	2.25	25 600
	1.6	165	264.0	2.56	27 225
	1.7	170	289.0	2.89	28 900
	2.1	173	363.3	4.41	29 929
	2.4	175	420.0	5.76	30 625
Totals	9.3	843	1576.3	17.87	142 279
Means	1.86	168.6			

To test whether b is significantly different from zero, calculate

$$E_{xy} = \sum (y - \bar{y})^2 - b^2 \sum (x - \bar{x})^2, \quad E_{xx} = (n-2) \sum (x - \bar{x})^2,$$

and hence

$$SE(b) = \sqrt{E_{xy}/E_{xx}}.$$

Then compare $t = b/SE(b)$ with the distribution of Table T3 with $df = n - 2$.

A 95% CI for the slope is given by

$$b - t_{n-2,0.05} \times SE(b) \text{ to } b + t_{n-2,0.05} \times SE(b).$$

Worked example: Linear regression

Using the data of Table 9.7 for a linear regression of FEV_1 on age, $b = 8.32/149.2 = 0.0558$ and $a = \bar{y} - b\bar{x} = 1.86 - (0.0558 \times 168.6) = -7.5479$. Thus the regression line is estimated by $FEV_1 = -7.55 + 0.056 \times$ Height.

The formal test of significance of the regression coefficient requires $E_{xy} = 0.1074$, $E_{xx} = 447.6$ and hence $SE(b) = (0.1074/447.6)^{1/2} = 0.0155$. From which $t = 0.056/0.0155 = 3.59$. We compare this with a t distribution with $df = 5 - 2 = 3$. Use of Table T3 gives the p-value as approximately 0.04 (more exactly 0.037) as we had in the correlation coefficient example above.

The 95% *CI* for the slope is given by $0.056 - 3.182 \times 0.0155$ to $0.056 + 3.182 \times 0.0155$. Finally, that is, 0.007 to 0.105 litres/cm.

Normal probability plots

Given a sample $y_1, y_2, \ldots, y_n$, we wish to see if they follow a Normal distribution. To do this:

1. Rank the data from smallest to largest, here labelled:

$$y_{(1)}, y_{(2)}, \ldots, y_{(n)}$$

   where $y_{(1)}$ represents the smallest observation and $y_{(n)}$ the largest.

2. Calculate the corresponding cumulative probability scores $(i - \frac{1}{2})/n$, for each $i = 1, 2, \ldots, n$.

3. From Table T5 obtain the Normal ordinates z_i, corresponding to the cumulative probability scores.

4. Plot the observed values y_i on the y-axis against the Normal ordinates, z_i, on the x-axis. Departures from linearity will indicate a lack of Normality. An estimate of the median is provided by the value of y_i corresponding to the z_i of zero.

Worked example: residual and normal ordinates

The residuals from the regression of FEV_1 on height of Table 9.7 are given in Table 9.8 and we wish to check if these follow a Normal distribution.

To do this the residuals are ordered, their corresponding cumulative probability scores calculated and the Normal ordinates, z_i determined from Table T5. Thus corresponding to the cumulative probabilities 0.1, $z = -1.28$, for probability 0.3, $z = -0.52$, and so on as given in the final column of Table 9.8. These are plotted in Figure 9.10.

Table 9.8 Residuals for the linear regression of FEV_1 and height in five patients with asthma

FEV_1 (litres) y	Height (cm) x	Predicted FEV_1	Residuals	Ordered residuals	$(i - \frac{1}{2})/5$	z_i
1.5	160	1.42	0.08	-0.28	0.1	-1.28
1.6	165	1.70	-0.10	-0.10	0.3	-0.52
1.7	170	1.98	-0.28	-0.05	0.5	0.00
2.1	173	2.15	-0.05	0.08	0.7	0.52
2.4	175	2.26	0.14	0.14	0.9	1.28

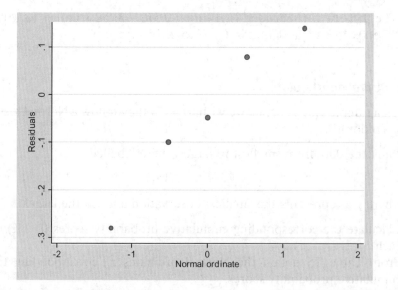

Figure 9.10 Plot of the residuals calculated from the regression of Table 9.7 against Normal ordinates. As this plot is approximately linear, we can see that there is no real evidence of a lack of Normality for these data

9.10 Exercises

1. A survey was conducted in 295 people asking about arthritic pain on a visual analogue scale (can be treated as continuous) in 295 people. Sex was coded 1 = male 0 = female. Medication was coded 1 = on medication 0 = not on medication.

   The output from a multiple linear regression computer program is shown in Table 9.8.

```
Table 9.8  Output from survey of 295 people
R-squared     = 0.0554
Adj R-squared = 0.0489
```

pain	Coef.	Std. Err.	t	P>|t|	[95% Conf. Interval]	
sex	-5.285991	3.294272	-1.60	0.110	-11.76952	A
medication	-9.489177	3.245583	B	0.004	-15.87688	-3.101475
_cons	94.18235	5.853297	16.09	0.000	82.66236	105.7024

```
{adjusted r-squared=1-(1-r-squared)(N-1)/(N-k-1) where N is number
of subjects and k is the number of predictors.}
```

   (i)   Deduce the values of A and B.
   (ii) Is the effect of medication significant? What is the assumption underlying this test?
   (iii) What is the expected value of the pain score in a woman not on medication?
   (iv) What is the expected value of the pain score for a man on medication?
   (v)   Is the model a good fit to the data?

2. A survey was conducted and asked 'do you consider your health to be poor?' This was coded 1 for 'yes' and 0 for 'no'. The effect of age (in decades) and sex on the outcome was examined using logistic regression.

```
Logit estimates
------------------------------------------------------------------------
ill |     Coef.      Std. Err.   z      P>|z|   [95% Conf. Interval]
--------+---------------------------------------------------------------
sex |    .037236     .2510687   0.15    0.882   -.4548497 .5293217
age |    .3310879    .2454655   A       0.177   -.1500157 B
_cons | -.5440707    .4480324  -1.21    0.225   -1.422198  .3340567
------------------------------------------------------------------------


------------------------------------------------------------------------
ill |  Odds Ratio   Std. Err.   z      P>|z|   [95% Conf. Interval]
--------+---------------------------------------------------------------
sex |  1.037938     .2605938   0.15    0.882   .6345433   1.69778
age |  C            .3418064   1.35    0.177   .8606945   2.25284
------------------------------------------------------------------------
```

  (i) Deduce the values of A B and C.
 (ii) Are either age or sex significant predictors of outcome?
(iii) Interpret the value of C.

10 Survival analysis

Medical Statistics Fourth Edition, David Machin, Michael J Campbell, Stephen J Walters
© 2007 John Wiley & Sons, Ltd

Summary

The major outcome variable in some clinical studies is the time measured from patient or subject entry into a study until a pre-specified 'critical event' has occurred. These times often have a rather skewed distribution. However, a key feature of 'survival-time' data is the presence of 'censored' observations. Censored observations arise in subjects that are included in the study but for whom the critical event of interest has not yet been observed. We describe the Kaplan–Meier survival curve, the Logrank test for comparing two groups, the use of the hazard ratio for data summary and the Cox proportional hazards regression model, which replaces linear regression when the continuous outcome data are survival times with censored observations.

10.1 Time to event data

The major outcome variable in some clinical trials is the time from randomisation, and start of treatment, to a specified critical event. The length of time from entry to the study to when the critical event occurs is called the survival time. Examples include patient survival time (time from diagnosis to death), the time a kidney graft remains patent, length of time that an indwelling cannula remains in situ, or the time a serious burn takes to heal. Even when the final outcome is not *actual* survival time, the techniques employed with such data are conventionally termed 'survival' analysis methods.

Example from the literature: Trial endpoints – children with neuroblastoma

Pearson et al (2007) describe a randomised clinical trial in children with neuroblastoma in which two chemotherapy regimens are compared. In brief, the object of therapy following diagnosis is first to reduce the tumour burden (to obtain a response); to maintain that response for as long as possible; then following any relapse to prolong survival. Key 'survival type' endpoints are therefore time from start of treatment to: response, progression and death; and duration of response as shown in Figure 10.1.

However a key feature of survival time studies is the distinction that needs to be made between calendar time and patient time-on-study that is illustrated in Figure 10.2. This shows a study including five patients who enter the study at different calendar times. This is typically the situation in any clinical trial in which the potential patients are those presenting at a particular clinic over a period of time and not all on the same date. The progress of patients recruited to the trial is then monitored for a period as is described in the appropriate trial protocol. Also at some future

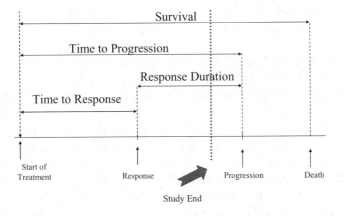

Figure 10.1 Endpoints or critical events relevant to a clinical trial in children with neuroblastoma

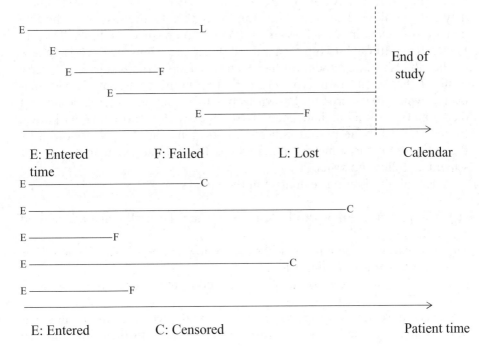

Figure 10.2 'Calendar time' when entering and leaving a study compared to 'Patient time' on the study

date (calendar time) the trial will close and an analysis conducted. For a patient recruited late in the trial, this may mean that some of their endpoint observations will not be made. Thus for such a patient, in the example of Figure 10.1, at the date of analysis only time to response may be observed, in which case time to progression and survival time will both be censored with the same *survival time* value, and response duration will also be censored. The calendar time on which these censorings occur will be the same date.

At this analysis (calendar) time, the patients will now be viewed as in the lower panel of Figure 10.2, that is, time will be measured from the start of entry to the study, that is by patient (follow-up) time rather than calendar time.

Although survival time is a continuous variable one often cannot use the standard *t*-test of Chapter 8 for analysis as the distribution of survival times is unlikely to be Normal and it may not be possible to find a transformation that will make it so. However, the major reason for the use of 'survival' methods is not the shape of the distribution but the presence of 'censored' observations. Censored observations arise in patients that are included in a study but for whom the critical event of interest has not yet been observed. For example, although some of the patients recruited to a particular trial may have died and their survival time is calculable, others may still be alive. The time from randomisation to the last date the live patient was examined is known as the censored survival time. Thus in Figure 10.2, although two patients 'Fail', three are 'Censored'. Here failure implies that the study endpoint has been reached (perhaps they have died), while of those censored, two were censored as the trial analysis was conducted while they were still known to be alive (they had therefore not yet died), and one patient had been 'Lost'. Essentially, 'Lost' means known to have lived for the period indicated, and then ceased to be followed by the study team for some reason. Perhaps the patient failed to return for scheduled follow-up visits.

Censored observations can arise in three ways:

(i) The patient is known to be still alive when the trial analysis is carried out.
(ii) Was known to be alive at some past follow-up, but the investigator has since lost trace of him or her.
(iii) Has died of some cause totally unrelated to the disease in question.

Clearly more survival time information would become available in situation (i) above if the analysis were delayed; possibly further time may be gained with (ii) if the patient was subsequently traced; while no further time is possible in situation (iii).

Example from the literature: No censored observations – duration of postoperative fever

Chant et al (1984) in a randomised trial including 108 adult patients undergoing appendicectomy compared two drugs, metronidazole and ampicillin, which are used to alleviate postoperative wound infection. One of the major outcome variables was the length of the postoperative fever actually experienced by the patients as measured from the date of surgery to the date of resolution of fever.

This period was observed in all patients so there were no censored observations and so the findings were summarised by use of the geometric mean number of days of fever in each group. The use of the geometric, rather than the arithmetic mean, implied that the logarithm of the fever duration has a more Normal-shaped distribution than the times themselves. The geometric mean in patients receiving ampicillin was 3.0 days, compared with 3.5 days for patients receiving metronidazole. This difference was statistically significant ($t = 2.45$, $df = 106$, p-value = 0.014) suggesting an advantage to ampicillin.

10.2 Kaplan–Meier survival curve

One method of analysis of survival data is to specify in advance a fixed time-point at which comparisons are to be made and then compare proportions of patients whose survival times exceed this time period. For example, one may compare the proportion of patients alive at 1 year in two treatment groups. However this ignores the individual survival times and can be very wasteful of the available information. Neither does it overcome the problem of observations censored at times less than 1 year from randomisation. However, techniques have been developed to deal with survival data that can take account of the information provided by censored observations. Such data can be displayed using a Kaplan–Meier (K-M) survival curve.

Example from the literature: Kaplan–Meier curves – ulcerative colitis

Hawthorne et al (1992) conducted a randomised trial in 67 patients with ulcerative colitis who had achieved a remission of at least 2 months when taking azathioprine. They were then randomised to either continue with azathioprine, or given a placebo.

The corresponding K-M survival curves of time from randomisation to recurrence of the disease are shown in Figure 10.3. The results revealed that continuing azathioprine treatment in ulcerative colitis was beneficial if patients have achieved remission while taking the drug.

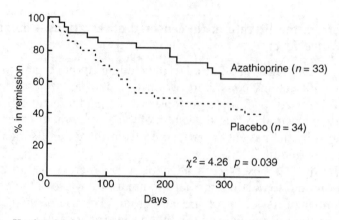

Figure 10.3 Kaplan–Meier survival curves for time from randomisation to recurrence of ulcerative colitis in 67 patients who had achieved remission by initially taking azathioprine. From Hawthorne et al (1992). Randomised controlled trial of azathioprine withdrawal in ulcerative colitis. *British Medical Journal*, **305**, 20–22: reproduced by permission of the BMJ Publishing Group

If there are no censored observations, then the K-M survival curve for n patients starts at time 0 with a value of 1 (or 100% survival) then continues horizontally until the time the first death occurs, it then drops by $1/n$ at this point. The curve then proceeds horizontally once more until the time of the second death when again it drops by $1/n$. This process continues until the time of the last death, when the survival curve drops by the final $1/n$ to take a value of 0 (0%). If two deaths happen to occur at the same time then the step down would be $2/n$.

The K-M estimate of the survival curve when there are censored observations mimics this process but essentially 'jumps' over the 'censored' observations which then leads to steps down of unequal sizes. The precise method of calculating the K-M survival curve is summarised below.

Procedure for calculating a Kaplan–Meier survival curve

1. First, order (rank) the survival times from smallest to largest. If a censored observation and a time to death are equal, then the censored observation is assumed to follow the death.
2. An event is a death. A censored observation has no associated event.
3. Determine the number at risk, n_i, as the number of patients alive immediately before the event at time t_i.
4. Calculate the probability of survival from t_{i-1} to t_i as $1 - d_i/n_i$. Note that we start at time zero with $t_0 = 0$.
5. The cumulative survival probability, $S(t_i)$, is the probability of surviving from 0 up to t_i. It is calculated as

6. $S(t_i) = (1 - d_i/n_i) \times (1 - d_{i-1}/n_{i-1}) \times \ldots \times (1 - d_1/n_1)$.
7. A censored observation at time t_i reduces the number at risk by one but does not change the cumulative survival probability at time t_i since $d_i = 0$.
8. A plot of the cumulative survival probability $S(t_i)$ against t_i, gives the K-M survival curve.

When comparing two or more survival curves, we usually assume that the mechanisms that result in censored observations occurring do not depend on the group concerned, that is, the censoring is 'non-informative' in that it tells us nothing relevant to the comparison of the groups. For example, in a randomised clinical trial, it is assumed that patients are just as likely to be lost to follow-up in one treatment group as in another. If there are imbalances in such losses then this can lead to spurious differences in survival between groups and false conclusions being drawn by the analysis.

Worked example: K-M survival curve

The calculations for the K-M survival curve are easiest to explain by example as in Table 10.1. There we consider a group of 16 patients randomised to a trial of two treatments A and B, where the outcome is survival time from start of treatment. Some patients are lost to follow-up while others have only been observed for short periods of time and so, in both cases, their observations are censored at the time of analysis.

For illustration of the K-M curve, we combine the data from both treatment groups and their ordered (or ranked) survival times are given in Table 10.1, Column 2. These range from the shortest survival time of 21 days to four patients still alive after 365 days on the trial and who therefore have censored survival times denoted 365+.

The resulting K-M curve is shown in Figure 10.4, from which it can be seen that the step sizes are unequal (caused by the censored values of 33+ and 100+, and the two deaths at 130 days). Further, the curve does not reach the time-axis as the longest survivors at 365 days are still alive.

On the K-M survival curve of Figure 10.4, the small spikes correspond to the censored observations. Above each spike, the number of patients censored at that time is given. In this example, all are marked '1' except for the longest censored observation at 365+ days where there is a '3'. When there are a large number of patients and perhaps a large number of censored observations, the 'spikes' may clutter the K-M curve. In which case the numbers at risk, which are a selection of the n_i of Table 10.1, are tabulated at convenient intervals beneath the K-M curves as illustrated.

Table 10.1 Illustration of calculations for the Kaplan–Meier survival curve and Logrank test in a clinical trial of 16 patients

| | | | Kaplan–Meier | | | | Logrank test | |
i	Ordered survival time t_i	Total number at risk n_i	Number of events at time t_i d_i	Probability of survival in t_{i-1}, t_i $1 - d_i/n_i$	Cumulative survival probability	Treatment	Number at risk in A n_{Ai}	Expected number of events in A e_{Ai}
0	0	16	–	1	1	–	8	0
1	21	16	1	0.938	0.938	A	8	0.500
2	33+	15	0	1	0.938	A	7	0
3	42	14	1	0.929	0.871	B	6	0.429
4	55	13	1	0.923	0.804	A	6	0.462
5	69	12	1	0.917	0.737	A	5	0.417
6	100+	11	0	1	0.737	B	4	0
7	130	10	2	0.800	0.590	A	4	0.800
8	130					A		
9	210	8	1	0.875	0.516	B	2	0.250
10	250+	7	0			B		*
11	290+	6	0			A		
12	310+	5	0			A		
13	365+	4	0			B		
14	365+					B		
15	365+					B		
16	365+					B		

*The expected number of events is not be calculated for times beyond the last recorded event – here 210 days.

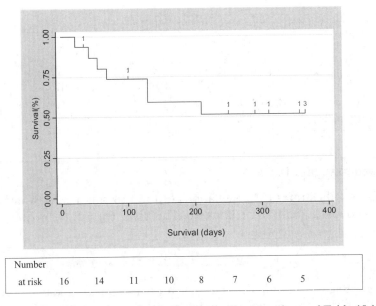

Figure 10.4   Kaplan–Meier survival curve for the 16 patients of Table 10.1

10.3   The Logrank test

To compare the survival times of two groups, the K-M survival curves for each are first calculated and then formally compared using the Logrank test. The null hypothesis of no difference between groups can be expressed by stating that the median survival times of the two groups are equal. The appropriate calculations are summarised below. The curious name, Logrank, for the test arises because it is related to another statistical test that uses the logarithms of the ranks of the data.

Procedure for calculating the Logrank test comparing two groups A and B

Using the notation summarised in Table 10.1

1. The total number of events observed in groups A and B are O_A and O_B.
2. Under the null hypothesis, the expected number of events in the group receiving treatment A at time t_i is
3. $e_{Ai} = (d_i n_{Ai})/n_i$.
4. The expected number of events should not be calculated beyond the last event (at time 210 days in this example).
5. The total number of events expected on A, assuming the null hypothesis of no difference between treatments, is $E_A = \Sigma e_{Ai}$.

---

6. The number expected on B is $E_B = \Sigma d_i - E_A$.
7. Calculate

$$\chi^2_{\text{Logrank}} = \frac{(O_A - E_A)^2}{E_A} + \frac{(O_B - E_B)^2}{E_B}.$$

8. This has a χ^2 distribution with $df = 1$ as two groups are being compared.

Worked example: Logrank test

Table 10.1 illustrates the calculations of the Logrank test in which treatment groups A and B are compared. This gives $O_A = 5$, $O_B = 2$, $E_A = 2.86$ and $E_B = 4.14$. From which

$$\chi^2_{\text{Logrank}} = \frac{(5 - 2.86)^2}{2.86} + \frac{(2 - 4.14)^2}{4.14} = 2.71.$$

Using Table T4 with $df = 1$ gives $p = 0.1$ (more precise calculations give 0.099) which suggests that we do not reject the null hypothesis.

10.4   The hazard ratio

We indicated earlier, that the median survival time may be a suitable summary for survival data as survival times often have rather skew distributions. However, there is an immediate problem if censored data are present. For example, if we were to ignore the censoring in the survival times of Table 10.1, we could calculate the median time, $M = (130 + 210)/2 = 170$ days. However, there are two censored values below this 'median' at 33+ and 100+ days, and these two observations have the potential to increase and may eventually both exceed the current median estimate of 170 days. In view of censored observations, the median is estimated by first calculating the K-M survival curve, then from the mid-point of the survival axis (survival of 50%) moving horizontally until the curve is met, then dropping vertically to the time axis.

Worked example: Median 'survival' time – recurrence of ulcerative colitis

Following the above process for the Placebo group of Figure 10.3 gives a median time to recurrence of approximately 210 days. However, that for the azathioprine group cannot be estimated as the K-M curve has not passed beneath the 50% recurrence value.

The hazard ratio (HR) has been specifically developed for survival data, and is used as a measure of the relative survival experience of two groups.

Procedure for calculating the HR when comparing two groups

1. Accumulate the observed number of events in each group, O_A and O_B.
2. Under the hypothesis of no survival difference between the groups, calculate the expected number of events in each group, E_A and E_B using the Logrank test.
3. The ratio O_A/E_A is the relative event rate in group A. Similarly O_B/E_B is the relative death rate in group B.
4. The *HR* is the ratio of these relative event rates, that is

$$HR = \frac{O_A/E_A}{O_B/E_B}.$$

When there is no difference between two groups, that is the null hypothesis is true, the value of $HR = 1$. It is important to note that for the *HR* the 'expected' deaths in each group are calculated using the Logrank method as described previously. This method allows for the censoring which occurs in nearly all survival data. It has parallels with the relative risk, RR, of Chapter 12 and has a similar interpretation. As a consequence, the term (not the calculation method) RR is often used rather than HR in a survival context also. In general, this is not good practice and we recommend the use of RR should be restricted so that one automatically knows it is *not* based on the *actual* survival times but perhaps on the proportions alive at a particular time-point.

Worked example: Hazard ratio

From the calculations summarised in Table 10.1, $O_A = 5$, $O_B = 2$, $E_A = 2.86$ and $E_B = 4.14$. From which

$$HR = \frac{O_A/E_A}{O_B/E_B} = \frac{5/2.86}{2/4.14} = 3.6.$$

Thus the risk of death with treatment A is almost four times that with treatment B. The corresponding survival curves are shown in Figure 10.5.

The HR gives an estimate of the overall difference between the survival curves. However, summarising the difference between two survival curves into one statistic can also have its problems. One particularly important consideration for its use is that the ratio of the relative event rates in the two groups should not vary greatly over time.

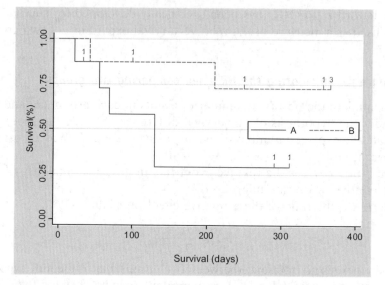

Figure 10.5   Kaplan–Meier survival curves by treatment group of the data of Table 10.1

It also turns out that if M_A and M_B are the respective median survival times of two groups, then the inverse of their ratio, that is $1/(M_A/M_B)$ or M_B/M_A, is approximately the HR.

Confidence interval for HR

Whenever an estimate of a difference between groups is given, it is useful to calculate a confidence interval (CI) for the estimate. Thus, for the HR obtained from any study, we would like to know a range of values which are not inconsistent with this estimate.

In calculating CIs, it is convenient if the statistic under consideration can be assumed to follow an approximately Normal distribution. However, the estimate of the HR is not Normally distributed. In particular it has a possible range of values from 0 to ∞, with the null hypothesis value of unity not located at the centre of this interval. To make the scale symmetric and to enable us to calculate CIs, we transform the estimate to make it approximately Normally distributed. We do this by using log HR, rather than HR itself, as the basis for our calculation.

95% confidence interval (CI) for a HR

1. Calculate the estimate: log HR.

2. Calculate: $SE(\log HR) = \sqrt{\left(\dfrac{1}{E_A} + \dfrac{1}{E_B}\right)}$, although this should strictly only be used if the number of events $E_A + E_B = O_A + O_B$ is relatively large.

3. Calculate the 95% CI for log *HR* as
   log *HR* – 1.96 × *SE*(log *HR*) to log *HR* + 1.96 × *SE*(log *HR*).
4. Calculate the 95% CI for HR as
   exp[log *HR* – 1.96 × *SE*(log *HR*)] to exp[log *HR* + 1.96 × *SE*(log *HR*)].

Worked example: – Confidence interval for the HR

Applying the calculation method to the data of Table 10.1 gives $O_A = 5$, $O_B = 2$, $E_A = 2.86$ and $E_B = 4.14$. From which log $(HR) = 0.71$ and

$$SE(\log HR) = \sqrt{\frac{1}{2.86} + \frac{1}{4.14}} = 0.7689.$$

A 95% CI for log (HR) sets $z_{0.975} = 1.96$ and gives a range from $0.71 - 1.96 \times 0.77$ to $0.71 + 1.96 \times 0.77$ or –0.8 to 2.2. Finally for the CI for the HR itself, we have to exponentiate these lower and upper limits to obtain exp(–0.8) = 0.4 to exp(2.2) = 9.0, that is 0.4 to 9.0. A 20-fold range of values!

The wide 95% CI emphasises that reliable conclusions could not be drawn from such data.

10.5 Modelling time to event data

If we think of our own lives for a moment, we are continually exposed to the possibility of our demise. However, having lived until now, we can think of the chance of our demise (say) in the next day, hour, or second as our hazard for the next interval be it, a second, hour or day. This can be thought of as our *instantaneous* death rate or failure rate conditional on living until now. Alternatively it expresses our hazard at time (our age), *t* (or now) which is denoted $h(t)$.

In general, suppose *n* people of a certain age group were alive at the start of a particular year, and *d* of these died in the following period of duration *D* units, then the risk of death per unit time in that period is $d/(nD)$. If we now imagine the width of the time interval, *D*, getting narrower and narrower then the number of deaths *d* will get fewer and fewer but the ratio *d/D* will stay constant. This gives the instantaneous death rate or the *hazard rate*. Thus at any particular time (say) *t*, we think of the hazard rate as applying to what is just about to happen in the next very short time period.

Now our own hazard may fluctuate with time and will certainly increase for all of us as, *t* (our age) increases. Similarly, if we become diseased, perhaps with a life-threatening illness, our hazard rate would unquestionably increase in which case the aim of therapy would be to restore it to the former (lower) value if possible. Individual hazards will differ, even in those of the precisely the same age, and it may be that particular groups may have (on average) higher values than others. Thus the hazard of developing dental caries may be greater in those who live in areas where fluoridation has not occurred. This leads us to quantify the benefit of fluoridation through the ratio of hazards (the HR) in those from fluoridation areas to those from non-fluoridation areas whose value may also be influenced by other factors such as dietary intake and tooth brushing frequency.

In Chapter 9 we described linear regression techniques for continuous data, logistic regression for binary data and both allowed the dependent variable to be related to one or more independent variables or covariates x_1, x_2, ...x_k. Although survival time is also a continuous variable the possibility of censored observations has to be taken account of in the regression modelling process. This leads us to the Cox proportional hazards regression model which models, as the dependent variable, the instantaneous hazard, $h(t)$, as it is the change in this that ultimately determines our survival time.

The multivariable Cox model links the hazard to an individual i at time t, $h_i(t)$ to a baseline hazard $h_0(t)$ by

$$\log[h_i(t)] = \log[h_0(t)] + \beta_1 x_1 + \beta_2 x_2 + \ldots + \beta_k x_k,$$

where x_1, x_2, ..., x_k are covariates associated with individual i. The baseline log hazard, $\log[h_0(t)]$, serves as a reference point, and can be thought of as the intercept, α, of a multiple regression equation of Chapter 9; for convenience often labelled β_0.

The Cox model is called the *proportional hazards* model because if we imagine two individuals i and j, then the equation assumes that the ratio of one hazard to the other, $h_i(t)/h_j(t)$, remains constant at whatever time, t, we consider their ratio. Thus irrespective of how $h_0(t)$ varies over time, the hazards of the two individuals remain proportional to each other.

The above expression for the Cox model can also be written as

$$h_i(t) = h_0(t)\exp(\beta_1 x_1 + \beta_2 x_2 + \ldots + \beta_k x_k).$$

More strictly $h_i(t)$ should be written $h_i(t; x_1, x_2, \ldots, x_k)$ as it depends both on t and the covariates x.

Cox proportional hazards regression model for two groups and no covariates

1. We wish to compare the survival time in two groups (control and intervention) denoted by $x = 0$ and $x = 1$.
2. The Cox model for the single covariate, x, denoting group is $h(t;x) = h_0(t)\exp(\beta x)$.
3. For the control group, $x = 0$, $h(t;0) = h_0(t)\exp(\beta \times 0) = h_0(t) \times 1 = h_0(t)$.

4. For the intervention group, $x = 1$, $h(t;1) = h_0(t)\exp(\beta \times 1) = h_0(t) \times \exp(\beta)$.
5. The ratio of these is the $HR = h(t;1)/h(t;0) = \exp(\beta)$ and this quantifies the effect of the intervention.
6. The regression coefficient of the model, β (= log HR) is estimated from the survival time data of both groups.

Technical example

Assume x is a binary variable taking values 0 and 1 for males and females respectively and the estimate of the regression coefficient, β, calculated from the survival data of both groups using the Cox model gives $b = 1.5$ say. With $x = 0$, $h_{Male} = \exp(1.5 \times 0) = 1.0$ while with $x = 1$, $h_{Female} = \exp(1.5 \times 1) = \exp(1.5) = 4.5$. The associated $HR = h_{Female}/h_{Male} = \exp(1.5 \times 1)/\exp(1.5 \times 0) = 4.5/1.0 = 4.5$. In this case, there is a greater risk of dying for females.

The Cox model, once fitted to the survival time data, provides a link to the Logrank test and the associated HR. In fact, since log $HR = \beta$, the regression coefficient itself is often referred to as the log hazard ratio.

Worked example: Cox model

Fitting the Cox model to the data of Table 10.1, using a computer package gives $HR = 3.7$. This is quite close to the value of 3.6 resulting from the Logrank test that we gave earlier. Such a small difference can be accounted for by the rounding during the respective calculations.

However, the 95% CI for the HR is given as 0.71 to 19.7, much wider than that given by the previous calculations. This disparity is caused by using the expression for the SE(log HR) given earlier which should really be confined to larger samples. Neither method is entirely reliable in the circumstances of our example.

The Cox analysis gives a p-value = 0.097 which compares with the Logrank p-value of 0.099 quoted previously.

When the Cox model includes several covariates, although the fitting procedure is straightforward using standard statistical packages, care should be taken to avoid including too many variables in the multivariable model. It has to be recognised that it is the number of events observed, rather than the number of subjects in the study that is important. In very broad terms, for every variable included in a multivariable Cox model a minimum of 10 (better 20) events should have been observed. This is to ensure that the regression coefficients estimated have reasonable precision.

Example from the literature: Cox multivariable regression – leg ulcers

Morell et al (1998) conducted a randomised controlled trial to compare healing times of patients with leg ulcers cared for at home or in the clinic. Their results are summarised in Figure 10.6, which suggests that those treated in the clinic group heal more quickly.

However, it is known that other factors such as patient age (Age), and features of the ulcer itself such as how long it has been present (Duration), the area at the time of randomisation (Area), and any history of deep vein involvement (DVI no or yes) will affect the healing times – perhaps more so than the intervention. The trial involved 213 patients and 129 ulcers were observed to heal (the critical event).

If a multivariable Cox regression model is to be used, then the five independent variables (Group, Age, Duration, Area, DVI) give 213/5 ≈ 40 patients per regression coefficient to be estimated and, more importantly, 129/5 ≈ 25 events. This is probably sufficient to obtain reliable estimates of the corresponding coefficients. The resulting Cox model is summarised in Table 10.2.

From this analysis, it is clear that even taking account of the possible influence of the potentially prognostic variables (Age, Area, Duration, DVI) the difference between the groups is significant (p-value = 0.006) and the effect substantial with $HR = \exp(0.5008) = 1.65$ (95% CI 1.16 to 2.36) in favour of the faster healing in those having a clinic visit.

Although Age, Duration and DVI were thought to be potentially prognostic this did not turn out to be the case as the corresponding 95% CIs all included the null value of $HR = 1$. In contrast, increasing Area is clearly adversely prognostic with $HR = 0.69$ (CI 0.58 to 0.83).

In the above example, the HR for the continuous covariate Area is expressed using units of $10\,cm^2$. This implies that a leg ulcer of (say) $30\,cm^2$ will heal 0.69 times less speedily than will one of $20\,cm^2$. The change could have been expressed in terms of $1\,cm^2$ in which case the regression coefficient would have been -0.03666 with $HR = \exp(-0.03667) = 0.964$. However, $0.964^{10} = 0.69$, as we have in Table 10.2 for the HR for Area.

The choice of units used in the calculations will depend on circumstances but for Age, for example, it is very unlikely even if age does indeed influence healing rate, that there will be much difference in healing between individuals of say 69 and 70 years, whereas a marked difference may be seen comparing individuals who are 60 as opposed to 70 years. This argues for decades as the unit for analysis rather than years. Nevertheless, whichever method is chosen, this choice does not affect the conclusions we draw but just how we express them.

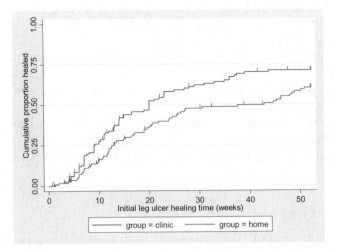

Figure 10.6   Healing times of initial leg ulcers by clinic and home care group From Morrell et al (1998). Cost effectiveness of community leg clinics. *British Medical Journal*, **316**, 1487–1491: reproduced by permission of the BMJ Publishing Group

Table 10.2   Cox multivariable proportional hazards regression model fitted to the healing times of 213 patients with leg ulcers (data from Morrell et al, 1998)

	b	$SE(b)$	z	p-value	$HR = \exp(b)$	95% CI
Group	0.5008	0.301	2.75	0.006	1.65	1.16 to 2.36
Age (per 10 years)	0.06976	0.080	0.82	0.41	1.07	0.91 to 1.26
Area (per 10 cm²)	−0.3666	0.090	−4.04	0.001	0.69	0.58 to 0.83
Duration (years)	−0.03605	0.002	−1.39	0.17	0.96	0.91 to 1.01
DVI (No vs. Yes)	−0.0866	0.202	−0.39	0.70	0.92	0.60 to 1.41

Further details of the Cox model are given by Walters (2003), Campbell (2006) and Machin et al (2006).

10.6   Points when reading the literature

Interpreting the results of a survival analysis

- Is the nature of the censoring specified? As far as possible check that the censoring is non-informative.
- Check that the total number of critical events is reported, as well as subjects and person-time of follow-up, with some measure of variability such as a range for the latter. In trials, are numbers of censored observations given by treatment group?
- Is the estimated survival rate at a conventional time point, by group, with confidence intervals given?

- Are the Kaplan–Meier survival curves by group displayed?
- Are the numbers at risk reported at regular time intervals?
- Is the regression model used specified?
- Is the proportional hazards assumption reasonable and has it been validated?
- If a multivariable Cox model is used, are the corresponding HRs and CIs reported for all the variables included?
- Are the conclusions drawn critically dependent on the statistical assumptions made?
- Is the computer program used for the analysis indicated?

10.7   Exercises

1. In the clinical trial of Hancock et al. (2004) to compare a new treatment for malignant melanoma (a form of skin cancer), patients were randomised to one of two groups: treatment with low-dose interferon alfa-2a as adjuvant therapy (Intervention – interferon), or no further treatment (Control – observation). They were followed up until the patient died or 5 years from randomisation. The survival times in years for a random sample of 10 patients from the Intervention group were as follows:

   0.91, 1.30, 1.56, 2.59*, 3.74, 3.76*, 4.28, 4.43, 5.0*, 5.0*

   (* A star indicates a censored observation.)

   (a) Explain what is meant by a *censored* observation. Also explain the meaning of the term *hazard function*.

   (b) Construct the Kaplan–Meier survival curve for this random sample of 10 patients from the Intervention group and show it on a suitable graph.

   (c) The full trial involved 674 patients, with 338 randomised to the Intervention group and 336 to the Control group. Figure 10.7 shows Kaplan–Meier estimates of survival functions for the overall survival times for the two treatment groups, and the results of a log-rank test.

   Use Figure 10.7 to estimate the median overall survival times for the two treatment groups. Is there a difference in the survival patterns of the two treatment groups? Comment on the results of the Logrank test.

   Previous studies have suggested that age, gender and histology are important factors in predicting overall survival time. Cox proportional hazards regression analysis was used to adjust survival times for these prognostic variables.

   Table 10.7 shows abbreviated computer output from two Cox regression models. In Analysis 1, a simple regression of overall survival time on

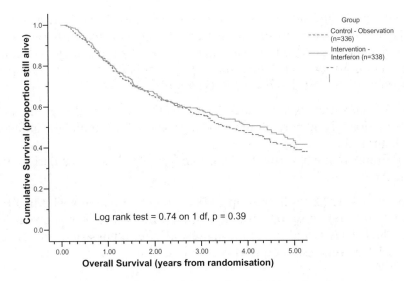

Figure 10.7 Kaplan–Meier estimate of overall survival functions by treatment group

Table 10.7 Computer analysis of survival data

Analysis 1: Cox regression – model: group

```
No. of subjects =       674
No. of failures =       351
```

	Haz.Ratio	Std.Err.	z	P>|z|	[95% Conf. Interval]
group	.912	.098	-0.86	0.391	.740 1.125

Analysis 2: Cox regression – model: age gender histology group

	Haz.Ratio	Std.Err.	z	P>|z|	[95% Conf. Interval]
age	1.002	.004	0.60	0.549	.994 1.010
gender	.739	.081	-2.76	0.006	.596 .916
histology	1.602	.240	3.15	0.002	1.195 2.149
group	.915	.098	-0.83	0.409	.741 1.130

treatment group alone was performed. Analysis 2 involved a multiple regression of survival time on age (years), gender and histology. (Note that gender was coded 0 = 'Male' and 1 = 'Female'; histology as 'localised non-metastatic' = 0 and 'metastatic' = 1. Similarly, treatment group was coded as 0 = Control and 1 = Intervention).

(d) Which variables are related to survival? Can one tell from the information given here if the model is good for predicting individual survival?
(e) Compare the hazard ratio for group from Analysis 2 that derived from Analysis 1.

2. Roche et al (2005) followed up 2448 consecutive patients who had been admitted to one hospital with an acute hip fracture. After one year 33% had died. They found the following results after a univariate and a multivariate Cox regression on deaths over one year.

Variable	Hazard ratio (95% CI)	
	Univariate	Multivariate (allowing for age, sex, and other covariates)
Comorbid cardiovascular disease	1.4 (1.2 to 1.6)	1.0 (0.8 to 1.2)
Comorbid respiratory disease	1.6 (1.3 to 1.9)	1.4 (1.1 to 1.7)
Post-operative chest infection	5.0 (4.2 to 6.0)	2.4 (1.9 to 3.0)
Parkinson's disease	1.4 (1.0 to 1.9)	1.1 (0.8 to 1.6)

(a) Interpret the hazard ratios for comorbid respiratory disease in the univariate and multivariate analysis.
(b) Is comorbid cardiovascular disease a significant risk factor? Discuss why the univariate and multivariate analyses differ. Is there any other variable that changes significance in the multivariate analysis?
(c) Why do you think the hazard ratio for post-operative chest infection is reduced?
(d) What assumption underlies the model for these variables? Do you think it equally likely for all the variables?

11 Reliability and method comparison studies

Medical Statistics Fourth Edition, David Machin, Michael J Campbell, Stephen J Walters
© 2007 John Wiley & Sons, Ltd

Summary

In the health sciences, often measurements are made which need to be validated. Physiotherapists may need a reliable method of measuring pain, an occupational therapist a reliable method of assessing whether someone is lifting a heavy weight correctly. In addition, different observers may come to different conclusions. Radiologists may disagree on the interpretation of an X-ray, physiotherapists on the level of pain actually experienced or pathologists on the histological grade of a tumour. Many projects start with a proposed method of measuring something, and the important question is: 'Does this instrument measure what it purports to measure?' In many disciplines new techniques evolve that are simpler or less invasive than earlier procedures and an important question is whether the new procedure can be used instead of the earlier one. This chapter has a different emphasis to preceding ones in that we are not *testing* whether something is reliable but rather *measuring* how reliable it is.

11.1   Introduction

Many measurements that are taken during any study require some degree of subjective judgement, whether this is when taking a temperature with a thermometer, assessing the results of diagnostic procedures or observing the effects of therapies. As a consequence, were the same observer to repeat, or different observers to appraise, the same outcome measure they may not obtain identical results. Observer agreement studies investigate the reproducibility of a single observer, and the level of the consensus between different observers, assessing the same unit, be it a specimen, radiograph or pathology slide.

Typically in observer agreement studies, several observers make assessments on each of a series of experimental units and these assessments are compared. For example, to examine the variation in measurements of the volume of intracranial gliomas from computed tomography, different observers might evaluate scans from a series of patients. The values of tumour volume so recorded could then be compared. In other circumstances, the assessments may be of binary form such as a conclusion with respect to the presence or absence of metastases seen on liver scintigraphy. Clearly, an ideal situation is one in which all the observers agree *and* the answer is correct. The correct answer can only be known if there is a 'gold' standard means of assessment available. For some diseases this may be only possible at autopsy but this is clearly too late for patient care purposes.

Assessment of *reliability* consists of determining that the process used for measurement yields reproducible and consistent results. Any measurement whether on a numerical scale or by more subjective means, should yield reproducible or similar values if it is used repeatedly on the same patient whilst the patient's condition has not changed materially. In these circumstances, reliability concerns the level of agreement between two or more repeated measures. This is sometimes known as the *test–retest* reliability.

Suppose the measuring instrument is a questionnaire, perhaps to measure patient quality of life. Then during the development stage of the questionnaire itself the reliability of the scales to be ultimately used is of particular concern. Thus for scales containing multiple items, all the items should have *internal reliability* and therefore be consistent in the sense that they should all measure the same thing. Just as with any quantitative measurement the final questionnaire should have test–retest reliability also.

It is important to note that tests of statistical significance are rarely appropriate for reliability studies. Thus Table 11.2 below looks like a standard (paired) 2×2 contingency table to be analysed by McNemar's test, but this will not tell us whether the reviewer is reliable.

11.2 Repeatability

A basic requirement of a measurement is that it is repeatable; if the same measurement is made on a second occasion, and nothing has changed then we would expect it to give the same answer, within experimental error.

Coefficient of variation

For a continuous observation which is measured more than once a simple measure of repeatability is the *coefficient of variation* (*CV*) which is the within subject standard deviation divided by the mean.

$$CV = \frac{100 \times (\text{Within subject } SD)}{Mean} = \frac{100 s_{\text{Within}}}{\bar{x}},$$

where $\bar{x}$ and s_{Within} are calculated from continuous data obtained from the same subject in a stable situation.

The CV is a measure of variation which is independent of the units in which the observation is measured. It is often used in, for example, clinical biochemistry where repeated assays are made on a substance with known concentration to test the assay method. Commonly a CV of <5% is deemed acceptable.

Example: CV – pulse rate

In the example of Section 3.3 in which the pulse rate in one subject was taken at 5 minute intervals on 12 occasions in 60 minutes, the mean rate was $\bar{x} = 63$ beats/min and the within–subject standard deviation, $s_{\text{Within}} = 2.2$ beats/min. Thus the $CV = (100 \times 2.2)/63 = 3.5\%$.

Intra-class correlation coefficient (ICC)

Rather than repeated measures being confined to only a single subject the more usual situation is to have repeated (often duplicate and by the same rater) measures on a number of subjects. In this case there are two sources of variability that must be taken into account when assessing repeatability. The first source, as with the CV, is the within patient standard deviation and the second, since we are now concerned with several individuals on which the duplicates are taken, is the between subject standard deviation, $s_{Between}$.

In these circumstances, repeatability can be assessed by the intra-class correlation coefficient (ICC). This measures the strength of agreement between repeated measurements, by assessing the proportion of the between-patient variance (the square of the standard deviation), to the total variance, comprising the sum of both the within and between variation.

$$ICC = \frac{s^2_{Between}}{s^2_{Within} + s^2_{Between}},$$

where s_{Within} and $s_{Between}$ are the within and between subject standard deviations.

If we only have one observation per person we cannot estimate the within person standard deviation. If we have more than one observation per person, we can estimate the standard deviation for each person and take the average variance as an estimate of s^2_{Within}. We can estimate the between person variance from the variance of the means for each person as shown in Section 11.5.

If the ICC is large (close to 1), then the within rater (or random error) variability is low and a high proportion of the variance in the observations is attributable to variation between raters. The measurements are then described as having high reliability. Conversely, if the ICC is low (close to 0), then the random error variability dominates and the measurements have low reliability. If the error variability is regarded as 'noise' and the true value of raters' scores as the 'signal', then the ICC measures the signal–noise ratio.

The ICC is the most commonly used method for assessing reliability with continuous data. It is also sometimes used for ordered categorical data that have more than four or five response categories. A value of at least 0.90 is often recommended if the measurements of concern are to be used for evaluating future patients for which therapeutic decisions are to be made.

In the context of a questionnaire, say to assess quality of life (QoL), if a patient is in a stable condition, an instrument should yield repeatable and reproducible results if it is used repeatedly on that patient. This is usually assessed using a test–retest study, with patients who are thought to have stable disease and who are not expected to experience changes due to treatment effects or toxicity. The patients are asked to complete the same QoL questionnaire on several occasions. The level of agreement between the occasions is a measure of the reliability of the instrument. It is important to select patients whose condition is stable, and to choose carefully a between-assessment time-gap that is neither too short nor too long. As would be the case for a pathologist making a diagnosis from slides, too short a period might allow subjects to recall their earlier responses, and too long a period might allow a true change in the status of the subject. However, problems associated with developing and using QoL and other instruments are often rather specialist in nature and readers are referred to Fayers and Machin (2007) for a more detailed discussion.

Example from the literature: ICC – Paediatric Asthma Quality of Life Questionnaire

Juniper et al (1996) evaluated the Paediatric Asthma Quality of Life Questionnaire (PAQLQ) by examining reliability in children aged 7 to 17 who had stable asthma. The corresponding ICC values are shown in Table 11.1, and all are above 0.80. These findings suggest that the PAQLQ has high test–retest reliability in stable patients.

Inappropriate method

Despite the ICC being the appropriate measure to use, the Pearson correlation coefficient, r, of Sections 9.2 and 9.9, is sometimes mistakenly used in this context. Clearly, if duplicate measures are made on n subjects, then r can be calculated. However, repeated measurements may have a value of r close to 1 and so be highly correlated *yet* may be systematically different. For example, if the observer records consistently higher values on the first occasion than on the second by (say) exactly 10 units on whatever measuring instrument is being used, then there would be zero agreement between the two assessments. Despite this, the correlation coefficient would be 1, indicating perfect association. So as well as good association, good agreement is required, which implies near equality of the measures being taken.

Table 11.1 ICC values for reliability of items in the PAWLQ

Item	Within-subject SD	Between-subject SD	Intraclass correlation ICC
Overall QoL	0.17	0.73	0.95
Symptoms	0.22	0.84	0.93
Activities	0.42	0.96	0.84
Emotions	0.23	0.64	0.89

From Juniper et al (1996). Measuring quality of life in children with asthma. *Quality of Life Research*, **5**, 35–46. © Springer. Reproduced by permission of Springer Science and Business Media.

11.3   Agreement

A common problem is measuring how well two observers make a binary (Yes/No) diagnostic decision, say after examining a patient or perhaps a specimen taken from a patient. A similar problem is how consistent does a single observer make the same decision. To assess the latter, we would require the same assessments to be repeated by the same observer. For example, the same slide would need to be reviewed by the pathologist on two occasions. The second review would need to be undertaken 'blind' to the results of the first review and clearly some time later. A 'wash-out' period long enough to ensure that the pathologist did not 'recognise' the slide but not too much later if the period may cause deterioration of the specimen or after the observer (now more experienced) changes his/her methods in a systematic way.

For a single observer examining the same specimen on two occasions, or two observers examining the same specimen but independently of each other, the degree of reproducibility is quantified by the probability of making a chance error. In the context of making a definitive (and binary) diagnosis, this is the probability of ascribing either absent (coded 0) to a diagnosis when it should be present (coded 1), or a 1 to a diagnosis that should be 0. For N_{Repeat} specimens this process is described in Table 11.2.

One method of measuring whether a reviewer agrees with themselves, or two reviewers agree, is simply to calculate the percentage of occasions the same response is obtained.

Observer(s) agreement   The estimated probability the observer(s) agree is

$$P_{Agree} = \frac{x_{00} + x_{11}}{N_{Repeat}}.$$

Observer(s) disagreement   The estimated probability observer(s) disagree is

$$P_{Disagree} = \frac{x_{10} + x_{01}}{N_{Repeat}}.$$

Table 11.2 The possible outcomes for a single observer reviewing the same material on two occasions, or two observers reviewing the same material independently of each other

Second Review(er)	First review(er)		
	Absent	Present	Total
Absent	x_{00}	x_{01}	n_0
Present	x_{10}	x_{11}	n_1
Total	m_0	m_1	N_{Repeat}

Cohen's kappa (κ)

If the diagnostic choice is binary, then there is a very limited number of options (only 2) for each specimen so that if observers made their repeated choices at random, rather than by careful examination, these will agree some of the time. Jacob Cohen developed the kappa (κ) statistic in 1960 to allow for chance agreements of this kind. It is essentially the proportion of cases that the raters agree minus the proportion of cases they are likely to agree by chance, scaled so that if the observers agree all the time, then κ is one. Thus if κ is equal to 1, there is perfect agreement, and when $\kappa = 0$ the agreement is no better than chance. Negative values indicate an agreement that is even less than what would be expected by chance.

Cohen's κ is given by:

$$\kappa = \frac{P_{Agree} - P_{Chance}}{1 - P_{Chance}},$$

where P_{Chance} is the proportion expected to show agreement by chance alone. The method of calculating P_{Chance} is given in Section 11.7.

Example from the literature: Cohen's κ – safety advice

Clamp and Kendrick (1998) used a telephone survey asking about safety to 165 families with children aged under 5 years who had been involved in a randomised trial concerning safety advice. They chose a random sample of 20 families from the survey who then received a home visit 2 weeks later to measure the consistency of the response to the questions posed. The investigators found that, for most questions, a high κ value (>0.59) was obtained and so concluded that the survey was valid.

The concept of a binary diagnostic division may be extended to that of an ordered categorical variable where, for example, a pathologist may grade patient material into different grades perhaps indicative of increasing severity of the disease. In which case the results may be summarised in a square $R \times R$ contingency table where R is the number of possible grades that can be allocated to the specimen.

Worked example: Cohen's κ – pathology review

Table 11.3 shows a comparison of two pathologists reviewing biopsy material from 118 patients with lesions of the uterine cervix. The grade categories were I = negative, II = tsquamous hyperplasia, III = carcinoma-in-situ and IV = squamous carcinoma.

The observed values in the diagonal (in bold) are $O_{11} = 22$, $O_{22} = 7$, $O_{33} = 36$ and $O_{44} = 7$. The corresponding expected values are $E_{11} = 26 \times 27/112 = 6.27$, $E_{22} = 2.79$, $E_{33} = 22.39$ and $E_{44} = 1.38$. Further, $p_{\text{Observed}} = (22 + 7 + 36 + 7)/112 = 0.64$ and $p_{\text{Expected}} = (6.27 + 2.79 + 22.39 + 1.38)/112 = 0.29$. Hence, $\kappa = (0.64 - 0.29)/(1 - 0.29) = 0.49$. This is only 'moderate' agreement and such a low value may then stimulate the pathologists concerned to review their classification methods in detail.

Kappa was developed for categorical classifications, where disagreement is equally likely between categories. When the categories are ordered, disagreement between more extreme categories is less likely. One can extend the concept of κ and give less weight to the more extreme disagreements. One set of weights (which weight the disagreement by the square of the distance between categories), leads to the equivalent of the ICC.

Kappa (κ) has a number of limitations:

1. The maximum value of $\kappa = 1$ is only obtainable when *unbiased* observers agree completely.
2. For a given level of agreement, κ increases when the number of categories decreases, and so should only be used for comparisons when the number of categories is the same.
3. κ depends on the marginal distributions, (the values of n_0, n_1, m_0 and m_1 in Table 11.2) so one can get the same values of κ, but different apparent agreements if, in one comparison one observer has a systematic bias, but in the other there is more random disagreement.
4. Some computer programs give p-value associated with κ. These should be ignored since the null hypothesis they are testing has no meaning.

Table 11.3 Pathologist agreement resulting from independent reviews of the same biopsy specimens from patients with lesions of the uterine cervix

Pathologist 1	Grade	Pathologist 2				Totals
		I	II	III	IV	
	I	**22**	2	2	0	26
	II	5	**7**	14	0	26
	III	0	2	**36**	0	38
	IV	0	1	14	**7**	22
Totals		27	12	66	7	112

11.4 Validity

Cronbach's alpha ($\alpha_{Cronbach}$)

Some questionnaires, such as those used to assess concepts such as anxiety and depression in patients often comprise a series of questions. Each question is then scored, and the scores combined in some way to give a single numerical value. Often this is done by merely summing the scores for each answer to give an overall scale score. The internal validity of each of the component questions of the scale is indicated if they are all positively correlated with each other; a lack of correlation of two such items would indicate that at least one of them was not measuring the concept in question. Alternatively, one might frame a question in two different ways, and if the answers are always similar, then the questions are internally consistent.

A measure of internal consistency is Cronbach's alpha, $\alpha_{Cronbach}$ (sometimes spelled Chronbach). It is essentially a form of correlation coefficient; a value of 0 would indicate that there was no correlation between the items that make up a scale, and a value of 1 would indicate perfect correlation.

If a questionnaire has k items, and this has been administered to a group of subjects, then the standard deviation, s_i, of the ith item and s_T the standard deviation of the sum score T of all the items is required. From which

$$\alpha_{Cronbach} = \frac{k}{k-1}\left(1 - \frac{\sum s_i^2}{s_T^2}\right).$$

A worked example is given in Section 11.7. For comparing groups, $\alpha_{Cronbach}$ values of 0.7 to 0.8 are regarded as satisfactory, although for clinical applications much higher values are necessary. However, a value of 1 would indicate that most of the questions could in fact be discarded, since all the information is contained in just one of them. Cronbach's α is essentially a measure of how correlated items are. Clearly, one would like items that all refer so a single concept such as pain to be related to each other. However, if they are too closely related then some of the questions are redundant. When constructing a questionnaire, one might omit items which have a weak or very strong correlation with other items in the domain of interest.

Example from the literature: $\alpha_{Cronbach}$ – patient satisfaction

McKinley et al (1997) used a questionnaire to measure patient satisfaction with out-of-hours calls made to general practitioners. They measured aspects such as satisfaction with communication, management and the doctor's attitude. They found values of $\alpha_{Cronbach}$ for each score ranging from 0.61 to 0.88 and concluded that the questionnaire had satisfactory internal validity.

11.5   Method comparison studies

A feature of laboratory work, and of many aspects of clinical work, is the evaluation of new instruments. It is usual in such studies to compare results obtained from the new method with that obtained from some standard. Alternatively, two devices may be proposed for measuring the same quantity and one may wish to determine which is the better. These may be, for example, a common paper tape measurement and a new plastic grid device to assess the extent of leg ulcer wounds as were compared by Liskay et al (2002).

Example: Method comparisons – two spirometers

Forced expiratory volume (FEV_1), which is the volume of air expelled in the first second of maximal forced expiration from a position of full inspiration, is measured by using a spirometer. Figure 11.1 displays the results of a study in which 56 subjects had their FEV_1 measured by both a Respiradyne and a Vitalograph spirometer (Jenkins et al, 1988). The purpose of the study was to see if the Respiradyne spirometer could be used in place of the Vitalograph.

As indicated above, a common method of analysis is first to calculate the correlation coefficient between the two sets of readings and then calculate a p-value on the null hypothesis of no association.

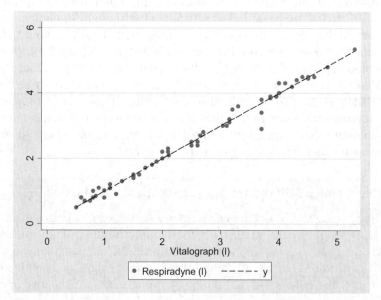

Figure 11.1 FEV_1 (litres) in 56 subjects by two different spirometers with the line of equality

Why calculating the correlation coefficient is inappropriate

1. The correlation coefficient is a measure of association. What is required here is a measure of agreement. We will have perfect association if the observations lie on any straight line, but there is only perfect agreement if the points lie on the line of equality $y = x$.
2. The correlation coefficient observed depends on the range of measurements used. so one can increase the correlation coefficient by choosing widely spaced observations. Since investigators usually compare two methods over the whole range of likely values (as they should), a good correlation is almost guaranteed.
3. Because of (2), data which have an apparently high correlation can, for individual subjects, show very poor agreement between the methods of measurement.
4. The test of significance is not relevant since it would be very surprising if two methods designed to measure the same thing were not related.

Bland and Altman (1986) argue that correlation coefficient is inappropriate and recommend an alternative approach. As an initial step one should plot the data as in Figure 11.1, but omit the calculation of the corresponding correlation coefficient and the associated test of significance. They then argue that a plot of the paired difference, d, between the two observations on each subject against their mean value is more likely to reveal features of these data in particular any systematic differences between methods.

Example: Bland and Altman plots – two spirometers

Figure 11.2 displays the scatter plot of the difference in FEV_1, as assessed by the Respiradyne and Vitalograph spirometers in each patient, against their mean value. From this plot it can be seen that there is no obvious relation between the size of the difference observed and the mean. Further, Figure 11.2 highlights the outlier (with d less than −0.5) whereas it is not so prominent in Figure 11.1.

The lack of agreement between methods is estimated by the mean difference, $\bar{d}$, and this provides an estimate of the systematic difference between the methods (ideally zero) which is termed the *bias* should one of the methods be a gold standard. Further the standard deviation of these differences allows the 'limits of agreement' to be set.

Method comparisons   If one method records as y and the other as x, then $d = y - x$ is calculated for each subject, and the corresponding mean, $\bar{d}$, and standard deviation, s, are calculated. Systematic difference or bias: $\bar{d}$, 95% 'limits of agreement' $\bar{d} - 2s$ to $\bar{d} + 2s$.

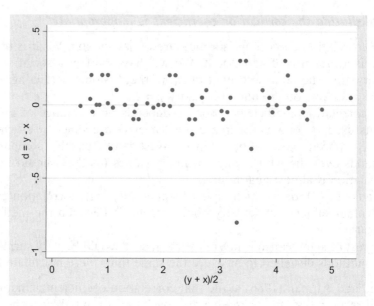

Figure 11.2 Scatter diagram of the difference between methods against the mean of both for the data of Figure 11.1

Example: Limits of agreement – two spirometers

For the FEV_1 data the mean difference $\bar{d} = 0.06\,\ell$ and $SD(d) = s = 0.15\,\ell$. The 'limits of agreement' are $-0.24\,\ell$ to $0.36\,\ell$ implying that one spirometer could give a reading as much as $0.36\,\ell$ above the other or $0.24\,\ell$ below it. Whether the bias observed or the limits of agreement are acceptable needs to be judged from a clinical viewpoint.

If an outlier is present it is good practice to check the results for this subject. Perhaps there has been a mistake entering the data, and if necessary that subject could be excluded from the calculations for the limits of agreement.

11.6   Points when reading the literature

1. When a new instrument has been used, has it been tested for reliability and validity?
2. When two methods of measurement have been compared, has correlation been used to assess whether one instrument can be used instead of another? If so are there systematic biases?
3. When Cohen's kappa is compared, are the marginal distributions similar? If not, then be careful about making comparisons.

11.7 Technical details

Calculation of the ICC

Suppose we measured FEV_1 on four patients with the following result (Table 11.4):

Our model is $y_{ij} = \mu + \tau_i + \varepsilon_{ij}$ where μ is the overall mean, τ_i is the additional effect of subject i and ε_{ij} is the random error from one measurement, j, to another. We assume τ and ε are random independent variables. The variance of τ is the *between subject variance* and the variance of ε is the *within subject variance*. It is important to note that we are not assuming an 'occasion' effect here. The calculations will give the same result if some of the observations on the two occasions are swapped. This is known as an *exchangeable error*.

With n pairs of observations x_{i1} and x_{i2}, $i = 1 \ldots n$, the within subject variance is estimated by $s^2_{\text{Within}} = \Sigma_{i=1}^{n}(x_{i1} - x_{i2})^2/2n$. Also if $\bar{x}_i = (x_{i1} + x_{i2}/2)$ then $\text{var}(\bar{x}_i) = s^2_{\text{Between}} + s^2_{\text{Within}}/2$

$$s^2_{\text{Within}} = \left[(-0.1)^2 + (-0.2)^2 + 0^2 + (0.1)^2\right]/8 = 0.0075 \text{ and } \text{var}(\bar{x}_i) = 0.0676.$$

Thus $s^2_{\text{Between}} = 0.0676 - 0.0075/2 = 0.06385$.

$$ICC = 0.06385/(0.0075 + 0.06385) = 0.895.$$

This is high and suggests the measurements of FEV_1 are repeatable.

Table 11.4 FEV_1 (in litres) for four patients measured on two occasions

Subject	FEV$_1$ (litres)			
	1st occasion	2nd occasion	Difference	mean
1	2.1	2.2	−0.1	2.15
2	2.3	2.5	−0.2	2.4
3	2.6	2.6	0.0	2.6
4	2.8	2.7	0.1	2.75

Calculation of Cronbach's alpha

Suppose a section of a questionnaire has three items, which measure pain say, each of which can have a score between 1 (no pain) and 5 (severe pain). The total of the three items make up the total pain score for a particular dimension of the questionnaire (Table 11.5).

If a questionnaire has k items, and this has been administered to a group of subjects, then if s_i is the *SD* of the ith item, T is the sum score of all the items, and s_T is the *SD* of T, then Cronbach's alpha, α_{Cronbach}, is

Table 11.5 Responses to three questions and total score
for four subjects

Subject	Q1	Q2	Q3	Total Score
1	1	1	2	4
2	3	3	2	8
3	5	5	4	14
4	3	2	3	8
SD	1.63	1.71	0.95	4.12

$$\alpha_{\text{Cronbach}} = \frac{k}{k-1}\left(1 - \frac{\sum s_i^2}{s_T^2}\right).$$

Thus for our data $k = 3$, and $\Sigma s_i^2 = 1.63^2 + 1.71^2 + 0.95^2 = 6.4835$, $s_T^2 = 16.9744$
and so $\alpha = 1.5(1 - 6.4835)/16.9744 = 0.927$.

The reason that α_{Cronbach} is a measure of correlation is as follows. If $X_1 \ldots X_k$
are independent random variables, and $T = X_1 + \ldots + X_k$ then $\text{Var}(T) = \text{Var}(X_1) + \ldots + \text{Var}(X_k)$ and so the numerator and denominator in the braces
in the equation for α_{Cronbach} are the same and so $\alpha_{\text{Cronbach}} = 0$. If $X_1 \ldots X_k$ are
perfectly correlated so that $X_1 = X_2 = \ldots = X_k$ then $T = kX_1$ and $\text{Var}(T) = k^2\text{Var}(X_1)$, whereas $\Sigma\text{Var}(X_i) = k\text{Var}(X_1)$. Thus the ratio in the braces is now
$1/k$ and so $\alpha_{\text{Cronbach}} = 1$.

Agreement by chance (P_{Chance})

From Table 11.2, $p_{\text{Agree}} = (x_{00} + x_{11})/N_{\text{Repeat}}$. To get the expected agreement
we use the row and column totals to estimate the expected numbers agreeing
for each category.

For negative agreement (Absent, Absent) the expected proportion is the
product of $(x_{01} + x_{00})/N_{\text{Repeat}}$ and $(x_{10} + x_{00})/N_{\text{Repeat}}$, giving $(x_{00} + x_{01})(x_{00} + x_{10})/N_{\text{Repeat}}^2$. Likewise for positive agreement the expected proportion is
$(x_{10} + x_{11})(x_{01} + x_{11})/N_{\text{Repeat}}^2$. The expected proportion of agreements for the
whole table is the sum of these two terms, that is

$$P_{\text{Chance}} = \frac{(x_{00} + x_{01})(x_{00} + x_{10})}{N_{\text{Repeat}}^2} + \frac{(x_{10} + x_{11})(x_{01} + x_{11})}{N_{\text{Repeat}}^2}.$$

Suppose we have an $R \times R$ contingency table, where $R > 2$, and the rows
contain the categories observed by one rater and the columns the categories
observed by the other rater. By analogy with Table 11.2, then the numbers
in the diagonals of the table, that is x_{ii}, are the numbers observed when the
two raters agree. The corresponding numbers expected by chance in category
i are labelled e_{ii}.

If N is the number of specimens classified and we denote $P_{Agree} = \Sigma x_{ii}/N$ and $P_{Chance} = \Sigma e_{ii}/N$, then

$$\kappa = \frac{P_{Observed} - P_{Chance}}{1 - P_{Chance}}.$$

11.8 Exercises

1. Collecting a urine sample in young non-toilet trained children can be challenging. The standard method is a urine collection bag device, but this is uncomfortable and can be contaminated. Farrell et al (2002) compare the bag, with the use of an absorbent sanitary pad. They studied 20 children and used the methods concurrently and their results are summarised in Table 11.6.

    Find Cohen's kappa and interpret.

Table 11.6 Presence or absence of bacteria in bags or pads for urinary incontinence

Pad	Bag		Total
	Bacteria present	Bacteria absent	
Bacteria present	2	0	2
Bacteria absent	3	15	18
Total	5	15	20

2. Bland and Altman (1997) describe the mini-HAQ that measures impairment in patients with cervical myelopathy. There are 10 items relating to activities of daily living: stand, get out of bed, cut meat, hold cup, walk, climb stairs, wash, use toilet, open a jar and enter/leave a car. The standard deviations from 10 questions in 2549 subjects are respectively: 1.04, 1.11, 1.12, 1.06, 1.04, 1.04, 1.01, 1.09, 1.02 1.03. The 10 items were summed for each subject and the SD of the total score was 8.80. Calculate and comment on the value of $\alpha_{Cronbach}$.

12 Observational studies

Medical Statistics Fourth Edition, David Machin, Michael J Campbell, Stephen J Walters
© 2007 John Wiley & Sons, Ltd

Summary

This chapter considers the design of observational studies: cross-sectional surveys, case–control studies and cohort studies together with the problems of inferring causality from such studies. A vital tool for eliciting information from subjects is the questionnaire and we discuss how these may be constructed and also how samples may be chosen.

12.1   Introduction

In an observational study one cannot determine which subjects get exposed to a risk, or given a new treatment. This is in contrast to the randomised controlled trial, to be described in Chapter 13. In many situations where an investigator is looking for an association between exposure to a risk factor and subsequent disease, it is not possible to randomly allocate exposure to subjects; you cannot insist that some people smoke and others do not, or randomly expose some industrial workers to radiation. Thus, studies relating exposure to outcome are often observational; the investigator simply observes what happens and does not intervene. The options under the control of the investigator are restricted to the choice of subjects, whether to follow them retrospectively or prospectively, and the size of the sample.

The major problem in the interpretation of observational studies is that although an association between exposure and disease can be observed, this does not necessarily imply a causal relationship. For example, many studies have shown that smoking is associated with subsequent lung cancer. Those who refuse to believe causation argue, however, that some people are genetically susceptible to lung cancer, and this same gene predisposes them to smoke! Factors that are related to both the exposure of a risk factor and the outcome are called confounding factors (see Figure 1.1 in Chapter 1). In observational studies it is always possible to think of potential confounding factors that might explain away an argument for causality. However, some methods for strengthening the causality argument are given later in the chapter.

12.2   Risk and rates

We introduced methods of summarising binary data in Chapter 2. We now provide more detail of these and some others.

Risk is defined as

$$\text{Risk} = \frac{\text{Number of events observed}}{\text{Number in the group}}$$

Thus if 100 people sat down to a meal and 10 suffered food poisoning, we would say the *risk* of food poisoning was 0.1 or 10%.

Often, however, we are interested in the number of events over a period of time. This leads to the definition of a *rate*, which is the number of events, for example deaths or cases of disease, per unit of population, in a particular time span. For example, Figure 4.1 shows that the crude United Kingdom mortality rate per person per year is about 0.010. Since this is a small number we usually multiply it by a larger number such as 1000, and express the mortality rate as 10 deaths per 1000 population per year.

To calculate a rate the following are needed:

- a defined period of time (for example, a calendar year);
- a defined population, with an accurate estimate of the size of the population during the defined period (for example the population of a city, estimated by a census);
- the number of events occurring over the period (for example the number of deaths occurring in the city over a calendar year).

The event could be a permanent one (like death) or a temporary one (like a cold). For a permanent event the person is no longer at risk of the event, and is removed from the 'at risk' population. Strictly, we should measure all the time that each member of the population is at risk.

Incidence is defined as

$$\text{Incidence} = \frac{\text{Number of events in defined period}}{\text{Total person-time at risk}} \times 1000$$

When the number of events is relatively small compared with the population at risk, then the total person-time at risk can be approximated by the mid-period population multiplied by the length of the period.

Crude mortality rate

When the length of the period is one year, an example of a rate is the crude mortality rate (CMR) for a particular year which is given by

$$\text{CMR} = \frac{\text{Number of deaths occurring in year}}{\text{Mid-year population}} \times 1000.$$

It is important to remember that rates must refer to a specific period of time.

Age-specific mortality rate

If a particular age group is specified, the age-specific mortality rate (ASMR) is obtained as

$$\text{ASMR} = \frac{\text{Number of deaths occurring in specified age group}}{\text{Mid-year number in that age group}} \times 1000.$$

The incidence rate refers to the number of new cases of a particular disease that develop during a specified time interval. The *prevalence* (which is strictly not a rate since no time period is specified) refers to the number of cases of disease that exist at a specified point in time.

Often the time period is implicit and risk and incidence are used synonymously.

12.3   Taking a random sample

For any observational studies, it is necessary to define the subjects chosen for the study in some way. For example, if a survey were to be conducted then a random sample of the population of interest would be required. In this situation, a simple random sample could be obtained first by numbering all the individual members in the target population, and then computer-generating random numbers from that list. Suppose the population totals 600 subjects, which are numbered 001 through to 600. If we use the first line of the random numbers in Table T2 and find the random sequence 534 55425 67. We would take the first three subjects as 534, 554 and 256, for example. These subjects are then identified on the list and sent a questionnaire. If the population list is not on computer file or is very large, the process of going backwards and forwards to write down addresses of the sample can be a tedious business. Suppose a list is printed on 1000 pages of 100 subjects per page, and a 10% sample is required, then one way is to choose a number between 1 and 100; from our sequence this would be 53, so we then take the 53rd member on every page as our sample from the population. This is clearly logistically easier than choosing a random sample of 1000 from a list of 100 000. A 0.5% sample would take someone from every second page after first choosing the entry at random between 001 and 200 comprising those of the first and second page. Such a device is known as *systematic random sampling*; the choice of starting point is random.

There are other devices which might be appropriate in specific circumstances. For example, to estimate the prevalence of menstrual flushing rather than sampling the national list containing millions of women, one may first randomly choose one county from a list of counties, from within each county a sample of electoral wards, and then obtain only lists for these wards from which to select the women. Such a device is termed *multi-stage random sampling*.

In other circumstances one may wish to ensure that equal numbers of men and women are sampled. Thus the list is divided into strata (men and women) and equal numbers sampled from each stratum.

12.4 Questionnaire and form design

Purpose of questionnaires and forms

It is important to distinguish between questionnaires and forms. Forms are used largely to record factual information, such as a subject's age, blood pressure or treatment group. They are commonly used in clinical trials to follow a patient's progress and are often completed by the responsible investigator. For forms, the main requirement is that the form be clearly laid out and all investigators are familiar with it. A questionnaire on the other hand, although it too may include basic demographic information, can be regarded as an instrument in its own right. For example, it may try to measure personal attributes such as attitudes, emotional status or levels of pain and is often completed by the individual concerned.

For questionnaires the pragmatic advice is, if possible, do not design your own, use someone else's! There are a number of reasons for this apparently negative advice. First, use of a standardised format means that results should be comparable between studies. Second, it is a difficult and time-consuming process to obtain a satisfactory questionnaire. Help with designing health measurement scales is given in Streiner and Norman (2003).

Types of questions

There are two major types of question: open or closed. In an open question respondents are asked to reply in their own words, whereas in a closed question the possible responses are given.

The advantages of open type questions are that more detailed answers are possible. They give the responders the feeling that they can express their own ideas. On the other hand, they take more time and effort to complete and they can be difficult to code and hence analyse since there may be a wide variety of disparate responses from different individuals. Closed questions can be answered by simply circling or ticking responses. When constructing responses to closed questions it is important to provide a suitable range of replies, or the responder may object to being forced into a particular category, and simply not answer the question. A useful strategy is to conduct a pilot study using open questions on a limited but representative sample of people. From their responses one can then devise suitable closed questions.

Another type of closed question is to make a statement and then ask whether the respondent agrees or disagrees. When a closed question has an odd number of responses, it is often called a Likert scale.

Some researchers prefer to omit central categories, such as 'average' or 'don't know' so as to force people to have an opinion. The danger is that if people do not wish to be forced, then they will simply not reply.

An alternative method of recording strength of feeling is by means of a visual analogue score (VAS). The VAS is scored by measuring the distance of the respondent's mark from the left-hand end of the scale.

Examples: Types of questions

Open question

'Please describe how do you feel about the treatment you have just received?'

Closed question

'How would you rate the treatment you have just received?'
(1) Excellent, (2) good, (3) average, (4) poor, (5) very poor.

Likert rating scales

'Medical statistics is not very interesting'
(a) Strongly agree, (b) agree, (c) don't know, (d) disagree, (e) strongly disagree.

Visual analogue score

'Please rate your pain by marking a line on the following scale:'

No Pain   **Worst possible pain**

12.5 Cross-sectional surveys

A cross-sectional study describes a group of subjects at one particular point in time. It may feature the proportion of people with a particular characteristic, which is a prevalence study. It may look at how the prevalence varies by other features such as by age or gender.

Suppose an investigator wishes to determine the prevalence of menstrual flushing in women in the ages 45–60. Then an appropriate design may be a survey of women in that age group by means of a postal questionnaire. In such a situation, this type of survey may be conducted at, for example, a town, county or national level. However, a prerequisite before such a survey is conducted is a list of women in the corresponding age groups. Once such a list is obtained it may be possible to send a postal questionnaire to all women on the list. More usually one may wish to draw a sample from the list and the questionnaire be sent to this sample. The sampling proportion will have to be chosen carefully. It is important that those who are selected be selected by an appropriate random sampling technique.

In some situations a visit by an interviewer to those included in the sample may be more appropriate. However, this may be costly both in time and money and will require the training of personnel. As a consequence this will usually involve a smaller sample than that possible by means of a postal questionnaire. On the other hand, response rates to postal questionnaires may be low. A low response rate can cause considerable difficulty in interpretation of the results as it can always be argued (whether true or not) that non-responders are atypical with respect to the problem being investigated and therefore estimates of prevalence, necessarily obtained from the responders only, will be inherently biased. Thus, in a well-designed survey, one makes every attempt to keep the numbers of non-responders to a minimum, and takes the potential response rate into account when estimating sample size.

Volunteers often present considerable problems in cross-sectional surveys. When the object of interest is a relationship within subjects, for example physiological responses to increasing doses of a drug, then one cannot avoid the use of volunteers. However, suppose one was interested in the prevalence of hypertension in the community. One approach would be to ask volunteers to come forward by advertising in the local newspaper. The difficulty here is that people may volunteer simply because they are worried about their blood pressure (this is known as *selection bias*) and also there is no way one can ascertain the response rate, or investigate reasons why people did not volunteer. A better approach would be to take a random sample from the community, either from an electoral roll, general practitioners' lists or a telephone list, and then invite each one individually to have their blood pressure measured. In that way the response rate is known and the non-responders identified.

Market research organisations have complex sampling schemes that often contain elements of randomisation. However, in essence they are grab or convenience samples, in that only subjects who are available to the interviewer can be questioned. So-called *quota samples* ensure that the sample is representative of the general population in say, age, gender and social class structure. Problems associated with the interpretation of quota samples are discussed in detail by Machin and Campbell (2005). They are not recommended, in general, for use in medical research.

Other biases are possible in cross-sectional studies. Consider a cross-sectional study that reveals a negative association between height and age. Possible interpretations include: people shrink as they get older, younger generations are getting taller, or tall people have a higher mortality than short people!

One of the differences between a cross-sectional study and other designs discussed in this chapter is that in the former subjects are included without reference to either their exposure or their disease. Cross-sectional studies usually deal with exposures that do not change, such as blood type or chronic smoking habit. However, in occupational studies a cross-sectional study might contain all workers in a factory, and their exposures determined by a retrospective work-history. Here the problem is the *healthy worker effect* in that people in work tend to be healthier than people not in work, even those in jobs which expose them to health hazards. A cross-sectional study resembles a case–control study (to be discussed in Section 12.8) except that the numbers of cases are not known in advance, but are simply the prevalent cases at the time of the survey.

Example from the literature: Prevalence of *Chlamydia*

Macleod et al (2005) sent questionnaires to 19773 people randomly selected from general practitioners lists and 14382 were successfully contacted (73%). They found the prevalence of *Chlamydia* to be 2.8%, (95% CI 2.2 to 3.4%) in men and 3.6% (3.1 to 4.9%) in women. They found people under the age of 25 had a higher prevalence (men 5.1%, women 6.2%). The authors indicate that selection bias may have affected their observations as it is thought that people who *know* they have *Chlamydia* may be less likely to respond.

12.6 Non-randomised studies

Pre-test/post-test studies

A pre-test/post-test study is one in which a group of individuals are measured, then subjected to an intervention, and then measured again. The purpose of the study is to observe the size of the resulting effect. The major problem is ascribing the change in the measurement to the intervention since other factors may also have changed in that interval.

Example from the literature: Before-and-after studies

Christie (1979) describes a consecutive series of patients admitted to a hospital with stroke in 1974 who were then followed prospectively until death and their survival time determined. Subsequently, a CT head scanner was installed in the hospital, and so in 1978 the study was repeated so that the scanner could be evaluated.

Successive patients in the 1978 series who had had a CT scan were matched by age, diagnosis and level of consciousness with patients in the 1974 series. A total of 29 matched pairs were obtained and their survival times compared. The results, given in Table 12.1, Column 2, appeared to show a marked improvement in the 1978 patients over those from 1974 with 31% with better survival and only 7% worse. This was presumed to be due to the CT scanner.

However, the study was then extended to an analysis of the 1978 patients who had not had a CT scan (Table 12.1, Column 3) compared with a matched group of 89 patients from 1974 using the same matching criteria. This second study again found an improvement; with 38% of the 1978 patients were doing better than the 1974 patients, and 19% doing worse. Taking the two components of the study together, then whether or not patients had received a CT scan, the outcome had improved over the years.

In the absence of the control study, the comparison of patients who had had no CT scan, the investigators may well have concluded that the installation of a CT head scanner had improved patient survival time. There are two possible explanations of the apparent anomaly. One is to suppose that other improvements in treatment, unrelated to CT scanning, had taken place between 1974 and 1978. The other is to ask what would a clinician do with a stroke patient even if he knew the outcome of a CT scan? The answer is, usually, very little. It is therefore possible that the patients in 1978 were, in fact, less seriously ill than those in 1974, despite the attempts at matching, and hence would live longer.

However, in certain circumstances before-and-after studies without control groups are unavoidable if the design is not in the direct control of the investigator. Such situations may arise when national policy legislates for a change, for example compulsory seat belt wearing, the value of which may still need to be evaluated.

Table 12.1   Data from Christie (1979)

Survival	CT scan in 1978	
	Yes	No
1978 better than 1974	9 (31%)	34 (38%)
1978 equal to 1974	18 (62%)	38 (43%)
1978 worse than 1974	2 (7%)	17 (19%)
	29	89

Example from the literature: Observational study – acute myocardial infarction

In June 2002 the town of Helena, Montana, USA imposed a law requiring smoke-free work places and public places but in December 2002 opponents won a court order suspending enforcement. Sargent et al (2004) found that there were 24 admissions to hospital for acute myocardial infarction in the 6 months of the smoking ban, compared with an average of 40 for the same six months in the years before and after the ban (difference 16 admissions, 95% CI 0.3 to 31.7). They concluded that the smoking ban may reduce morbidity from heart disease, which encouraged smoking bans in other areas.

Quasi-experimental designs

A prospective study that has both a test group and a control group, but in which the treatment is not allocated at random, is known as a quasi-experimental design. It is often used to take advantage of information on the merits of a new treatment which is being implemented in one group of patients, but where randomisation is difficult or impossible to implement.

The main disadvantage of a quasi-experimental study is that, because treatments are not randomised to the subjects, it is impossible to state at the outset that the subjects are comparable in the two groups. Thus, for example, when comparing survival rates in patients undergoing different types of surgery, each performed by different surgeons, it is possible that different surgeons will have different selection thresholds of risk for admitting patients to surgery. As a consequence, any difference in mortality observed between types of surgical intervention may be clouded by systematic patient differences, and hence not reflect the relative mortality of the surgical alternatives.

Example from the literature: Quasi experimental study – cancer in Gulf War veterans

Macfarlane et al (2003) compared the incidence rates of cancer in UK service personnel who were deployed in the Gulf War of 1990 to the incidence rate for service personnel not employed in the gulf war. They followed up 51 721 Gulf War veterans for 11 years, and chose a control group of 50 755 personnel matched for age, gender, rank, service and level of fitness. There were 270 incident cancers in those who went to the Gulf, compared with 269 in the control, an incidence rate ratio for all cancers of 0.99 (95% CI 0.83 to 1.17). It was concluded that there was no excess risk of cancer in Gulf war veterans.

Clearly it is impossible to randomly choose whether people went to the Gulf or not, but there is no reason to suppose that people selected for Gulf service were at any different risk of cancer at the time than those not selected, when age, gender and other factors are controlled for.

12.7 Cohort studies

A cohort is a component of a population identified so that its characteristics for example, causes of death or numbers contracting a certain disease can be ascertained as it ages through time.

The term 'cohort' is often used to describe those born during a particular year but can be extended to describe any designated group of persons who are traced over a period of time. Thus, for example, we may refer to a cohort born in 1950, or to a cohort of people who ever worked in a particular factory. A cohort study, which may also be referred to as a follow-up, longitudinal or prospective study, is one in which subsets of a defined population can be identified who have been exposed (or will be exposed) to a factor which may influence the probability of occurrence of a given disease or other outcome. A study may follow two groups of subjects, one group exposed to a potential toxic hazard, the other not, to see if the exposure influences, for example, the occurrence of certain types of cancers. Cohort studies are usually confined to studies determining and investigating aetiological factors, and do not allocate the equivalent of treatments. They are termed observational studies, since they simply *observe* the progress of individuals over time.

Design

The progress of a cohort study is described in Figure 12.1 and Table 12.2 provides the corresponding notation. Thus members of the 'without' disease group are first identified (clearly those who already have the disease of interest are not of concern here) and their 'exposure' status determined. They are then followed for a pre-specified duration after which time their disease status (Present/Absent) is determined.

Relative risk From Table 12.2, the risk of developing the disease within the follow-up time is $a/(a + c)$ for the exposed population and $b/(b + d)$ for the unexposed population.

The relative risk (RR) is the ratio of these two, that is

$$RR = \frac{a/(a+c)}{b/(b+d)} = \frac{a(b+d)}{b(a+c)}.$$

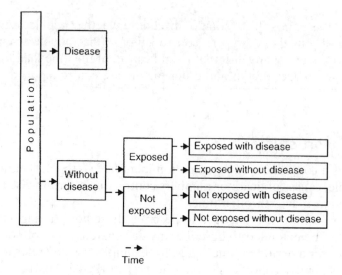

Figure 12.1   Definition and progress of a cohort study

Table 12.2   Notation for a cohort study

Number of subjects who develop the disease in the follow-up period	Risk factor		Total
	Exposed	Not exposed	
Yes	a	b	$a + b$
No	c	d	$c + d$
Total	$a + c$	$b + d$	N

Example from the literature: Cohort study – mortality in slate workers

Campbell et al (2005) studied a cohort of people living in towns in North Wales associated with slate mining. Over a period of 24 years they followed up a group of men who worked or had worked with slate and a control group comprising men who had never been exposed to slate dust. The slate workers and controls were well matched for age and smoking habit. The results are given in Table 12.3.

The risk of death to slate-workers is 379/726 = 0.52 while that for the non-slate workers is 230/529 = 0.43, giving $RR = 0.52/0.43 = 1.21$ with 95% CI 1.07 to 1.36 (see Section 12.11).

In fact the published report took note of the actual survival times and so analysed this study using the survival techniques of Chapter 10. They found a hazard ratio $HR = 1.24$, (95% CI 1.04 to 1.47, $p = 0.015$) and concluded that exposure to slate increases a man's risk of death at any point in time by about 25%.

It is useful to note that in this study the RR and HR are numerically close.

Table 12.3 Results of a slate workers study

Outcome	Exposure or risk factor – occupation	
	Slate worker	Non – slate worker
Died in follow-up period	379	230
Survived follow-up period	347	299
Total	726	529

From Campbell et al (2005). A 24 year cohort study of mortality in slate workers in North Wales. *Journal of Occupational Medicine*, **55**, 448–453: by permission of Lippincott Williams & Wilkins, WoltersKluwer Health.

The population attributable risk

If very few men were exposed to slate dust, the effect of slate exposure on the health of the population is not going to be large, however serious the consequences to the individual. The effect of a risk factor on community health is related to both relative risk and the percentage of the population exposed to the risk factor and this can be measured by the attributable risk (AR).

Attributal risk   The terminology is not standard, but if $I_{\text{Population}}$ is the incidence of a disease in the population and I_{Exposed} and $I_{\text{Non-Exposed}}$ are the incidence in the exposed and non-exposed respectively. Then the excess incidence attributable to the risk factor is simply $I_{\text{Population}} - I_{\text{Non-Exposed}}$ and the population attributable risk is

$$AR = (I_{\text{Population}} - I_{\text{Non-Exposed}})/I_{\text{Population}}.$$

that is the proportion of the population risk that can be associated with the risk factor.

Some authors define the *excess risk* (or *absolute risk difference*) as $I_{\text{Exposed}} - I_{\text{Non-Exposed}}$ and the population attributable risk as $(I_{\text{Exposed}} - I_{\text{Non-Exposed}})/I_{\text{Non-Exposed}}$, but the definition given above has the advantage of greater logical consistency.

If we define, from Table 12.2, $\theta_{\text{Exposed}} = (a + b)/N$ to be the proportion of the population of size N exposed to the risk factor, then it can be shown that

$$AR = \frac{\theta_{\text{Exposed}}(RR - 1)}{1 + \theta_{\text{Exposed}}(RR - 1)}.$$

The advantage of this formula is that it enables us to calculate the attributable risk from the relative risk, and the proportion of the population exposed to the risk factor. Both of these can be estimated from cohort studies and also from case–control studies in certain circumstances when the controls are a random sample of the population.

Worked example: Attributable risk

Suppose the miners represented 5% of the population in the towns in North Wales where they lived, then $AR = 0.05 \times 0.21/(1 + 0.05 \times 0.21) = 0.01$, or about 1%. Thus one might conclude that slate mining increased overall mortality by about 1% in those towns.

Why quote a relative risk?

The relative risk provides a convenient summary of the outcome of a cohort study. It is in many cases independent of the incidence of the disease and so is more stable than the individual risks. For example, if we studied the effect of slate exposure on a different population of men, the death rate in the unexposed group may be different, say for illustration half that of the original population. The incidence or death rate in the exposed group is also likely to be half that of the first group, and so the relative risk of slate exposure compared with non-exposure remains unaltered.

Also, it is often the case that if a factor, in addition to the principal one under study, acts independently on the disease process, then the joint relative risk is just the product of the two relative risks. Thus if smokers, had a relative risk of 2 of dying compared with non-smokers, then the risk of dying amongst smokers who are also exposed to slate is likely to be $2 \times 1.2 = 2.4$.

The interpretation of cohort studies is often that much more difficult than a randomised trial as bias may influence the measure of interest. For example, to determine in a cohort study if the rate of cardiovascular disease is raised in men sterilised by vasectomy, it is necessary to have a comparison group of non-vasectomised men. However, comparisons between these two groups of men may be biased as it is clearly not possible to randomise men to sterilisation or non-sterilisation groups. Men who are seeking sterilisation would certainly not accept the 'no sterilisation' option. Thus the comparison that will be made here is between those men who opt for sterilisation against those who do not, and there may be inherent biases present when comparisons are made between the two groups. For example, the vasectomised men may be fitter or better educated than the non-vasectomised men and this may influence cardiovascular disease rates.

In the design of a cohort study, careful consideration before commencement of the study must be taken to identify and subsequently measure important prognostic variables that may differ between the exposure groups. Provided they are recorded, differences in these baseline characteristics between groups can be adjusted for in the final analysis.

Size of study

The required size of a cohort study depends not only on the size of the risk being investigated but also on the incidence of the particular condition under investigation. In the vasectomy example, cardiovascular events are not particularly rare among a cohort of men aged 40–50, and this may determine that the cohort of middle-aged men be investigated. On the other hand, if a rare condition were being investigated very few events would be observed amongst many thousands of subjects, whether exposed to the 'insult' of interest or not. This usually prevents the use of cohort studies to investigate aetiological factors in rare diseases.

Problems in interpretation of cohort studies

When the cohort is made up of employed individuals, the risk of dying in the first few years of follow-up is generally less than that of the general population and so we have the 'healthy worker' effect. It is due to the fact that people who are sick are less likely to be employed. It is also known that people who respond to questionnaires are likely to be fitter than those who do not. Both these effects can lead to problems in the interpretation of risks from populations of employed individuals. Another problem arises when follow-up is poor, or when it is more complete for the exposed group than for the unexposed group. We are then led to ask: Are the people lost to follow-up different in any way and could a poor follow-up bias the conclusions?

Post-marketing surveillance

Post-marketing surveillance is a particular type of cohort study carried out on a population of people receiving an established drug. In such an example a drug that is in routine use nationwide may be monitored; not for its efficacy but for any untoward medical event happening to patients receiving the drug. The incidence of such adverse events with the new drug is then compared with the incidence in patients receiving alternatives to the new medicine.

12.8 Case–control studies

Design

A case–control study, also known as a case-referent study or retrospective study, starts with the identification of persons with the disease (or other outcome variable) of interest, and a suitable control (reference) group of persons without the disease. The relationship of a risk factor to the disease is examined by comparing the diseased and non-diseased with regard to how frequently the risk factor is present. If the variable under consideration is quantitative, the average levels of the risk factor in the cases and controls are utilised.

The design and progress of a case–control study is shown in Figure 12.2. Here we identify people with a disease and select a group of controls who do not have the disease. We then retrospectively determine whether, in the past, how much exposure to the risk factor of interest each group has had.

There are two possible variations in design. The control subjects can be chosen to match individual cases for certain important variables such as age and gender, leading to what is known as a matched design. Alternatively, the controls can be a sample from a suitable non-diseased population, leading to an unmatched design. It is a common misconception that there must be matching criteria in all case–control studies, but this is not so. However, it is important that the statistical analysis utilised reflects the chosen design.

Unmatched study

As just indicated, in an unmatched design the controls can be a sample from a suitable non-diseased population and Table 12.4 gives the notation for this situation.

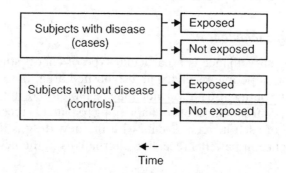

Figure 12.2 Design and progress of a case–control study

Table 12.4 Notation for an unmatched case–control study

Risk factor	Cases (with disease)	Controls (without disease)
Exposed	a	b
Not exposed	c	d
Total	a + c	b + d

Example from the literature: Case–control study – mobile phone use and glioma

Hepworth et al (2006) describe a case–control study of mobile phone use and glioma. The cases were 966 people with diagnosed with a glioma between certain dates. The controls were randomly selected from general practitioner lists. Telephone use was defined as regular use for at least 6 months in the period up to 1 year before diagnosis.

The controls were interviewed in exactly the same way as the cases, using a computer-assisted personal interview. The results of the study are summarised in Table 12.5.

We are interested in the relative risk of glioma in people who regularly use mobile phones. We cannot estimate it directly in a case–control study because, as discussed below, a case–control study is retrospective, and relative risk is measured in a prospective cohort study. Instead we calculate the odds ratio for exposure and disease (as defined in Chapter 2).

Odds ratio   From Table 12.4, given that a subject has a disease, the odds of having been exposed are a/c; given that a subject does not have a disease, the odds of having been exposed are b/d. Then the odds ratio is

$$OR = \frac{a/c}{b/d} = \frac{ad}{bc}.$$

An *OR* of unity means that cases are no more likely to be exposed to the risk factor than controls.

Worked example: Odds ratio – mobile phone use and glioma

From Table 12.5 the odds ratio for mobile phone use and glioma is

$$OR = (508 \times 818)/(456 \times 898) = 1.01$$

The corresponding 95% CI is 0.87 to 1.19 (see Section 12.11). This shows that regular phone users are no more at risk of glioma than never or non-regular users. As the confidence interval is narrow we have good evidence that there is little or no effect as the null hypothesis value of $OR = 1$ is within this narrow interval.

Table 12.5   Results from a case–control study on glioma and mobile phone use (Hepworth et al, 2006)

Mobile phone use	Cases	Controls
Regular	508	898
Never/non-regular	456	818
Total	964	1716

Matched studies

In some case–control studies each case is matched on an individual basis with a particular control. In this situation the analysis should take matching into account. The notation for a matched case–control study is given in Table 12.6.

In this situation we classify each of the N case–control pairs by exposure of the case and the control. An important point here is that the concordant pairs, that is, situations where the case and control are either both exposed or both not exposed, tell us nothing about the risk of exposure separately for cases or controls. Consider a situation where it was required to discriminate between two students in tests that resulted in either a simple pass or fail. If the students are given a variety of tests, in some they will both pass and in some they will both fail. However, it is only by the tests where one student passes and the other fails, that a decision as to who is better can be given.

The odds ratio for a matched case–control study is given by

$$OR = f/g.$$

The main purpose of matching is to permit the use of efficient analytical methods to control for confounding variables that might influence the case–control comparison. In addition it can lead to a clear identification of appropriate controls. However, matching can be wasteful and costly if the matching criteria lead to many available controls being discarded because they fail the matching criteria. In fact if controls are too closely matched to their respective cases, the odds ratio may be underestimated. Usually it is worthwhile matching at best only one, or at most two or three, variables which are presumed or known to influence outcome strongly, common variables being age, gender and social class.

Table 12.6 Notation for a matched case–control study

Cases	Controls		Total
	Exposed	Not exposed	
Exposed	e	f	a
Not exposed	g	h	c
Total	b	d	N

> ## Example from the literature: Matched case–control study – suicide after discharge from a psychiatric hospital
>
> King et al (2001) matched 293 people who committed suicide after being discharged from mental hospitals with people discharged from the same hospital at the same time who were alive on the day the case had died. One variable of interest was whether a key worker was on holiday at the time of the reference case's death. The results are given in Table 12.7.

The odds ratio for a key worker on holiday as a risk for suicide is given by $OR = 19/7 = 2.7$, with 95% CI 1.09 to 7.64 (details beyond this book but available in Altman et al (2000) suggesting that this may be an important, albeit quite uncommon risk factor.

Analysis by matching?

In many case–control studies matching is not used with the control of bias or increase of precision of the odds ratio in mind, but merely as a convenient criterion for choosing controls. Thus for example, a control is often chosen to be of the same sex, of a similar age and with the same physician as the case for convenience. The question then arises whether one should take this matching into account in the analysis. The general rule is that the analysis should reflect the design. Matched and unmatched analyses will give similar results if, in the notation of Table 12.6, $f \times g$ is close to $e \times h$. This is clearly not the case in the suicide example of Table 12.7.

Selection of controls

The general principle in selecting controls is to select subjects who *might* have been cases in the study, and to select them independently of the exposure

Table 12.7 Results of matched case–control study

Case	Control		
Key worker on holiday	Key worker on holiday?		
	Yes	No	Total
Yes	0	19	19
No	7	267	274
Total	7	286	293

From King et al (2001). The Wessex Recent Inpatient Suicide Study: a case control study of 234 recently discharged psychiatric patient suicides. *British Journal of Psychiatry*, **178**, 531–536: by permission of The Royal College of Psychiatrists.

variable. Thus if the cases were all treated in one particular hospital the controls should represent people who, had they developed the disease, would also have gone to the same hospital. Note that this is not the same as selecting hospital controls (see the example below). Since a case–control study is designed to estimate relative, and not absolute, risks, it is not essential that the controls be representative of all those subjects without the disease, as has been sometimes suggested. It is also not correct to require that the control group be alike in every respect to the cases, apart from having the disease of interest. As an example of this 'over-matching' consider a study of oestrogens and endometrial cancer. The cases and controls were both drawn from women who had been evaluated by uterine dilatation and curettage. Such a control group is inappropriate because agents that cause one disease in an organ often cause other diseases or symptoms in that organ. In this case it is possible that oestrogens cause other diseases of the endometrium, which requires the women to have dilatation and curettage and so present as possible controls.

The choice of the appropriate control population is crucial to a correct interpretation of the results.

Confounding

Confounding arises when an association between an exposure and an outcome is being investigated, but the exposure and outcome are both strongly associated with a third variable. An extreme example of confounding is 'Simpson's paradox', when the third factor reverses the apparent association between the exposure and outcome.

Example from the literature: Simpson's Paradox

As an illustration of Simpson's paradox, Julious and Mullee (1994) give an example describing a cohort study of patients with diabetes which is shown in Table 12.8.

It would appear from the top panel of the table that a higher proportion of patients (40%) with non-insulin diabetes died, implying that non-insulin diabetes carried a higher risk of mortality. However, non-insulin diabetes usually develops after the age of 40. Indeed when the patients are split into those aged <40 years and those aged ≥40, it is found that in both age groups a smaller proportion of patients with non-insulin diabetes died compared with those with insulin diabetes (0% versus 1% and 41% versus 46%). Thus as might be expected, in fact the insulin-dependent patients had the higher mortality.

Table 12.8 Simpson's paradox

Vital status	Insulin dependent	
	No	Yes
Alive	326	253
Dead	218	105
Total	544	358
Percentage dead	40%	29%

Vital status	Patients aged ≤ 40 Insulin dependent		Patients age >40 Insulin dependent	
	No	Yes	No	Yes
Alive	15	129	311	124
Dead	0	1	218	104
	15	130	529	228
Percentage dead	0%	1%	41%	46%

From Julious & Mullee (1994). Confounding and Simpson's Paradox. *British Medical Journal*, **309**, 1480–1481: reproduced by permission of the BMJ Publishing Group.

Limitations of case–control studies

Ascertainment of exposure in case–control studies relies on previously recorded data or on memory, and it is difficult to ensure lack of bias between the cases and the controls. Since they are suffering a disease, cases are likely to be more motivated to recall possible risk factors. One of the major difficulties with case–control studies is in the selection of a suitable control group, and this has often been a major source of criticism of published case–control studies. This has led some investigators to regard them purely as a hypothesis-generating tool, to be corroborated subsequently by a cohort study.

12.9 Association and causality

Once an association between a risk factor and disease has been identified, a number of questions should be asked to try to strengthen the argument that the relationship is causal. These are known as the *Bradford Hill* criteria.

1. *Consistency*. Have other investigators and other studies in different populations led to similar conclusions?
2. *Plausibility*. Are the results biologically plausible? For example, if a risk factor is associated with cancer, are there known carcinogens in the risk factor?
3. *Dose–response*. Are subjects with a heavy exposure to the risk factor at greater risk of disease than those with only slight exposure?

4. *Temporality*. Does the disease incidence in a population increase or decrease following increasing or decreasing exposure to a risk factor? For example, lung cancer in women is increasing some years after the numbers of women taking up smoking increased.
5. *Strength of the relationship*. A large relative risk may be more convincing than a small one (even if the latter is statistically significant). The difficulty with statistical significance is that it is a function of the sample size as well as the size of any possible effect. In any study where large numbers of groups are compared some statistically significant differences are bound to occur.
6. *Reversibility*. If the putative cause is removed, the effect should diminish. For example lung cancer in men is diminishing, some time after the prevalence of smoking in men declined.
7. No other convincing explanations are available. For example, the result is not explained by confounding.

12.10   Points when reading the literature

1. In a cohort study, have a large percentage of the cohort been followed up, and have those lost to follow-up been described by their measurements at the start of the study?
2. How has the cohort been selected? Is the method of selection likely to influence the variables that are measured?
3. In a case–control study, are the cases likely to be typical of people with the disease? If the cases are not typical, how generalisable are the results likely to be?
4. In a matched case–control study, has allowance been made for matching in the analysis?
5. In any observational study, what are the possible biases? How have they been minimised and have the Bradford Hill criteria been considered?

12.11   Technical details

Confidence interval for a relative risk

Given the notation of Table 12.1 the standard error of the log relative risk for large samples is given by

$$SE(\log RR) = \sqrt{\left(\frac{1}{a} - \frac{1}{a+c} + \frac{1}{b} - \frac{1}{b+d}\right)}$$

The reason for computing the standard error on the logarithmic scale is that this is more likely to be Normally distributed than the RR itself. It is important to note that when transformed back to the original scale, the confidence interval so obtained will be asymmetric about the RR. There will be a shorter distance from the lower confidence limit to the RR than from the RR to the upper confidence limit.

Worked example

From the data of Table 12.3

$$SE(\log RR) = \sqrt{\left(\frac{1}{379} - \frac{1}{726} + \frac{1}{230} - \frac{1}{529}\right)} = 0.061.$$

Thus a 95% CI for $\log(RR)$ is $0.191 - 1.96 \times 0.061$ to $0.191 + 1.96 \times 0.061$ or 0.071 to 0.310.

The corresponding 95%CI for the RR is 1.07 to 1.36.

CI for an odds ratio

Using the notation of Table 12.4 the standard error of the log OR, in large samples, is given by

$$SE(\log OR) = \sqrt{\frac{1}{a} + \frac{1}{b} + \frac{1}{c} + \frac{1}{d}}.$$

Worked example

For the data of Table 12.5, $OR = 1.01$ and so log $OR = 0.01$, while

$$SE(\log OR) = \sqrt{\frac{1}{537} + \frac{1}{534} + \frac{1}{639} + \frac{1}{622}} = 0.083.$$

This gives a 95% CI of −0.14 to 0.17.

The corresponding 95% CI for the OR is exp(−0.14) to exp(0.17) or 0.87 to 1.19.

12.12 Exercises

1. What type of study is being described in each of the following situations?

   (a) All female patients over the age of 45 on a general practitioner's list were sent a questionnaire asking whether they had had a cervical smear in the last year.

(b) A group of male patients who had had a myocardial infarction (MI) were asked about their egg consumption in the previous month. A similar-sized group of males of the same age who had not had an MI were also asked about their egg consumption in the last month, to investigate whether egg consumption was a risk factor for MI.

(c) A secondary school's records from 50 years previously were used to identify pupils who were active in sport and those who were not. These were traced to the present day, and if they had died, their death certificates were obtained to see whether the death rates were different in the two groups.

(d) A new method of removing cataracts (phacoemulsification) has been developed. Eye surgeons are randomised to receive training in the new technique immediately or after one year. The outcome of patients in the two groups is compared in the 6 months following randomisation.

(e) A new centre for chiropractic opens in town. An investigator compares the length of time off work after treatment for patients with back pain who attend the chiropractic centre and those who attend the local hospital physiotherapy centre over the same period.

2. Many observational studies have shown that women taking hormone replacement therapy (HRT) are at lower risk of heart disease. What biases might be involved in these conclusions?

3. Yates and James (2006) conducted a case–control study of students who struggled at medical school (dropped out or attended the academic progress committee). Over five successive cohorts they identified 123 strugglers and for each struggler chose four controls at random from the same year group. They obtained 492 controls. They found that 61 of the strugglers were male compared with 168 of the controls. Obtain an odds ratio for struggling for males and a 95% confidence interval.

13 The randomised controlled trial

Summary

This chapter emphasises the importance of randomised clinical trials in evaluating alternative treatments or interventions. The rationale for, and methods of, randomising patients are given. We delineate the 'ABC' of clinical trials: Allocation at random, Blindness and Control. The value of a study protocol is stressed. Different types of randomised trials, such as factorial, cluster and cross-over trials are described and we distinguish between those to established superiority from those that seek equivalence. Checklists of points to consider when designing, analysing and reading the reports describing a clinical trial are included. We also discuss the use of the summary statistic Number Needed to Treat (NNT).

13.1   Introduction

A clinical trial is defined as a prospective study to examine the relative efficacy of treatments or interventions in human subjects. In many applications one of the treatments is a standard therapy (control) and the other a new therapy (test).

Even with well established and effective treatments it is well recognised that individual patients may react differently once these are administered. Thus aspirin will cure some with headache speedily whilst others will continue with their headache. The human body is a very complex organism, whose functioning is far from completely understood, and so it is not surprising that it is often difficult to predict the exact reaction that a diseased individual will have to a particular therapy. Even though medical science might suggest that a new treatment is efficacious, it is only when it is tried in practice that any realistic assessment of its efficacy can be made and the presence of any adverse side-effects identified. Thus it is necessary to do comparative trials to evaluate the new treatment against the current standard.

Although we are concerned with the use of statistics in all branches of medical activity, this chapter is focussed primarily on the randomised clinical trial because it has a central role in the development of new therapies. It should be emphasised, however, that randomised controlled trials are relevant to other areas of medical problems and not just therapeutic interventions; for example, in the evaluation of screening procedures, alternative strategies for health education and in the evaluation of contraceptive efficacy.

13.2   Why randomise?

Randomisation

Randomisation is a procedure in which the assignment of a subject to the alternatives under investigation is decided by chance, so that the assignment cannot be predicted in advance. It is probably the most important innovation that statisticians have given to medical science. It was introduced in agriculture by the founder of modern statistics, RA Fisher (1890–1962) and developed in medicine by Austin Bradford Hill (1897–1991). Chance could mean the toss of a coin, the draw of a card, or more recently a computer generated random number. The main point is that the investigator does not influence who gets which of the alternatives. It may seem a perverse method of allocating treatment to an ill person. In the early days of clinical trials, when treatment was expensive and restricted, it could be justified as being the only fair method of deciding who got treated and who did not. More recently it has been shown that it is the *only* method, both intellectually and practically, that can ensure there is no bias in the allocation process. In other methods an investigator has the potential, consciously or subconsciously, to bias the allocation of treatments. Bitter experience has shown that other methods are easily subverted, so that, for example, sicker patients get the new treatment. It is important to distinguish *random* from *haphazard* or *systematic* allocation. A typical systematic allocation method is where the patients are assigned to test or control treatment alternately as they enter the clinic. The investigator might argue that the factors that determine precisely which subject enters the clinic at a given time are random and hence treatment allocation is also random. The problem here is that it is possible to predict which treatment the patients will receive as soon as or even before they are screened for eligibility for the trial. This knowledge may then influence the investigator when determining which patients are admitted to the trial and which are not. This in turn may lead to bias in the final treatment comparisons.

The main point of randomisation is that *in the long run* it will produce study groups comparable in *unknown* as well as known factors likely to influence outcome apart from the actual treatment being given itself. Sometimes one can balance treatment arms for known prognostic factors (see Section 13.3 on how to conduct randomisation). But suppose after the trial, it was revealed that (say) red-haired people did better on treatment. Randomisation will ensure that in a large trial, red-haired people would be equally represented in each arm. Of course, any trial will only be of finite size, and one would always be able to find factors that don't balance, but at least randomisation enables the investigator to put 'hand-on-heart' and say that the design was as bias free as possible.

Randomisation also guarantees that the probabilities obtained from statistical tests will be valid, although this is a rather technical point.

Random assignment and the protocol

The trial protocol will clearly define the patient entry criteria for a particular trial. After the physician has determined that the patient is indeed eligible for the study, there is one extra question to answer. This is: 'Are each of the treatments under study appropriate for this particular patient?' If the answer is 'Yes' the patient is then randomised. If 'No' the patient is not included in the trial and would receive treatment according to the discretion of the physician. It is important that the physician does not know, at this stage, which of the treatments the patient is going to receive if they are included in the trial. The randomisation list should therefore be prepared and held by separate members of the study team or distributed to the clinician in charge in sealed envelopes to be opened only once the patient is confirmed as eligible for the trial.

The ethical justification for a physician to randomise a patient in a clinical trial is his or her uncertainty as to the best treatment for the particular patient.

Historical controls

In certain circumstances, however, randomisation is not possible; one classic example is the first studies involving heart transplantation and the subsequent survival experience of the patients. At that time, it would have been difficult to imagine randomising between heart transplantation and some other alternative, and so the best one could do in such circumstances was to compare survival time following transplant with previous patients suffering from the same condition when transplants were not available. Such patients are termed historical controls. A second possibility is to make comparisons with those in which a donor did not become available before patient death. There are difficulties with either approach. One is that those with the most serious problems will die more quickly. The presence of any waiting time for a suitable donor implies only the less critical will survive this waiting time. This can clearly bias comparisons of survival experience in the transplanted and non-transplanted groups. For this reason one should interpret studies which use historical controls with care.

13.3　Methods of randomisation

Simple randomisation

The simplest randomisation device is a coin, which if tossed will land with a particular face upwards, with probability one-half. Thus, one way to assign treatments of patients at random would be to assign treatment A whenever a particular side of the coin turned up, and B when the obverse arises. An alternative might be to roll a six-sided die; if an even number falls A is given, if an odd number, B. Such procedures are termed simple randomisation. It is usual to generate the randomisation list in advance of recruiting the first patient. This has several advantages: it removes the possibility of the physician not randomising properly; it will usually be more efficient in that a list may be computer generated very quickly; it also allows some difficulties with simple randomisation to be avoided.

To avoid the use of a coin or die for simple randomisation one can consult a table of random numbers such as Table T2. Although Table T2 is in fact computer generated, the table is similar to that which would result from throwing a 10-sided die, with faces marked 0 to 9, on successive occasions. The digits are grouped into blocks merely for ease of reading. The table is used by first choosing a point of entry, perhaps with a pin, and deciding the direction of movement, for example along the rows or down the columns. Suppose the pin chooses the entry in the 10th row and 13th column and it had been decided to move along the rows; the first 10 digits then give 534 55425 67; even numbers assigned to A and odd to B then generate BBA BBAAB AB. Thus of the first 10 patients recruited four will receive A and 6 B.

Although simple randomisation gives equal probability for each patient to receive A or B it does not ensure, as indeed was the case with our example, that at the end of patient recruitment to the trial equal numbers of patients received A and B. In fact even in relatively large trials the discrepancy from the desired equal numbers of patients per treatment can be quite large. In small trials the discrepancy can be very serious perhaps, resulting in too few patients in one group to give acceptable statistical precision of the corresponding treatment effect.

Blocked randomisation

To avoid such a problem, balanced or restricted randomisation techniques are used. In this case the allocation procedure is organised in such a way that equal numbers are allocated to A and B for every block of a certain number of patients. One method of doing this, say for successive blocks of four patients, is to generate all possible combinations but ignoring those, such as AAAB, with unequal allocation. The valid combinations are:

1	AABB	4	BABA
2	ABAB	5	BAAB
3	ABBA	6	BBAA

These combinations are then allocated the numbers 1 to 6 and the randomisation table used to generate a sequence of digits. Suppose this sequence was 534 55425 67 as before, then reading from left to right we generate the allocation BAAB ABBA BABA BAAB for the first 16 patients. Such a device ensures that for every four successive patients recruited balance between A and B is maintained. Should a 0, 7, 8 or 9 occur in the random sequence then these are ignored as there is no associated treatment combination in these cases. It is important that the investigating physician is not aware of the block size, otherwise he or she will come to know, as each block of patients nears completion, the next treatment to be allocated. This foreknowledge can introduce bias into the allocation process since the physician may subconsciously avoid allocating certain treatments for particular patients. Such a difficulty can be avoided by changing the block size at random as recruitment continues.

In clinical trials which involve recruitment in several centres, it is usual to use a randomisation procedure for each centre to ensure balanced treatment allocation within centres. Another important use of this stratified randomisation in clinical trials is if it is known that a particular patient characteristic may be an important prognostic indicator perhaps good or bad pathology then equal allocation of treatments within each prognostic group or strata may be desirable. This ensures that treatment comparisons can be made efficiently, allowing for prognostic factors. Stratified randomisation can be extended to more than one stratum, for example, centre and pathology, but it is not usually desirable to go beyond two strata.

One method that can balance a large number of strata is known as minimisation. One difficulty with the method is that it requires details of all patients previously entered into the trial, before allocation can be made.

Carrying out randomisation

Once the randomised list is made, and it is usually best done by an impartial statistical team and *not* by the investigator determining patient eligibility, how is randomisation carried out? One simple way is to have it kept out of the clinic but with someone who can give the randomisation over the telephone or electronically. The physician rings the number, gives the necessary patient details, perhaps confirming the protocol entry criteria, and is told which treatment to give, or perhaps a code number of a drug package. Once determined, treatment should commence as soon as is practicable.

Another device, which is certainly more common in small-scale studies, is to prepare sequentially numbered sealed envelopes that contain the appropriate treatment. The attending physician opens the envelope only when they have decided the patient is eligible for the trial and consent has been obtained. The name of the patient is also written on the card containing the treatment allocation and the card returned to the principal investigator immediately. Any unused envelopes are also returned to the responsible statistical team once the recruitment to the trial is complete as a check on the randomisation process.

The above discussion has used the example of a randomised control trial comparing two treatments as this is the simplest example. The method extends relatively easily to more complex designs, however. For example, in the case of a 2×2 factorial design involving four treatments, the treatments, labelled A, B, C and D, could be allocated the pair of digits 0-1, 2-3, 4-5 and 6-7 respectively. The random sequence 534 55425 67 would then generate CBC CCCBC DD; thus in the first 10 patients none would receive A, two B, six C and two D. Balanced arrangements to give equal numbers of patients per group can be produced by first generating the combinations for blocks of an appropriate size.

13.4 Design features

The need for a control group

In Chapter 12 we discussed the hazards of conducting 'before-and-after' type studies, in which physicians simply stop using the standard treatment and start using the new. In any situation in which a new therapy is under investigation, one important question is whether it is any better than the currently best available for the particular condition. If the new therapy is indeed better then, all other considerations being equal, it would seem reasonable to give all future patients with the condition the new therapy. But how well are the patients doing with the current therapy? Once a therapy is in routine use it is not generally monitored to the same rigorous standards as it was during its development. So although the current best therapy may have been carefully tested many years prior to the proposed new study, changes in medical practice may have ensued in the interim. There may also be changes in patient characterisation or doctors' attitudes to treatment. It could well be that some of these changes have influenced patient outcomes. The possibility of such changes makes it imperative that the new therapy be tested alongside the old. In addition, although there may be a presumption of improved efficacy, the new therapy may turn out to be not as good as the old. It therefore becomes very important to re-determine the performance of the standard treatment under current conditions.

Treatment choice and follow-up

When designing a clinical trial it is important to have firm objectives in view and be sure that the therapeutic question concerned is of sufficient importance to merit the undertaking. Thus, clearly different and well-defined alternative treatment regimens are required. The criteria for patient entry should be clear and measures of efficacy should be pre-specified and unambiguously determined for each patient. All patients entered into a trial and randomised to treatment should be followed up in the same manner, irrespective of whether or not the treatment is continuing for that individual patient. Thus a patient who refuses a second injection in a drug study should be monitored as closely as one who agreed to the injection. From considerations of sample size (see Chapter 14) it is often preferable to compare at most two treatments, although, clearly, there are situations in which more than two can be evaluated efficiently.

Blind assessment

Just as the physician who determines eligibility to the study should be blind to the actual treatment that the patient would receive, any assessment of the patient should preferably be 'blind'! Thus one should separate the assessment process from the treatment process if this is at all possible. To obtain an even more objective view of efficacy it is desirable to have the patient 'blind' to which of the treatments he is receiving. It should be noted that if a placebo or standard drug is to be used in a double-blind trial, it should be packaged in exactly the same way as the test treatment. Clinical trials are concerned with real and not abstract situations so it is recognised that the ideal 'blind' situation may not be possible or even desirable in all circumstances. If there is a choice, however, the maximum degree of 'blindness' should be adhered to. In a 'double-blind' trial, in which neither the patient nor the physician know the treatment, careful monitoring is required since treatment-related adverse side-effects are a possibility in any trial and the attendant physician may need to be able to have immediate access to the actual treatment given should an emergency arise.

'Pragmatic' and 'explanatory' trials

One can draw a useful distinction between trials that aim to determine the exact pharmacological action of a drug ('explanatory' trials) and trials that aim to determine the efficacy of a drug as used in day-to-day clinical practice ('pragmatic' trials). There are many factors besides lack of efficacy that can interfere with the action of a drug; for example, if a drug is unpalatable, patients may not like its taste and therefore not take it.

Explanatory trials often require some measure of patient compliance, perhaps by means of blood samples, to determine whether the drug was actually taken by the patient. Such trials need to be conducted in tightly controlled situations. Patients found not to have complied with the prescribed dose schedule may be excluded from analysis.

On the other hand, pragmatic trials lead to analysis by 'intention to treat' or 'ITT'. Thus once patients are randomised to receive a particular treatment they are analysed as if they have received it, whether or not they did so in practice. This will reflect the likely action of the drug in clinical practice, where even when a drug is prescribed there is no guarantee that the patient will take it. In general we would recommend that trials be analysed on an ITT basis although there are situations where a so-called 'per protocol' analysis is best. For example, a trial in which blood levels of the drugs were also to be monitored where it is important that only those actually taking the drugs (rather than allocated to the drug and possibly not taking it) are used to summarise the profiles.

Superiority and equivalence trials

Implicit in a comparison between two treatments is the presumption that if the null hypothesis is rejected then there is a difference between the treatments being compared. Thus one concludes that one treatment is 'superior' to the other irrespective of the magnitude of the difference observed. However in certain situations, a new therapy may bring certain advantages over the current standard, possibly in a reduced side-effects profile, easier administration or cost but it may not be anticipated to be better with respect to the primary efficacy variable. For example, if the treatments to compare are for an acute (but not serious) condition then perhaps a cheaper but not so efficacious (within quite wide limits) alternative to the standard may be acceptable. However, if the condition is life-threatening then the limits of 'equivalence' would be narrow as any advantages of the new approach must not be offset by an unacceptable increase in (say) death rate. Under such conditions, the new approach may be required to be at least 'equivalent' to the standard in relation to efficacy if it is to replace it in future clinical use. This implies that 'equivalence' is a pre-specified maximum difference between treatments which, if observed to be less after the clinical trial is conducted, would render the two treatments equivalent.

One special form of equivalence trial is that termed a 'non-inferiority' trial. Here we only wish to be sure that one treatment is 'not worse than' or is 'at least as good as' another treatment: if it is better, that is fine (even though superiority would not be required to bring it into common use). All we need is to get convincing evidence that the new treatment is not worse than the standard.

Design features of equivalence trials

- Decide on whether equivalence or non-inferiority is required;
- Decide the limits for equivalence or non-inferiority;
- Ensure very careful attention to detail in trial conduct especially patient compliance;
- Plan for a per protocol analysis.

Although analysis and interpretation can be quite straightforward, the design and management of equivalence trials is often much more complex.

In general, careless or inaccurate measurement, poor follow-up of patients, poor compliance with study procedures and medication all tend to bias results towards no difference between treatment groups. This implies that an ITT analysis is not likely to be appropriate since we are trying to offer evidence of equivalence, poor study design and logistical procedures may therefore actually help to hide treatment differences. In general, therefore, the quality of equivalence trials needs especially high compliance of the patients with respect to the treatment protocol.

Example: Non-inferiority – adjuvant treatment of post-menopausal women with early breast cancer

The ATAC Trialists' Group (2002) conducted a three-group randomised trial of anastrozole (arimidex) (**a**), tamoxifen (**t**) and the combination (**at**) in postmenopausal women with early breast cancer. The trial was designed to test two hypotheses. One was that that the combination (**at**) was superior to tamoxifen alone (**t**) and the second that anastrozole (**a**) was either non-inferior or superior to tamoxifen alone (**t**). This latter comparison comprises the 'equivalence' component to the trial.

The trial report quotes: 'Disease-free survival at 3 years was 89.4% on anastrozole and 87.4% on tamoxifen (hazard ratio 0.83 [95% CI 0.71 to 0.96] $p = 0.013$).' Thus with a better disease-free survival (DFS) at 3 years there was no evidence of inferiority with anastrozole as compared to tamoxifen. One can be confident of non-inferiority but this does not imply a conclusion of superiority even though the 3-year DFS rate is higher by 2.0%.

13.5 Design options

Parallel designs

In a parallel design, one group receives the test treatment, and one group the control as represented in Figure 13.1.

Example from the literature: Parallel group trial – patient consultations

Thomas (1987) randomly allocated patients who consulted him for minor illnesses to either a 'positive' or a 'negative' consultation. After two weeks he found that 64% of those receiving a positive consultation got better compared with only 39% of those who received a negative consultation, despite the fact that each group got the same amount of medication! Statistical analysis was used to show that these differences were unlikely to have arisen by chance. The conclusion was therefore that a patient who received a positive consultation was more likely to get better.

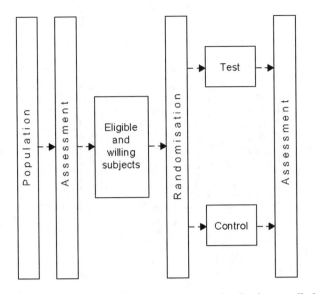

Figure 13.1 Stages of a parallel two group randomised controlled trial

Cross-over designs

In a cross-over design the subjects receive both the test and the control treatments in a randomised order. This contrasts with the parallel group design in that *each* subject now provides an estimate of the difference between test and control. Situations where cross-over trials may be useful are in chronic diseases that remain stable over long periods of time, such as diabetes or arthritis, where the purpose of the treatment is palliation and not cure. The two-period cross-over design is described in Figure 13.2.

Example from the literature: Cross-over trial – non-insulin dependent diabetes

Scott et al (1984) conducted a trial of Acarbose or placebo (an inactive treatment) in non-insulin dependent diabetics. After a 2-week run-in period to allow patients to become familiar with details of the trial, 18 patients were allocated by random draw (a method not recommended) to either Acarbose or placebo tablets. After 1 month individuals were crossed over to the alternative tablet, for a further month. In the final week of each of the 1-month treatment periods the percentage glycosolated haemoglobin (HbA1%) was measured.

The difference between HbA1% levels after placebo and Acarbose was calculated for each patient. The average difference was 0.3% with standard deviation of 0.5% indicating an effect of moderate size of Acarbose over placebo of 0.3/0.5 = 0.6.

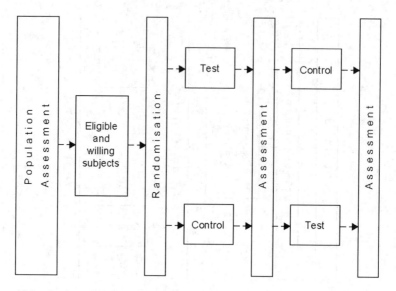

Figure 13.2   Stages of a two group two period cross-over randomised controlled trial

The two-period, two-treatment (2 × 2) cross-over trial has the advantage over a parallel group design testing the same hypothesis in that, because subjects act as their own controls, the number of subjects required is considerably less.

There are, however, a number of problems. One difficulty with cross-over designs is the possibility that the effect of the particular treatment used in the first period will carry over to the second period. This may then interfere with how the treatment scheduled for the second period will act, and thus affect the final comparison between the two treatments (the carry-over effect). To allow for this possibility, a washout period, in which no treatment is given, should be included between successive treatment periods. Other difficulties are that the disease may not remain stable over the trial period, and that because of the extended treatment period, more subject drop-outs will occur than in a parallel group design.

A cross-over study results in a paired (or matched) analysis. It is incorrect to analyse the trial ignoring this pairing, as that analysis fails to use all the information in the study design.

Cluster randomised trials

In some cases, because of the nature of the intervention planned, it may be impossible to randomise on an individual subject basis in a trial. Thus an investigator may have to randomise communities to test out different types of health promotion or different types of vaccine, when problems of contamination or logistics, respectively, mean that it is better to randomise a group rather than an individual. Alternatively, one may wish to test different ways of counselling patients, and it would be impossible for a health professional once trained to a new approach to then switch methods for different patients following randomisation. For example, 10 health professionals may be involved and these are then randomised, five to each group, to be trained or not in new counselling techniques. The professionals each then recruit a number of patients who form the corresponding cluster all receiving counselling according to the training (or not) of their health professional. The simplest way to analyse these studies is by group, rather than on an individual subject basis.

Example from the literature: Cluster design – diabetes

Kinmonth et al (1998) describe a trial of 'patient-centred care' in newly diagnosed patients with diabetes. Forty-one primary care practices were randomised to receive either a 3-day course in this new patient-centred method, or only the Diabetic Association guidelines. The outcome measures were the individual patient body-mass indices and HbA1c levels after 1 year. In this case it was impossible for a general practitioner to revert to old methods of patient care after having received the training, and so a cluster design was chosen with the general practitioner as the unit of randomisation.

Factorial trials

A factorial trial is used to evaluate two or more interventions simultaneously. Note that a factorial trial is not a study which merely balances prognostic factors, such as age or gender, but which are not interventions, as has been stated in several textbooks!

Example from the literature: 2 × 2 factorial design – breast self examination

McMaster et al (1985) describe a randomised trial to evaluate breast self-examination teaching materials. Four different experimental conditions were evaluated in health centre waiting rooms in which women were waiting to see their general practitioner. These were:

(A) No leaflets or tape/slide programme available (control)
(B) Leaflets displayed
(C) Tape/slide programme
(D) Leaflets displayed and tape/slide programme

Here the two types of treatment are leaflets and the tape/slide programme. The evaluation of the four experimental conditions was conducted
on four weekdays (Monday to Thursday) for 4 weeks. In order to eliminate
bias, a Latin square experimental procedure was employed, in which each
experimental condition was evaluated on each of the four weekdays.

In general the treatments in a factorial design are known as factors and
usually they are applied at only one level, that is, a particular factor is either
present or absent. For example, one factor may be radiotherapy for patients
with a certain cancer and the options are to give or not give. Factorial designs
are useful in two situations: first the clinician may believe that the two treatments together will produce an effect that is over and above that anticipated
by adding the effects of the two treatments separately (synergy), and is often
expressed statistically as an interaction. Alternatively, the clinician may
believe that an interaction is most unlikely. In this case, one requires fewer
patients to examine the effects of the two treatments, than the combined
number of patients from two separate parallel group trials, each one examining the effect of one of the treatments.

The use of this 2×2 factorial design enabled two questions to be asked
simultaneously. Thus, groups A and B versus C and D measured the value
of the tape/slide programme while groups A and C versus B and D measured
the value of the leaflets.

13.6   Meta-analysis

In many circumstances randomised trials have been conducted that are unre-
alistically small, some unnecessarily replicated while others have not been
published as their results have not been considered of interest. It has now
been recognised that to obtain the best current evidence with respect to a
particular therapy that all pertinent clinical trial information needs to be
obtained, and if circumstances permit, the overview is completed by a formal
combination of all the trials by means of a (statistical) meta-analysis of all
the trial data. This recognition has led to the Cochrane Collaboration and a
worldwide network of overview groups addressing numerous therapeutic
questions (Chalmers et al 1993). In certain situations this has brought definitive statements with respect to a particular therapy. For others it has lead to
the launch of a large-scale confirmatory trial.

Although it is not appropriate to review the methodology here, it is clear
that the 'overview' process has led to many changes to the way in which
clinical trial programmes have developed. They have provided the basic
information required in planning new trials, impacted on an appropriate trial
size (see Chapter 14), publication policy and very importantly raised reporting standards. They are an integral part of evidence-based medicine and are

impacting directly on decisions that affect patient care and questioning conventional wisdom in many areas.

13.7 The protocol

The protocol is a formal document specifying how the trial is to be conducted. It will usually be necessary to write a protocol if the investigator is going to submit the trial to a grant-giving body for support and/or to an ethical committee for approval. However, there are also good practical reasons why one should be prepared in any case. The protocol provides the reference document for clinicians entering patients into clinical trials. Furthermore some medical journals insist that every trial they consider for publication should be pre registered (and before patent entry) with an appropriate body.

The main content requirements of a study protocol are:

1. Introduction, background and general aims. This would describe the justification for the trial and, for example, the expected pharmacological action of the drug under test and its possible side-effects.
2. Specific objectives. This should describe the main hypothesis or hypotheses being tested. For example, the new drug may be required to achieve longer survival than the standard sufficient to offset the possibly more severe side-effects.
3. Patient selection. Suitable patients need to be clearly identified. It is important to stress that all treatments under test must be appropriate for the patients recruited.
4. Personnel and roles. The personnel who have overall responsibility for the trial and who have the day-to-day responsibility for the patient management have to be identified. The respective roles of physician, surgeon, radiotherapist, oncologist and pathologist may have to be clarified and organised in a trial concerned with a new treatment for cancer. The individual responsible for the coordination of the data will need to be specified.
5. Adverse events. Clear note should be made of who to contact in the case of a clinical emergency and arrangements made for the monitoring of adverse events.
6. Trial design and randomisation. A brief description of the essential features of the design of the trial should be included preferably with a diagram (such as Figures 13.1 and 13.2). It is useful also to include an indication of the time of visits for treatment, assessment and follow-up of the patients. There should also be a clear statement of how randomisation is carried out.
7. Trial observations and assessments. Details of the necessary observations and their timing need to be provided. The main outcome variables should

be identified so that the clinician involved can ensure that these are assessed in each patient.

8. Treatment schedules. Clear and unambiguous descriptions of the actual treatment schedules need to be provided. These could be very simple instructions in the case of prescribing a new antibiotic for otitis media, or be very complex in a chemotherapy regimen for osteosarcoma.

9. Trial supplies. It is clearly important that there be sufficient supplies of the new drug available and that those responsible for dispensing the drug and other supplies are identified.

10. Patient consent. The method of obtaining patient consent should be summarised and, if appropriate, a suggested consent form included.

11. Required size of study. The anticipated treatment effect, the test size and power (see Chapter 14) should be specified and the number of patients that need to be recruited estimated. It is often useful to include an estimate of the patient accrual rate.

12. Forms and data handling. Details of how the data are to be recorded should be provided. It is usual for a copy of the data forms to be attached to the protocol.

13. Statistical analysis. This would give a brief description of how the data are to be analysed. It would include the tests that are to be used and whether one- or two-sided comparisons are to be utilised.

14. Protocol deviations. Treatment details are required for patients who deviate from or refuse the protocol therapy. Clearly, a particular therapy may be refused by a patient during the course of the trial so alternative treatment schedules may be suggested. This section may also describe dose modifications permitted within the protocol which are dependent on patient response or the appearance of some side-effect.

13.8 Checklists for design, analysis and reporting

A guide to the useful points to look for when considering a new trial is given by checklists such as those of Gardner et al (2000). Although these lists were developed primarily for assessing the quality of manuscripts submitted for publication, each contain items that cover aspects worthy of consideration at the planning stage of a trial.

Design

The main consideration here is that should the design not be suitable to answer the trial questions(s) posed no amount of 'statistical juggling' at the analysis stage can correct any basic faults. For example, if a cross-over trial design is used without an adequate washout period then this cannot be rectified by the analysis. A major consideration at the planning stage is whether there is a reasonable expectation that sufficient patients can be recruited to the proposed trial. Most of the points covered here should be clearly answered in the protocol but many of these may not be made so explicit in any subsequent publication.

Checklist of design features

1. Are the trial objectives clearly formulated?
2. Are the diagnostic criteria for entry to the trial clear?
3. Is there a reliable supply of patients?
4. Are the treatments (or interventions) well defined?
5. Is the method and reason for randomisation well understood?
6. Is the treatment planned to commence immediately following randomisation?
7. Is the maximum degree of blindness being used?
8. Are the outcome measures appropriate and clearly defined?
9. How has the study size been justified?
10. What arrangements have been made for collecting, recording and analysis of the data?
11. Has appropriate follow-up of the patients been organised?
12. Are important prognostic variables recorded?
13. Are side-effects of treatment anticipated?
14. Are many patient drop-outs anticipated?

Analysis and presentation

Provided a good design is chosen, then once completed the statistical analysis may be relatively straightforward and will have been anticipated at the planning stage. However, there are always nuances and unexpected features associated with data generated from every clinical trial that will demand careful detail at the analysis stage. Perhaps there are more missing values than anticipated, or many more censored survival observations through patient loss in one group than the other, or many of the assumptions made at the design stage have not been realised. In contrast to the choice of a poor design, a poor analysis can be rescued by a second look at the same data although this necessity will be wasteful of time and resource and delay dissemination of the 'true' trial results.

In many situations, the final trial report published in the medical literature can only concentrate on the main features and there may be a limit on the detail which can be presented. This may lead to difficult choices of exactly what to present. However, guidance for the 'key' features should be in the trial protocol itself.

Checklist for analysis and presentation

1. Are the statistical procedures used adequately described or referenced?
2. Are the statistical procedures appropriate?
3. Have the potential prognostic variables been adequately considered?
4. Is the statistical presentation satisfactory?
5. Are any graphs clear and the axes appropriately labelled?
6. Are confidence intervals given for the main results?
7. Are the conclusions drawn from the statistical analysis justified?

CONSORT

It is widely recognised that randomised controlled trials are the only reliable way to compare the effectiveness of different therapies. It is thus essential that randomised trials be well designed and conducted, and it is also important that they be reported adequately. In particular, readers of trial reports should not have to infer what was probably done – they should be told explicitly. To facilitate this, the CONSORT statement of Altman et al (2001) has been published and includes a list of 22 items which should be covered in any trial report and a suggested flow chart to describe the patient progress through the trial. The checklist applies principally to trials with two parallel groups. Some modification is needed for other situations, such as cross-over trials and those with more than two treatment groups.

In essence the requirement is that authors should provide enough information for readers to know how the trial was performed so that they can judge whether the findings are likely to be reliable.

The CONSORT recommendations have been adopted by many of the major clinical journals, and together with the use of checklists similar to those above, these will impact on the design and conduct of future trials by increasing awareness of the requirements for a good trial.

13.9   Number needed to treat (*NNT*)

A summary measure which is sometimes used to present the results of a clinical trial is the *number needed to treat* (*NNT*). The *NNT* is derived by supposing the proportions of subjects having a success on the Test and Control groups are p_{Test} and $p_{Control}$. Then, if we treat n patients with Test and n patients with Control group, then we would expect np_{Test} successes in the Test group and $np_{Control}$ in the Control. If we had just 1 extra success with the Test over the Control group then $np_{Test} - np_{Control} = 1$. From this the number treated in each group in order to obtain *one extra* success is $n = 1/(p_{Test} - p_{Control})$. We call this the *NNT*, thus

$$NNT = \frac{1}{|p_{\text{Test}} - p_{\text{Control}}|}.$$

The vertical straight brackets mean take the absolute value of $(p_{\text{Test}} - p_{\text{Control}})$, that is, ignore whether the difference is positive or negative. The value obtained in the calculation is rounded to the nearest whole number above.

Example from the literature

Sackett et al (1997) show that the use of anti-hypertensive drugs to prevent death, stroke or myocardial infarction over 1.5 years in patients with a diastolic blood pressure between 115 and 129 mmHg has an *NNT* of 3. However, the use of the same drugs in patients with a diastolic blood pressure between 90 and 109 mmHg with the same outcome over 5.5 years has an *NNT* of 128.

This illustrates one of the problems of the *NNT*; namely that it depends on the baseline incidence. A treatment with the same relative risk reduction will have vastly different *NNT*s in populations with differing baseline rates.

It is also possible to calculate a confidence interval for an *NNT*, but this is difficult to understand when the treatments are not statistically significantly different, and we recommend confidence intervals for the difference $(p_{\text{Test}} - p_{\text{Control}})$ instead.

Example from the literature: NNT – labour in water

Table 2.8 contained results from a trial by Cluett et al (2004) to test the value of labour in water and the outcome was need for an epidural anaesthetic. The proportions not needing epidurals were $26/49 = 0.53$ and $17/50 = 0.34$ for the Test and Control groups respectively. Thus the difference in these proportions that favours labour in water is $0.53 - 0.34 = 0.19$. Thus *NNT* $= 1/0.19 = 5.26$ or 6 to the nearest whole number above. Thus we would need to treat six patients with a labour in water and six in the control, to expect one fewer woman in labour to need an epidural anaesthetic.

13.10 Points when reading the literature

1. Go through the checklists described in Section 13.8.
2. Check whether the trial is indeed truly randomised. Alternate patient allocation to treatments is not randomised allocation.

3. Check the diagnostic criteria for patient entry. Many treatments are tested in a restricted group of patients even though they could then be prescribed for other groups. For example, one exclusion criterion for trials of non-steroidal anti-inflammatory drugs (NSAIDs) is often extreme age, yet the drugs once evaluated are often prescribed for elderly patients.
4. Was the analysis conducted by 'intention to treat' or 'per protocol'?
5. Is the actual size of the treatment effect reported, and the associated confidence interval reported?
6. Does the Abstract correctly report what was found in the paper?
7. Have the CONSORT suggestions been followed?

13.11   Exercises

The authors of this book have been involved in the design of many clinical trials. We suggest, as an exercise for the reader in judging how well we as authors put into practice what we have advocated in this chapter, that some of our papers are subjected to critical appraisal in a systematic way. Some are published before the CONSORT statement and some after and so one might judge whether reporting on our part has improved.

1. Kinmonth AL, Woodcock A, Griffin S, Spiegal N and Campbell MJ (1998). Randomised controlled trial of patient centred care of diabetes in general practice: impact on current well-being and future disease risk. *British Medical Journal*, **317**, 1202–1208.

2. McMaster V, Nichols S and Machin D (1985). Evaluation of breast self-examination teaching materials in a primary care setting. *J. Royal College of General Practitioners*, **35**, 578–580.

3. Poon C-Y, Goh B-T, Kim M-J, Rajaseharan A, Ahmed S, Thongprasom K, Chaimusik M, Suresh S, Machin D, Wong H-B and Seldrup J (2006). A randomised controlled trial to compare steroid with cyclosporine for the topical treatment of oral lichen planus. *Oral Surgery, Oral Pathology, Oral Radiology and Endodontology*, **102**, 47–55.

4. Morrell CJ, Spiby H, Stewart P, Walters S and Morgan A (2000). Costs and effectiveness of community postnatal support workers: randomised controlled trial. *British Medical Journal* 2000; **321**: 593–598.

5. Thomas KJ, MacPherson H, Thorpe L, Brazier J, Fitter M, Campbell MJ, Roman M, Walters SJ, Nicholl J (2006). Randomised controlled trial of a short course of traditional acupuncture compared with usual care for persistent non-specific low back pain. *British Medical Journal*, **333**, 623–625.

14 Sample size issues

Medical Statistics Fourth Edition, David Machin, Michael J Campbell, Stephen J Walters
© 2007 John Wiley & Sons, Ltd

Summary

We cover the rationale for sample size calculations. Calculations when the objective is to estimate a prevalence, or to compare two groups with binary or continuous outcomes are described.

14.1   Introduction

Why sample size calculations?

There are a number of reasons for requiring investigators to perform a power-based sample size calculation before the start of a study. A study that is too small may be unethical, since it subjects people to procedures that may turn out to be of no value, if the study is not powerful enough to demonstrate a worthwhile difference. Similarly, a study that is too large may also be unethical since one may be giving people a treatment that could already have been proven to be inferior. On more pragmatic grounds, funding agencies will require a sample size estimate since the cost of a study is usually directly proportional to the size, and the agency will want to know that its money is well spent. Many journals now have checklists that include a question on whether a sample size is included (and to be reassured that is was carried out *before* the study and not in retrospect!). For example, the statistical guide-lines for the *British Medical Journal* in Altman et al (2000) state that: 'Authors should include information on . . . the number of subjects studied and why that number of subjects was used.' Such a question often forms part of measures of quality of papers.

Why not sample size calculations?

A cynic once said that sample size calculations are a guess masquerading as mathematics. To perform such a calculation we often need information on factors such as the standard deviation of the outcome which may not be available. Moreover the calculations are quite sensitive to some of these assumptions.

One could argue that any study, whatever the size, contributes information, and therefore could be worthwhile and several small studies, pooled together in a meta-analysis are more generalisable than one big study. Rarely is a single study going to answer a clinically important question. Often, the size of studies is determined by practicalities, such as the number of available patients, resources, time and the level of finance available. Finally, studies, including clinical trials, often have several outcomes, such as benefit and adverse events, each of which will require a different sample size and yet sample size calculations are focussed on one outcome.

Summing up

Our experience is that sample size calculations are invaluable in forcing the investigator to think about a number of issues before the study commences. The mere fact of the calculation of a sample size means that a number of fundamental issues have been thought about: (i) What is the main outcome variable and when it is to be measured? (ii) What is the size of effect judged clinically important? (iii) What is the method and frequency of data analysis? Some medical journals now require protocols to be lodged in advance of the study being conducted, and it can be instructive to see whether the outcomes reported in a paper coincide with those highlighted in the protocol. A study may declare two treatments equivalent, but a glance at the protocol may show that the confidence interval for the difference includes values deemed clinically important prior to the study.

An investigator should not expect a single number carved in stone, from a medical statistician, rather the statistician can supply two answers. First, whether the study is worth attempting, given the time and resources available. Second, a range of numbers which would indicate what size sample would be required under different scenarios.

It is important to know that the number of patients required depends on the type of summary statistic being utilised. In general, studies in which the outcome data are continuous and can be summarised by a mean require fewer patients than those in which the response can be assessed only as either a success or failure. Survival time studies (see Chapter 10) often require fewer events to be observed than those in which the endpoint is 'alive' or 'dead' at some fixed time after allocation to treatment.

14.2   Study size

In statistical terms the objective of any medical study is to estimate from a sample the corresponding population parameter or parameters. Thus if we were concerned with blood pressure measurements, the corresponding population mean is μ which is estimated by $\bar{x}$, whereas if we were concerned with the response rate to a drug the population parameter is π which we estimate by p. When planning a study, we clearly do not know the population values and neither do we have the corresponding estimates. However, what we do need is some idea of the *anticipated* values that the population parameters may take. We denote these with the subscript 'Plan' in what follows. These anticipated values need to be derived from detailed discussions within the design team by extracting relevant information from the medical literature and their own experience. In some cases, the team may be reasonably confident in their knowledge while in other circumstances the plan values may be very tentative.

For illustrative purposes, we will assume we are planning a two group randomised trial of Test (T) versus Control (C) and we consider the situations of continuous (say blood pressure) and binary (response rate) outcomes. In which case the main parameter of interest is the true difference in efficacy of the treatments, δ, which we anticipate to be δ_{Plan}.

The appropriate number of patients to be recruited to a study is dependent on four components, each of which requires careful consideration by the investigating team.

Fundamental ingredients for a sample size calculation:

1. Type I error rate α
2. Type II error rate β
3. (i) For continuous outcomes – anticipated standard deviation of the outcome measure, σ_{Plan}
   (ii) For binary outcomes – proportion of events anticipated in the control group $\pi_{Plan, C}$
4. (i) For continuous outcomes, anticipated effect size $\delta_{Plan} = \mu_{Plan,T} - \mu_{Plan,C}$
   (ii) For binary outcomes, anticipated effect size $\delta_{Plan} = \pi_{Plan,T} - \pi_{Plan, C}$.

Type I and Type II error rates

In Chapter 7 we discussed the definition of Type I and Type II errors. The error rates are usually denoted by α and β and are the false positive and false negative error rates respectively. We have argued earlier against, and it is worth repeating, the rigid use of statistical significance tests. Thus we have discouraged the use of statements such as: 'The null hypothesis is rejected p-value <0.05', or worse, 'We accept the null hypothesis p-value >0.05'. However, in calculating sample size it is convenient to think in terms of a significance test and to specify the test size α in advance. It is conventional to set $\alpha = 0.05$. We also require is the acceptable false negative or Type II error rate, β, that is judged to be reasonable. This is the probability of not rejecting the null hypothesis of no difference between treatments, when the anticipated benefit in fact exists. The *power* of the study is defined by $1 - \beta$, which is the probability of rejecting the null hypothesis when it is indeed false. Experience of others suggests that in practice the Type II error rate is often set at a maximum value of $\beta = 0.2$ (20%). More usually this is alternatively expressed as setting the *minimum* power of the test as $1 - \beta = 0.8$ (80%). Why is the allowable Type I error (0.05) less than the Type II error (0.20) error? Investigators are innately conservative. They would prefer to accept an established treatment against the evidence that a new treatment is better, rather than risk going over to a new treatment, will all its possible attendant problems such as long-term side effects, and different procedures.

Standard deviation of the outcome measure

For continuous data is it necessary to specify the standard deviation of the outcome measure, σ_{Plan}. This may be obtained from previous studies that used this measure. Note that we need the standard deviation, not the standard error, and that it is the standard deviation of the outcome measure, not the difference in outcome measure between intervention and control. When comparing two treatments, as here, it is commonly assumed that the standard deviation is the same in the two groups.

> *Tips on finding the anticipated standard deviation of an estimate.*   Often papers only give estimate of an effect with a 95% CI.
>   We need the standard deviation, SD.
>
> - Let U be upper limit of the CI and L the lower limit.
> - Use the fact that $U - L$ is about 4 times the standard error, SE.
> - Use the fact that $SE = SD/\sqrt{n}$ to obtain $SD = SE \times \sqrt{n}$.

Control group response

For binary data it is necessary to postulate the response of patients to the control or standard therapy. As already indicated, we denote this by $\pi_{Plan,C}$ to distinguish it from the value that will be obtained from the trial, denoted p_C. Experience of other patients with the particular disease or the medical literature may provide a reasonably precise value for this figure in many circumstances.

The (anticipated) effect size

The effect size is the most important variable in sample size calculations. It sometimes called the anticipated benefit, but is generally considered the size of an effect that would make it worthwhile adopting the new treatment to replace the old. Thus for a binary outcome we must postulate the size of the anticipated response in patients receiving the new treatment, which we denote by $\pi_{Plan,T}$. Thus one might know that approximately 40% of patients are likely to respond to the control therapy, and if this could be improved to 50% by the new therapy then a clinically worthwhile benefit would have been demonstrated. Thus the anticipated benefit or effect size $\delta_{Plan} = \pi_{Plan,T} - \pi_{Plan,C}$ $= 0.1$ (10%). Of course it is not yet known if the new therapy will have such

benefit, but the study should be planned so that if such an advantage does
exist there will be a good chance of detecting it.

Relationship between type I error, type II error and effect size

The distribution of the population mean difference, δ, under the null and
alternative hypotheses is given in Figure 14.1.

Suppose the outcome is continuous and we look at the difference in mean
values between the treatment and control arms. Figure 14.1 shows the
expected distribution of the mean difference under the null (H_0) and alternative hypotheses (H_A). If the mean difference exceeds a certain value determined by the test statistic then we reject the null hypothesis, and accept the
alternative. Where does the sample size come in? The width of the curves is
determined by the standard error of the estimate, $SE(d)$, which is proportional to the inverse of the square root of the sample size. Thus as the sample
size gets bigger the curves become narrower. If α and δ remain the same the
value of β will diminish and the power will increase. If we keep the sample
sizes fixed, but increase δ then again β will diminish and the power will
increase.

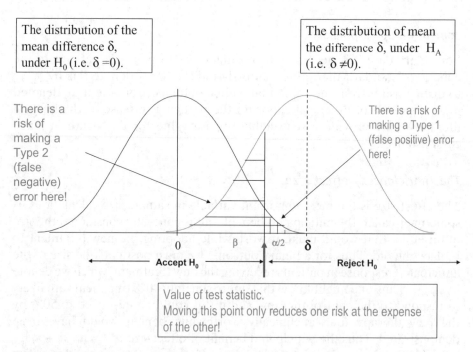

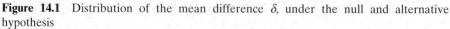

Figure 14.1 Distribution of the mean difference δ, under the null and alternative
hypothesis

> *Directions of sample size estimates*
>
> - Goes up for smaller α;
> - Goes up for smaller β (that is, larger power);
> - Goes up for smaller δ_{Plan};
> - Goes *down* for smaller σ_{Plan}.

14.3 Continuous data

A simple formula, for comparing the mean difference in outcomes between two groups, for two-sided significance of 5% and power of 80% is given by

$$m = 16\left(\frac{\sigma_{Plan}}{\delta_{Plan}}\right)^2 = \frac{16}{\Delta_{Plan}^2}, \qquad (14.1)$$

where m is the number of patients required per group.

In equation 14.1, $\Delta_{Plan} = \delta_{Plan}/\sigma_{Plan}$ is termed the standardised effect size since the anticipated difference is expressed relative to the anticipated standard deviation of each treatment group. The formula shows immediately why the effect size is the most important parameter – if one halves the effect size, one has to quadruple the sample size.

For clinical trials, in circumstances where there is little prior information available about the (standardised) effect size, Cohen (1988) has proposed that a value of $\Delta_{plan} \leq 0.2$ is considered a 'small' standardised effect, $\Delta_{Plan} \approx 0.5$ as 'moderate', and $\Delta_{Plan} \geq 0.8$ as 'large'. Experience has suggested that in many areas of clinical research these can be taken as a good practical guide for design purposes.

Worked example: Simple formula for a continuous variable – behavioural therapy

Suppose we wished to design a trial of cognitive behavioural therapy for subjects with depression. The outcome is the Hospital Anxiety and Depression scale (HADS), which is measured on a 0 (not anxious or distressed) to 21 (very anxious or distressed) scale and we regard a change of 2 points as being clinically important. We know from previous published studies in this patient population that the standard deviation of HADS score is 4 points.

Thus the anticipated standardised effect size is, $\Delta_{Plan} = \delta_{Plan}/\sigma_{Plan} = 2/4 = 0.5$, which Cohen would suggest is a 'moderate' effect. Using equation 14.1, for 80% power and two-sided 5% significance, we would require $m = 64$ patients per group or 128 patients in all.

As this calculation is based on 'anticipated' values the calculated sample size should be rounded upwards sensibly – in this case to 130 patients or possibly even 150 depending on circumstances.

14.4   Binary data

For binary data, Table 14.1 shows how the number of patients required per treatment group changes as $\pi_{\text{Plan,C}}$ (denoted π_1 for brevity) changes for fixed $\alpha = 0.05$ and $1 - \beta = 0.8$.

Thus for $\pi_1 = 0.5$ (50%), the number of patients to be recruited to each treatment decreases from approximately 400, 100, 40 and 20 as δ_{Plan} (denoted $\delta = \pi_2 - \pi_1$) increases from 10, 20, 30 to 40%. If α or β are decreased then the necessary number of subjects increases. The eventual study size depends on these arbitrarily chosen values in a critical way.

Example from the literature: Trial size – labour in water

The trial by Cluett et al (2004) found that 47% of those pregnant women giving birth who had a labour in water needed an epidural, compared with 66% in those with standard management.

Suppose that the trial is to be conducted again but now with the benefit of hindsight. The response to labour in water approximately 50% and that to standard care 65%. These provide the anticipated response rate for the control treatment as $\pi_{\text{Plan,C}} = 0.65$ and an expected benefit, $\delta_{\text{Plan}} = \pi_{\text{Plan,T}} - \pi_{\text{Plan,C}} = -0.15$. Here the benefit is a *reduction* in the proportion requiring epidurals but we ignore the sign as it is the magnitude of the difference which is relevant for sample size calculations.

Setting $\alpha = 0.05$ and $1 - \beta = 0.8$, then Table 14.1 suggests approximately $m = 170$ patients per group. Thus a total of 340 patients would be required for the confirmatory study. This calculation indicates that the reported trial of 99 patients was too small, or at least that the investigators had postulated a much larger (and unrealistic) value for δ_{Plan}.

Formulae for more precise calculations for the number of patients required to make comparisons of two proportions and for the comparison of two means are given in Section 14.8. The book by Machin et al (2008) gives extensive examples, tables and computer software for this and other situations.

It is usual at the planning stage of a study to investigate differences that would arise if the assumptions used in the calculations are altered. In particular we may have over-estimated the response rate of the controls. If $\pi_{\text{Plan,C}}$ is set to 0.60 rather than 0.65, then, keeping $\pi_{\text{Plan,T}} = 0.50$, $\delta_{\text{Plan}} = 0.10$, and there is a change in our estimate of the required number of patients from $m = 170$ to approximately 388 per group. As a consequence we may have to be concerned about the appropriate value to use for the response rate for the controls as it is so critical to the final choice of sample size.

Table 14.1 Sample size m per group required for a given response rate in the control group (π_1) and the effect size anticipated ($\delta = \pi_2 - \pi_1$) with 80% power ($1 - \beta = 0.80$) and 5% ($\alpha = 0.05$) two-sided significance

π_2	π_1 0.05	0.10	0.15	0.20	0.25	0.30	0.35	0.40	0.45	0.50	0.55	0.60	0.65	0.70	0.75	0.80	0.85	0.90
0.10	435																	
0.15	141	686																
0.20	76	199	906															
0.25	49	100	250	1094														
0.30	36	62	121	294	1251													
0.35	27	43	73	138	329	1377												
0.40	22	32	49	82	152	356	1471											
0.45	18	25	36	54	89	163	376	1534										
0.50	15	20	27	39	58	93	170	388	1565									
0.55	12	16	22	29	41	61	96	173	392	1565								
0.60	11	14	17	23	31	42	62	97	173	388	1534							
0.65	9	11	14	18	24	31	43	62	96	170	376	1471						
0.70	8	10	12	15	19	24	31	42	61	93	163	356	1377					
0.75	7	8	10	12	15	19	24	31	41	58	89	152	329	1251				
0.80	6	7	8	10	12	15	18	23	29	39	54	82	138	294	1094			
0.85	5	6	7	8	10	12	14	17	22	27	36	49	73	121	250	906		
0.90	4	5	6	7	8	10	11	14	16	20	25	32	43	62	100	199	686	
0.95	4	4	5	6	7	8	9	11	12	15	18	22	27	36	49	76	141	435
1.00	3	4	4	5	6	6	7	8	10	11	13	15	18	22	27	35	48	74

The cells in the table give the number of patients required in each treatment arm.

In certain situations an investigator may have access only to a restricted number of patients for a particular trial. In this case the investigator reasonably asks: 'With an anticipated response rate $\pi_{\text{Plan,C}}$ in the controls, a difference in efficacy postulated to be δ_{Plan}, and assuming $\alpha = 0.05$, what is the power $1 - \beta$ of my proposed study?' If the power is low, say 50%, the investigator should decide not to proceed further with the trial, or seek the help of other colleagues, perhaps in other centres, to recruit more patients to the trial and thereby increase the power to an acceptable value. This device of encouraging others to contribute to the collective attack on a clinically important question is used by, for example, the British Medical Research Council, the US National Institutes of Health, and the World Health Organization.

14.5 Prevalence

We described surveys in Chapter 12 and one might be designed to find out, for example, how many people wear dentures. Such a study is non-comparative and therefore does not involve hypothesis testing, but does require a sample size calculation. Here, what we need to know is how accurately we should estimate the prevalence of people wearing dentures in the population. Recall from Chapter 6 that, if m (rather than n) is the sample size, then the estimated standard error of the proportion p estimated from a study is $SE(p) = \sqrt{\dfrac{p(1-p)}{m}}$. This expression can be inverted to give $m = \dfrac{p(1-p)}{SE^2}$.

Thus if we state that we would like to estimate a prevalence, which is anticipated to have a particular value π_{Plan}, and we would like to have a 95% confidence interval of $\pi_{\text{Plan}} \pm 1.96 SE_{\text{Plan}}$, we have the ingredients for a sample size calculation if we specify a required magnitude for the SE in advance. Specifically

$$m = \frac{\pi_{\text{Plan}}\left(1 - \pi_{\text{Plan}}\right)}{SE_{\text{Plan}}^2}.$$

Here, there is no explicit power value. The type I error is reflected in the width of the confidence interval. If we do carry out a survey of the prescribed size, m, *and* the prevalence is about the size π_{Plan} we specified, then we would expect our calculated confidence interval to be wider than the specified 50% of the time, and narrower than the specified 50% of the time.

Worked example: Sample size – prevalence

Suppose we wished to estimate the prevalence of left-handed people in a population, using a postal questionnaire survey. We believe that it should be about 10% and we would like to have a final 95% confidence interval of 4% to 16%.

Here $\pi_{Plan} = 0.1$ and the anticipated width of the confidence interval is $0.16 - 0.04 = 0.12$, suggesting $SE_{Plan} = 0.12/(2 \times 1.96) \approx 0.03$. Thus $m = [0.1(1 - 0.1)]/(0.03^2) = 100$. This implies the upper and lower limits of the confidence interval are ± 0.06 away from the estimated prevalence, π_{Plan}. Using Table 14.2, this leads to a more accurately estimated sample size of $m = 97$.

Note m is the number of responders to the survey. We may have to survey more patients to allow for non-response. If we assume a 50% response rate to the postal survey then we actually need to mail out $2 \times 100 = 200$ questionnaires to get the required number of responders.

14.6 Subject withdrawals

One aspect of a clinical trial, which can affect the number of patients recruited, is the proportion of patients who are lost to follow-up during the course of the trial. These withdrawals are a particular problem for trials in which patients are monitored over a long period of follow-up time.

Table 14.2 Sample size m required to estimate the anticipated prevalence (π_{Plan}) with upper and lower confidence limits of ± 0.01, ± 0.02, ± 0.05, ± 0.06, or ± 0.10 away from the anticipated value

π_{plan}	Required precision for the upper and lower confidence limits for the anticipated prevalence π_{Plan}				
	± 0.01	± 0.02	± 0.05	± 0.06	± 0.10
0.05	1825	457	73		
0.10	3458	865	139	97	35
0.15	4899	1225	196	137	49
0.20	6147	1537	246	171	62
0.25	7203	1801	289	201	73
0.30	8068	2017	323	225	81
0.35	8740	2185	350	243	88
0.40	9220	2305	369	257	93
0.45	9508	2377	381	265	96
0.50	9604	2401	385	267	97
0.55	9508	2377	381	265	96
0.60	9220	2305	369	257	93
0.65	8740	2185	350	243	88
0.70	8068	2017	323	225	81
0.75	7203	1801	289	201	73
0.80	6147	1537	246	171	62
0.85	4899	1225	196	137	49
0.90	3458	865	139	97	35
0.95	1825	457	73		

In these circumstances, as a precaution against such withdrawals, the planned number of patients is adjustment upwards to $N_W = N/(1 - W)$ where W is the anticipated withdrawal proportion. The estimated size of W can often be obtained from reports of studies conducted by others. If there is no such experience to hand, than a pragmatic value may be to take $W = 0.1$.

Example from the literature: Withdrawals – labour in water

For the planned confirmatory trial following that of Cluett et al (2004) the sample size calculations from Table 14.1 suggested approximately $m = 170$ patients per group. Thus with an anticipated withdrawal rate of 10% this might then be increased to 189, or a total of $N = 378$ or 380 mothers.

14.7   Internal pilot studies

As we have indicated, in order to calculate the sample size of a study one must first have suitable background information together with some idea as to what is a realistic difference to seek. Sometimes such information is available as prior knowledge from the literature or other sources, at other times, a pilot study may be conducted.

Traditionally, a pilot study is a distinct preliminary investigation, conducted before embarking on the main trial. However, Birkett and Day (1994) have explored the use of an internal pilot study. The idea here is to plan the clinical trial on the basis of best available information, but to regard the first patients entered as the 'internal' pilot. When data from these patients have been collected, the sample size can be re-estimated with the revised knowledge so generated.

Two vital features accompany this approach: first, the final sample size should only ever be adjusted upwards, *never* down; and second, one should only use the internal pilot in order to improve the components of the sample size calculation that are independent of the anticipated effect size. This second point is crucial. It means that when comparing the means of two groups, it is valid to re-estimate the planning standard deviation, σ_{Plan} but not δ_{Plan}. Both these points should be carefully observed to avoid distortion of the subsequent significance test and a possible misleading interpretation of the final study results.

14.8   Points when reading the literature

1. Check if the sample size in the study is justified, either by a power based calculation or by availability. If not, consider the paper to be of lower quality.

2. Check if the variable used in the sample size calculation is the main outcome in the analysis
3. If a study is not significant, and the authors are claiming equivalence, look at the size of the effect considered clinically important in the sample size calculation and see if the confidence intervals reported in the analysis contain this effect. If so, the equivalence is not proven.

14.9 Technical details

As described earlier, to compute sample sizes we need to specify a significance level α and a power $1 - \beta$. The calculations depend on a function $\theta = (z_{\alpha/2} + z_{1-\beta})^2$, where $z_{\alpha/2}$ and $z_{1-\beta}$ which are the ordinates for the Normal distribution of Table T1. Some convenient values of θ are given in Table 14.3.

Comparison of proportions

Suppose we wished to detect a difference in proportions $\delta_{\text{Plan}} = \pi_{\text{Plan,T}} - \pi_{\text{Plan,C}}$ with two-sided significance level α and power $1 - \beta$. For a χ^2 test, the number in each group should be at least

$$m = \theta \left[\frac{\pi_{\text{Plan,T}} \left(1 - \pi_{\text{Plan,T}}\right) + \pi_{\text{Plan,C}} \left(1 - \pi_{\text{Plan,C}}\right)}{\delta_{\text{Plan}}^2} \right].$$

We can also use Table 14.1, if we only require a significance level of 5% and a power of 80%.

Worked example: Comparison of proportions

In a clinical trial suppose the anticipated placebo response is 0.25, and a worthwhile response to the drug is 0.50. How many subjects are required in each group so that we have an 80% power at 5% significance level?

With $\alpha = 0.05$ and $\beta = 0.2$, then from Table 14.3, $\theta = 7.8$. The design team suggest $\delta_{\text{Plan}} = \pi_{\text{Plan,T}} - \pi_{\text{Plan,C}} = 0.25$, $m = 7.8 \times [(0.25 \times 0.75 + 0.5 \times 0.5)/0.25^2] = 54.6$. Thus we need at least 55 patients per group or $N = 2m = 110$ patients in all. From Table 14.1, we would be able to say that the required number of patients is 58 per group.

Table 14.3 Table to assist in sample size calculations

Two-sided significance level	Power	$\theta = (z_{\alpha/2} + z_{1-\beta})^2$
5%	80%	7.8
5%	90%	10.5
1%	80%	11.7
1%	90%	14.9

Comparison of means (unpaired data)

Suppose on the control drug we expect the mean response to be $\mu_{Plan,C}$ and on the test we expect it to be $\mu_{Plan,T}$. If the standard deviation, σ_{Plan}, of the response is likely to be the same with both drugs, then for two-sided significance level α and power $1 - \beta$ the approximate number of patients per group, is

$$m = 2\theta \frac{\sigma^2_{Plan}}{\delta^2_{Plan}}.$$

Worked example: comparison of means

Suppose in a clinical trial to compare two treatments to reduce blood pressure one wished to detect a difference of 5 mmHg, when the standard deviation of blood pressure is 10 mmHg, with power 90% and 5% significance level.

Here $\delta_{Plan} = 5$, $\sigma_{Plan} = 10$ giving an anticipated standardised effect size of $\Delta_{Plan} = 5/10$. Use of Table 14.3 with $\alpha = 0.05$ and $\beta = 0.1$ gives $\theta = 10.5$, hence $m = 2 \times 10.5 \times 10^2/5^2 = 84$ per treatment group or approximately $N = 170$ patients in total.

14.10   Exercises

1. Suppose we wish to estimate the prevalence of nurses dissatisfied with their job. We think it will be about 20%, and we would like to estimate this to within 5%. How many subjects do we need?

2. Hippisley-Cox et al (2003) described a survey of the results of various statins on serum cholesterol in general practice. They found that the serum cholesterol for 554 patients on atorvastatin to be 4.99 mmol/l (95% CI 4.90 to 5.09). Suppose a new statin came on the market and we wished to design a trial to see if it was an improvement on this. Assume a difference of 0.5 mmol in serum cholesterol is worthwhile. How many patients would be needed for a two-sided significance of 5% and 80% power?

3. Suppose we are planning an exercise trial in 50–74-year-old men, to see if a daily exercise regime for a year will lead to improved quality of life compared to a control group. We know from published data on the SF-36 quality of life measure that at this age men have a mean score on the Physical Function dimension of 73.0, with a standard deviation of 27.0. Suppose the effect of the daily exercise regime on physical function will be considered important if it increases the Physical Function Dimension of the SF-36 by at least 10 points. How many patients would be needed for a two-sided significance of 5% and 90% power?

4. Suppose we are planning an exercise trial in 50–74-year-old men identified as at high risk of a heart attack, to see if a daily exercise regime for a year will lead to a reduction in the number of heart attacks. One group will be given the daily exercise regime and the other control group will receive no help. On the basis of published evidence we expect that in the control group 20% of the men will have suffered a heart attack within the year. We would be interested in detecting a reduction of heart attacks to 15% in the exercise group. How many patients would be needed for a two-sided significance of 5% and 80% power?

15 Common pitfalls

Summary

Some common errors found in the medical literature are described. They comprise problems in using the *t*-test, repeated measure studies, plotting the change of a variable in time against the initial value, regression to the mean and confusing statistical and clinical significance.

15.1   Introduction

Many of the statistical errors that occur in the medical literature are frequently not very major and could be overcome with a little more care by the writing team and by more vigilance from any reviewers (Cole et al 2004). For example, using a *t*-test when it is dubious that the data are Normally distributed, or failing to provide enough information for the reader to discover exactly how a test was carried out. There are frequent examples of poor presentation, or of presentation in the Abstract of results irrelevant to the problem being tackled by the paper. These errors do not usually destroy a paper's total credibility; they merely detract from its quality and serve to irritate the reader. However, some errors stem from a fundamental misunderstanding of the underlying reasoning in statistics, and these can produce spurious or incorrect analyses. One of these we discussed in Chapter 11, which is the inappropriate use of the correlation coefficient in method comparison studies.

15.2   Using the *t*-test

We give a fictitious example, which is based, however, on a number of published accounts. Thirty patients with chronic osteoarthritis were entered into a randomised double-blind two-group trial that compared a non-steroidal anti-inflammatory drug (NSAID) with placebo. The trial period was one month. Table 15.1 summarises the change in the visual analogue scale (VAS) rating for pain, the number of tablets of paracetamol taken during the study and the haemoglobin levels at the end of the study.

Table 15.1   Results of a two-group trial of an NSAID in patients with chronic osteoarthritis

	Placebo		NSAID			
Number of patients (*n*)	15		15			
Observation	Mean	SD	Mean	SD	*t*	*p*
Change in VAS (cm)	1.5	2.0	3.5	2.5	2.41	0.02
Paracetamol (number of tablets)	20.1	19.7	15.1	14.7	0.79	NS
Haemoglobin (g/dl)	13.2	1.00	12.5	1.10	1.82	NS

The first problem encountered with Table 15.1 is that the degrees of freedom for the *t*-statistic are not given. If it is a straightforward two-sample *t*-test then they can be assumed to be $2n - 2 = 28$. However, it is possible that the design is that of a crossover trial and hence is paired, in which case a paired *t*-test used with $df = n - 1 = 14$, or the results come from an adjusted comparison, using multiple regression as described in Chapter 9. In both these cases the degrees of freedom will be less than the presumed 28. Of course, some clue to which is appropriate may be given in the supporting text.

The second problem is that the comparison of interest is the difference in response between the NSAID and placebo, together with an estimate of uncertainty or precision of this difference, and yet this comparison is not given. Two extra columns should therefore be added to Table 15.1. The first would give the mean difference in the observations between placebo and NSAID, and the second a measure of the precision of this estimate, such as a 95% confidence interval. We cannot obtain these with the information given in Table 15.1 without knowledge of the full design and/or type of analysis conducted.

From the data it can be seen that for both the change in VAS and the number of tablets taken, the SDs in each treatment group are similar in size as their respective means. Since a change in VAS can be either positive or negative, this need not be a problem. However, the number of tablets cannot be negative, it must be zero or a positive number, and so the large SD indicates that these data must be markedly skewed. This calls into question the validity of the use of the *t*-test on data which is non-Normal. Either a transformation of the original data, perhaps by taking the logarithm of the number of tablets, or perhaps the use of the non-parametric Mann–Whitney test of Chapter 8 would be more appropriate.

For the number of tablets of paracetamol and haemoglobin the table gives $p = \text{NS}$. The abbreviation means 'not significant' and is usually taken to mean a *p*-value >0.05, but the notation is uninformative and should not be used. Its use gives no indication of how close *p* is to 0.05. For the number of tablets of paracetamol taken, if $df = 28$ then from Table T1, $p > 0.20$ (more precise value 0.42) and for haemoglobin $0.05 < p < 0.10$ (more precise value 0.08). Both are larger than the conventional value of 0.05 for formal statistical significance. However, the *p*-values suggest that a larger trial may have produced a 'significant' difference for haemoglobin but not for the number of tablets although for the latter, since the analysis is clearly incorrect, this may not be the case. Further, if we assume the unpaired *t*-test with $df = 28$ is appropriate for comparing the mean haemoglobin values, the corresponding 95% CI for the difference is -0.09 to $1.49\,\text{g/dl}$. This indicates the possibility of the existence of quite a large effect of the NSAID on haemoglobin. A large (clinically important) effect is usually taken as a difference in excess of about 0.8 of the SD. Here the SD for the NSAID group is 2.5 and the upper limit of the 95% CI about 1.5, so the possible effect may be as much as $1.5/2.5 = 0.6$. This may be thought of as a moderate difference and may be of clinical importance were it found to be the case.

15.3   Plotting change against initial value

Adjusting for baseline

In many clinical studies, baseline characteristics of the subjects themselves may be very influential on the value of the subsequent endpoint assessed. For example, in the context of clinical trials in children with neuroblastoma it is known that prognosis in those with metastatic disease is worse than in those without. Indeed the difference between these two groups is likely to exceed any difference observed between alternative treatments tested within a randomised trial. In other situations, the outcome measure of interest may be a repeat value of that assessed at baseline. Thus in the example of Table 15.1, pain was measured at the beginning and end of study, so that it was the change in VAS (end of study minus baseline) for each patient that was subsequently summarised in order to compare treatments. In such circumstances, investigators are often tempted to graph this change against the baseline; the logic being to correct in some way for different baseline levels observed (which may be considerable).

Worked example: Weight change

The birthweight and weight at one month of 10 babies randomly selected from a larger group is given in Table 15.2.

The research question is: 'Do the lighter babies have a different rate of growth early in life than the heavier ones?' The graph of the change in weight or growth over the 1-month period against the birthweight is shown in Figure 15.1. It would appear from this figure that the smaller babies grow fastest because the growth (the y-axis) declines as the birth-weight increases (the x-axis). Indeed the correlation between birthweight and weight gain is $r = -0.79$ which has $df = 8$ and $p = 0.007$.

The negative correlation observed in Figure 15.1 appears to lead to the conclusion that weight gain is greatest in the 'smallest at birth' babies but this is a fallacious argument.

In fact, if we took any two equal sized sets of *random* numbers (say) A and B and plotted $A - B$ on the y-axis against B on the x-axis we would obtain a negative association. This is because we have $-B$ in the y-term and $+B$ in the x-term and as a consequence we are guaranteed a negative correlation. The presence of this intrinsic correlation makes the test of significance for an association between a change and the initial value invalid. Thus in the above example with $r = -0.79$, we do not know how much of this negative value is due to the phenomenon we have just described.

However, provided that the two sets of data have approximately the same variability, a valid test of significance can be provided by correlating $(A - B)$ with $(A + B)/2$. Somewhat surprisingly, if we took any two equal sets of *random* numbers (say) A and B as before and plotted $A - B$ on the y-axis against $(A + B)/2$ on the x-axis we would not get an intrinsic negative correlation but one close to zero of any sign; its magnitude differing from zero only by the play of chance.

Worked example: Weight change

Figure 15.2 shows weight gain plotted against the mean of birth- and 1-month weights. The corresponding correlation coefficient is $r = -0.13$ and with $df = 8$ this yields $p = 0.70$. Although the negative relationship is still apparent, the evidence for a relationship is much weaker using this approach.

Regression to the mean

Imagine an individual with a randomly varying resting carotid pulse rate, as was observed in the example of Figure 3.6, and that this rate has an approximately Normal distribution about the mean level for that individual with a certain SD. Suppose we wait until an observation occurs which is two SDs above the mean, perhaps the third last in Figure 3.6 then the chance that the next value is smaller than a quite extreme observation with value close to (mean + 2SD) is about 0.975 or 97.5%. We are assuming here that the

Table 15.2 Birthweight and 1-month weight of 10 babies – data ordered by increasing birthweight for convenience

Birthweight (g)	1-month weight (g)	Weight gain (1-month – Birth)	Mean (1-month + Birth)/2
2566	3854	1288	3210
2653	4199	1546	3426
2997	5492	2495	4244
3292	5317	2025	4304
3643	4019	375	3831
3888	4685	787	4286
4065	4576	512	4320
4202	4293	91	4247
4219	4569	350	4394
4369	3700	−669	4035

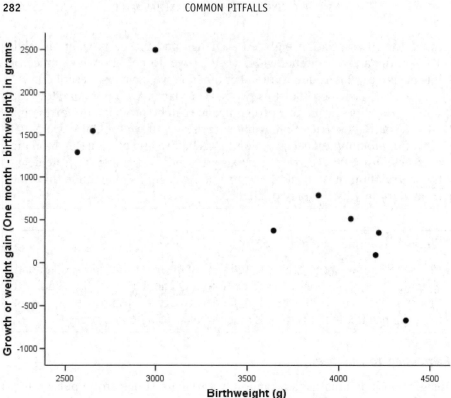

Figure 15.1   Growth of 10 babies in 1 month against birthweight

successive values are independent of each other and this may not be entirely
the case. Nevertheless the chance of the next observation being less than this
quite extreme observation will be high. This phenomenon is termed *regression to the mean* but, as we have illustrated, despite its name it is not confined
to regression analysis. It also occurs in intervention studies which target
individuals who have a high value of a risk variable, such as cholesterol. In
such a group, the values measured later will, by chance, often be lower even
in the absence of any intervention effect.

In intervention studies having the same entry requirement for both groups
can compensate for the regression to the mean. In this situation, if the interventions were equally effective then both groups would regress by the same
amount. Thus it would not be a problem in a trial in which the interventions
are randomised. However, it can appear in more insidious guises, for example
by choosing a locality which for 1 year only has had a high cot death rate;
even if nothing is done, the cot death rate for that district is likely to fall in
the next. In randomised studies, where we have *a priori* evidence that the
baseline results should be comparable, then the correct method to adjust for
baseline is multiple regression as described in Chapter 9. The dependent

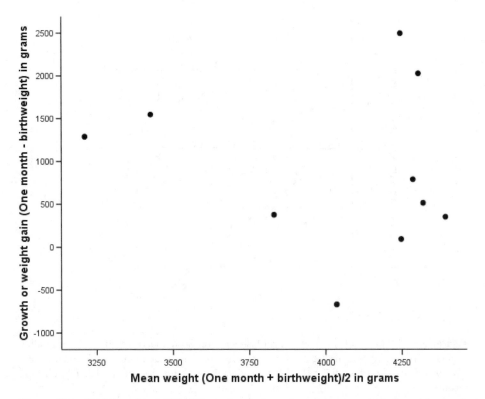

Figure 15.2 Weight gain of 10 babies in 1 month against the mean of birth and 1-month weight

variable is the outcome, and the independent variables include the baseline and a dummy variable for the intervention. One would get the same result if the dependent variable is the difference between outcome and baseline, but the former is easier to understand and more generalisable.

Example from the literature: Change in serum cholesterol

Findlay et al (1987) give in the graph of Figure 15.3 the change in fasting serum cholesterol against their initial cholesterol level in 33 men after 30 weeks of training.

The correlation of $r = -0.57$, with quoted $p < 0.001$, suggests strongly that those with high initial levels changed the most. However, after extracting the date from this graph, the resulting correlation of the change cholesterol with the mean of the initial and final levels is $r = 0.28$, $df = 31$ and $p = 0.11$. This implies that the association could well have arisen by chance, although if any relationship does exist it is more likely to be positive since the observed $r > 0$!

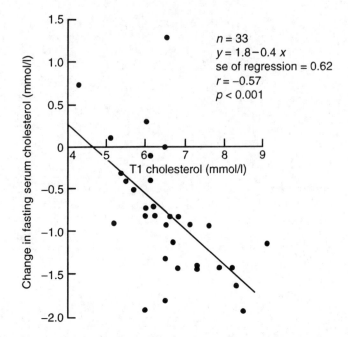

Figure 15.3 Change in fasting serum cholesterol after 30 weeks of training. From Findlay et al (1987). Cardiovascular effects of training for a marathon run in unfit middle-aged men. *British Medical Journal*, **295**, 521–524: reproduced by permission of the BMJ Publishing Group.

15.4   Repeated measures

A common design used in the collection of clinical data is one in which a subject receives a treatment and then a response is measured on several occasions over a period of time. Thus in the early development stage of a new drug, subjects may receive a single injection of the compound under study then blood samples are taken at intervals and tested in order to determine the pharmacokinetic profile.

Example: Metabolic rates in pregnant women

Figure 15.4 shows a graph of the metabolic rate measured over a 2-hour period in seven women following a test meal. The study was repeated at 12–15, 25–28 and 34–36 weeks of pregnancy. The corresponding values in the same women following lactation were used as controls.

The numerous significance tests would appear to imply, for example, that at 25–28 weeks of pregnancy the metabolic rate of a woman 60 minutes after ingesting a meal was not significantly different from control, but that it was significantly different at 45 and 75 minutes.

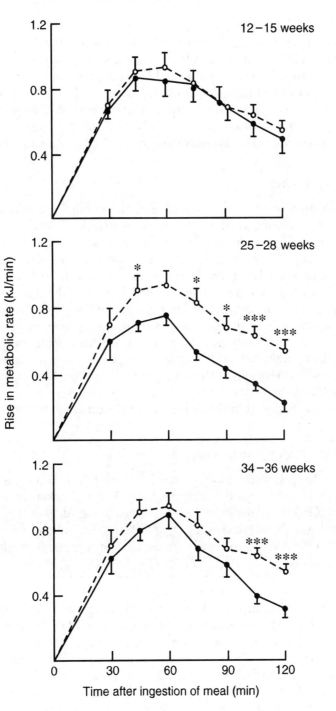

Figure 15.4 Rise in metabolic rate in response to test meal. Female subjects after lactation (dotted line) and at 12–15, 25–28 and 34–36 weeks of pregnancy (solid line). Points are means. Bars are SEM (standard error of mean). * $p < 0.05$, *** $p < 0.001$

In addition, although the use of *, ** and *** notation to summarise differences as statistically significant with p-values less than 0.05, 0.01 and 0.001, respectively, gives a quick impression of differences between groups, their use is not encouraged. One reason is that exact probabilities for the p-values are more informative than, for example, merely implying the p-value < 0.05 by use of *. Also, and usually more importantly, the magnitude of the p-values for comparisons which are not 'statistically significant' are not indicated by this device. This is equivalent to the 'NS' problem of Table 15.1.

Invalid approaches

The implication of the error bars used in the graphs is that the true curve could be plausibly drawn through any point that did not take it outside the ranges shown. This is not true for several separate reasons. Since the error bars are in fact 68% confidence intervals (one standard error either side of the mean), then crudely there is a 68% chance that the true mean is within the limit. If we had 10 independent observations, then the chances of the true line passing through each set of intervals is $0.68^{10} = 0.02$. This is small and hence true line is very unlikely to passing through them all. However, the observations are certainly not independent, so this calculation gives only a guide to the true probability that the curve passes through all the intervals. Nevertheless it does suggest that this probability is likely to be small.

Additionally, the average curve calculated from a set of individual curves may differ markedly from the shape of these individual curves.

Example: – Average response over time

To illustrate this, three response curves labelled A, B and C are shown in Figure 15.5, together with their average. The individual responses are simply a sudden change from Level 1 values to Level 2 but these occur at different times for the three subjects. Plotting the average response at each time point a, b and c, gives the impression of a gradual change for the whole group.

Often the stated purpose of the significance test is to ask the question, 'When does the response under one treatment differ from the response under another?' It is a strange logic that perceives the difference between two groups of continuous variables changing from not significantly different to significantly different between two adjacent time points. Thus suppose the time points in Figure 15.4 had been only 1 minute (or 1 second) apart rather than 15 minutes, then it would certainly seem very strange to test for a difference between successive time points – yet in reality, if the curve is truly

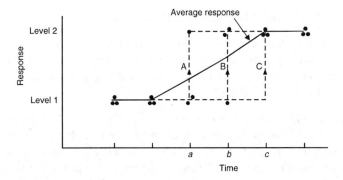

Figure 15.5 Response curves from three individuals and their a average response at each time point. The three subjects change from level 1 to level 2 at times, *a*, *b* and *c* respectively

changing, then they will be different but it is not sensible to say they are significantly different even if two values (far apart) are very different. Similarly it is the whole curve that one wishes to compare between groups not individual points along the profiles.

Valid approaches

Having plotted the individual response curves, a better approach is to try to find a small number of statistics that effectively summarise the data. For example in Figure 15.5, each individual can be summarised by the time at which they change from Level 1 to Level 2. These are times *a*, *b* and *c*. Similarly in Figure 15.4 the area under the curve from 0 to 120 minutes will effectively summarise the change in metabolic rate over the period.

Summary statistics for repeated measure curves:

- area under the curve (AUC);
- maximum (or minimum) value achieved;
- time taken to reach the maximum (or minimum);
- slope of the line.

The above statistics can then be used in an analysis as if they were raw observations; one for each subject. Thus in the example of Figure 15.4, one could compare the area under the metabolic rate curve for the four periods: after lactation, 12–15, 25–28 and 34–36 weeks, In general the analysis of repeated measures is quite tricky, and a statistician should be consulted early in the process.

15.5 Clinical and statistical significance

Once a study has been designed, conducted, the data collected and ultimately analysed the conclusions have to be carefully summarised. There are two aspects to consider, depending on whether or not the result under consideration is statistically significant.

1. Given a large enough study, even small differences can become statistically significant. Thus in a clinical trial of two hypotensive agents, with 500 subjects on each treatment, one treatment reduced blood pressure on average by 30 mmHg and the other by 32 mmHg. Suppose the pooled standard deviation was 15.5 mmHg, then the two-sample z-test, which can be used since the samples are very large, gives $z = 2.04$, $p = 0.04$. This is a statistically significant result which may be quoted in the Abstract of the report as 'A was significantly better than B, p-value = 0.04', without any mention that it was a mere 2 mmHg better. Such a small difference is unlikely to be of any practical importance to individual patients. Thus the result is *statistically significant* but not *clinically important*.

2. On the other hand, given a small study, quite large differences fail to be statistically significant. For example, in a clinical trial of a placebo versus a hypotensive agent, each group with only 10 patients, the change in blood pressure for the placebo was 17 mmHg and for the hypotensive drug it was 30 mmHg. If the pooled standard deviation were 15.5 mmHg, by the two-sample t-test: $t = 1.9$, $df = 18$ and $p = 0.06$. This fails to reach the conventional 5% significance level and may be declared *not statistically significant*. However, the potential benefit from a reduction in blood pressure of 13 mmHg is substantial and so the result should not be ignored. In this case, it would be misleading to state in the Abstract 'There was no significant difference between the drug A and B', and it would be better to quote the extra gain achieved of 13 mmHg, together with a 95% CI of –2 to 28 mmHg. In this way the reader can truly judge if the trial results are indicative of no difference or that, in a larger trial, the clinically important benefit of 17 mmHg indicated may be proven to be so.

15.6 Exploratory data analysis

'Fishing expeditions'

There is an important distinction to be made between studies that test well-defined hypotheses and studies where the investigator does not specify the hypotheses in advance. It is human nature to wish to collect as much data as possible on subjects entered in a study and, having once collected the data, it is incumbent on the investigator to analyse it all to see if new and unsuspected relationships are revealed.

In these circumstances it is important, *a priori*, to separate out the main hypothesis (to be tested) and subsidiary hypotheses (to be explored). Within the 'to be explored' category of so-called 'fishing expeditions' or 'data-dredging exercises' the notion of statistical significance, as discussed in Chapter 7, plays no part at all. It can be used only as a guide to the relative importance of different results. As one statistician has remarked: 'If you torture the data long enough it will eventually confess!' Subsidiary hypotheses that are statistically significant should be presented in an exploratory manner, as results needing further testing with other studies. For clinical trials, this is particularly the case for subgroup analysis. Doctors are always interested to see whether a particular treatment works only for a particular category of patient. The difficulty is that the subgroup is not usually specified in advance. Results of subgroup analysis, where the subgroups are discovered during the data processing, should always be treated with caution until confirmed by other studies.

If the data set is large, a different approach to 'fishing' is to divide it into two, usually equal and randomly chosen, sets. One set is used for the exploratory analysis. This then generates the hypotheses that can be tested in the second set of data.

Multiple comparisons

In some cases, it may be sensible to carry out a number of hypothesis tests on a single data set. Clearly if one carried out a large number of such tests, each with significance level set at 5%, then, even in the absence of any real effects, some of the tests would be significant by chance alone.

There are a number of solutions to controlling the consequentially inflated (above 5%) Type I error rate. A simple ad-hoc method is to use a Bonferroni correction. The idea is that if one were conducting k significance tests, then to get an overall Type I error rate of α, one would only declare any one of them significant if the p-value was less than α/k. Thus, if a clinician wanted to test five hypotheses in a single experiment (say five different treatments against a control) then he/she would not declare a result significant unless the p-value for any one of the tests was less that 0.01. The test tends to be rather conservative; that is the true Type I error rate will now be less than 0.05, because the hypothesis tests are never truly independent. Thus it would miss detecting a significant result for an uncertain number of the tests conducted. However, it can be useful to temper enthusiasm when a large number of comparisons are being carried out!

There is no general consensus on what procedure to adopt allow for multiple comparisons (Altman et al, 2000). We would therefore recommend the reporting unadjusted p-values (to three decimal places/significant figures) and confidence limits with a suitable note of caution with respect to interpretation. As Perneger (1998) concludes: 'simply describing what tests of significance have been performed, and why, is generally the best way of dealing with multiple comparisons.'

15.7   Points when reading the literature

1. Are the distributional assumptions underlying parametric tests such as the *t*-test satisfied? Is there any way of finding out?
2. If a correlation coefficient is tested for significance is the null hypothesis of zero correlation a sensible one?
3. Is the study a repeated measures type? If so, beware! Read the paper by Matthews et al (1990) for advice on handling these types of data.
4. Are the results clinically significant as well as statistically significant? If the results are statistically *not* significant, is equivalence between groups being claimed? If the result is statistically significant, what is the size of the effect? Is there a confidence interval quoted?
5. Have a large number of tests been carried out that have not been reported? Were the hypotheses generated by an exploration of the data set, and then confirmed using the same data set?
6. Have the subjects been selected because of a high or low value of a particular variable, and this variable subsequently remeasured? If so beware!

15.8   Exercises

1. A police authority installed speed cameras at accident black spots. In the following year they noted that the number of accidents at these sites had fallen from the year before the cameras were installed. Can one thus conclude that speed cameras are successful in reducing accidents?

2. A group of children were identified as slow learners. They were then randomly allocated to take either a cod liver oil capsule or a dummy placebo in a double blind trial. After 6 months the group allocated cod-liver oil appeared to have improved in terms of reading ability, relative to the dummy group and this difference was statistically significant (*p*-value < 0.01). Can one say this was a causal effect? Should one recommend all slow learners take cod liver oil?

References

Altman DG (1991). *Practical Statistics for Medical Research*. London, Chapman & Hall.

Altman DG, Machin D, Bryant TN and Gardner MJ (2000). *Statistics with Confidence*, 2nd edition. London, British Medical Journal.

Altman DG, Schultz KF, Moher D, Egger M, Davidoff F, Elbourne D, Gotzsche PC and Lang T (2001) The revised CONSORT statement for reporting randomised trials: Explanation and Elaboration. *Annals of Internal Medicine*, **134**, 663–694.

ATAC (Arimidex, Tamoxifen Alone or in Combination) Trialists' Group (2002). Anastrozole alone or in combination with tamoxifen versus tamoxifen alone for adjuvant treatment of postmenopausal women with early breast cancer: first results of the ATAC randomised trial. *Lancet*, **359**, 2131–2139.

Armitage P, Berry G and Matthews JNS (2002). *Statistical Methods in Medical Research*, 4th edition. Oxford, Blackwell Science.

Bell BA, Smith MA, Kean DM, McGhee CN, MacDonald HL, Miller JD, Barnett GH, Tocher JL, Douglas RH and Best JJ (1987). Brain water measured by magnetic resonance imaging. Correlation with direct estimation and changes after mannitol and dexamethasone. *Lancet*, **i**, 66–69.

Birkett MA and Day SJ (1994). Internal pilot studies for estimating sample size. *Statistics in Medicine*, **13**, 2455–2463.

Bland M (2000). *An Introduction to Medical Statistics*, 3rd edition. Oxford, Oxford University Press.

Bland JM and Altman DG (1986). Statistical methods for assessing agreement between two methods of clinical measurement. *Lancet*, **1**, 307–310.

Bland JM and Altman DG (1997) Statistics notes: Cronbach's alpha. *British Medical Journal*, **314**, 572.

Brown LM, Pottern LM and Hoover RN (1987). Testicular cancer in young men: the search for causes of the epidemic increase in the United States. *Journal of Epidemiology and Community Health*, **41**, 349–354.

Burke D and Yiamouyannis J (1975). Letters to Hon. James Delany. *Congressional Record*, **191**, H7172–7176 and H12731–12734.

Campbell MJ (1985). Predicting running speed from a simple questionnaire. *British Journal of Sports Medicine*, **19**, 142–144.

Campbell MJ (2006). *Statistics at Square Two: Understanding Modern Statistical Applications in Medicine*, 2nd edition. Oxford, Blackwell BMJ Books.

Campbell MJ, Hodges NG, Thomas HF, Paul A and Williams JG (2005). A 24 year cohort study of mortality in slate workers in North Wales. *Journal of Occupational Medicine*, **55**, 448–453.

Chalmers I (1993). The Cochrane collaboration: preparing, maintaining and disseminating systematic reviews of the effects of health care. *New York Academy of Sciences*, **703**, 156–163.

Chant ADB, Turner DTL and Machin D (1984). Metrionidazole v ampicillin: differing effects on postoperative recovery. *Annals of the Royal College of Surgeons of England*, **66**, 96–97.

Christie D (1979). Before and after comparisons: a cautionary tale. *British Medical Journal*, **279**, 1629–1630.

Clamp M and Kendrick D (1998). A randomised controlled trial of general preventative safety advice for families with children under 5 years. *British Medical Journal*, **316**, 1576–1579.

Cluett ER, Pickering RM, Getliffe K and Saunders NJSG (2004). Randomised controlled trial of labouring in water compared with standard augmentation for management of dystocia in first stage of labour. *British Medical Journal*, **328**, 314.

Cohen J (1988). *Statistical Power Analysis for the Behavioral Sciences*, 2nd edition. New Jersey, Lawrence Earlbaum.

Cole TJ, Altman DG, Ashby D, Campbell MJ, Deekes J, Evans S, Inskip H, Morris J and Murray G (2004). BMJ Statistical errors. *British Medical Journal*, **329**, 462. [Letter]

Cox IM, Campbell MJ and Dowson D (1991). Red blood cell magnesium and chronic fatigue syndrome. *Lancet*, **337**, 757–760.

Doll R, Peto R, Boreham J and Sutherland I (2004). Mortality in relation to smoking: 50 years' observations on male British doctors. *British Medical Journal*, **328**, 1519.

Elwood PC and Sweetnam PM (1979). Aspirin and secondary mortality after myocardial infarction. *Lancet*, **ii**, 1313–1315.

Enstrom JE and Kabat GC (2003). Environmental tobacco smoke and tobacco related mortality in a prospective study of Californians, 1960–98. *British Medical Journal*, **326**, 1057–1067. [1]

Farrell M, Devine K, Lancaster G and Judd B (2002). A method comparison study to assess the reliability of urine collection pads as a means of obtaining urine specimens from non-toilet trained children for microbiological examination. *Journal of Advanced Nursing*, **37**, 387–393.

Fayers PM and Machin D (2007) *Quality of Life: The Assessment, Analysis and Interpretation of Patient-Reported Outcomes*, 2nd edition. Chichester, John Wiley & Sons.

Findlay IN, Taylor RS, Dargie HJ, et al (1987). Cardiovascular effects of training for a marathon run in unfit middle-aged men. *British Medical Journal*, **295**, 521–524.

Furness S, Connor J, Robinson E, Norton, R, Ameratunga S and Jackson R (2003). Car colour and risk of car crash injury: population based case control study. *British Medical Journal*, **327**, 1455–1456.

Gaffney G, Sellars S, Flavell V, Squier M and Johnson A (1994). Case–control study of intrapartum care, cerebral palsy, and perinatal death. *British Medical Journal*, **308**, 743–750.

Glazener CMA, Herbison GP, Wilson PD, MacArthur C, Lang GD, Gee H and Grant AM (2001). Conservative management of persistent postnatal urinary and faecal incontinence: randomised controlled trial. *British Medical Journal*, **323**, 1–5.

Gardner MJ, Machin D and Campbell MJ (2000). Use of checklists for the assessment of the statistical content of medical studies. In: Altman DG, Machin D, Bryant TN and Gardner MJ (eds) *Statistics with Confidence*. London, BMJ Books.

Griffiths TL, Burr ML, Campbell IA, Lewis-Jenkins V, Mullins J, Shiels K, Turner-Lawlor PJ, Payne N, Newcombe RG, Lonescu AA, Thomas J and Tunbridge J (2000). Results at 1 year of outpatient multidisciplinary pulmonary rehabilitation: a randomised controlled trial. *Lancet*, **355**, 362–368.

Hancock BW, Wheatley K, Harris S, Ives N, Harrison G, Horsman JM, Middleton MR, Thatcher N, Longman PC, Marsden JR, Borrows L, Gore M (2004). Adjuvant interferon in high-risk melanoma: the AIM HIGH study. *Journal of Clinical Oncology*, **22**, 53–61.

Hawthorne AB, Logan RFA, Hawkey CJ, Foster PN, Axon AT, Swarbrick ET, Scott BB and Lennard-Jones JE (1992). Randomised controlled trial of azathioprine withdrawal in ulcerative colitis. *British Medical Journal*, **305**, 20–22.

Henquet C, Krabbendam L, Spauwen J, Kaplan C, Lieb R, Wittchen H and Van Os J (2005). Prospective cohort study of cannabis use, predisposition for psychosis and psychotic symptoms in young people *British Medical Journal*, **330**, 11–14.

Hepworth SJ, Schoemaker MJ, Muir KR, Swerdlow AJ, Tongeren MJ and McKinney PA (2006). Mobile phone use and risk of glioma in adults: case-control study. *British Medical Journal*, **332**, 883–887.

Hippisley-Cox J, Cater R, Pringle M and Coupland C. (2003) Cross-sectional survey of effective lipid lowering drugs in reducing serum cholesterol concentrations in patients in 17 general practices. *British Medical Journal*, **326**, 689–692.

Hobbs FDR, Davis RC, Roalfe AK, Hare R, Davies MK and Kenkre JE (2002). Reliability of N-terminal pro-brain natriuretic peptide assay in diagnosis of heart failure: cohort study in representative and high risk community populations. *British Medical Journal*, **324**, 1498–1500.

Jenkins SC, Barnes NC and Moxham J (1988). Evaluation of a hand held spirometer, the Respirodyne, for the measurement of forced expiratory volume in the first second (FEV1), forced vital capacity (FVC) and peak expiratory flow rate (PEFR). *British Journal of Diseases of the Chest*, **82**, 70–75.

Johnson CD, Toh SKC and Campbell MJ (2004). Comparison of APACHE-II score and obesity score (APACHE-O) for the prediction of severe acute pancreatitis. *Pancreatology*, **4**, 1–6.

Julious SA and Mullee MA (1994) Confounding and Simpson's paradox. *British Medical Journal*, **309**, 1480–1481.

Juniper EF, Guyatt GH, Feeny DH, Ferrie PJ, Griffith LE and Townsend M (1996). Measuring quality of life in children with asthma. *Quality of Life Research*, **5**, 35–46.

King EA, Baldwin DS, Sinclair JMA, Baker N, Campbell MJ and Thompson C (2001). The Wessex Recent Inpatient Suicide Study: a case control study of 234 recently discharged psychiatric patient suicides *British Journal of Psychiatry*, **178**, 531–536.

Kinmonth AL, Woodcock A, Griffin S, Spiegal N and Campbell MJ (1998). Randomised controlled trial of patient centred care of diabetes in general practice: impact on current well-being and future disease risk. *British Medical Journal*, **317**, 1202–1208.

Kristensen J, Langhoff-Roos J and Kristensen FB (1995). Idiopathic preterm deliveries in Denmark. *Obstetrics & Gynecology*, **85**, 549–552.

Liskay AM, Mion LC and Davis BR (2002). Comparison of two devices for wound measurement. *Dermatology Nursing*, **5**, 437–441.

Macfarlane GJ, Biggs A-M, Maconochie N, Hotopf M, Doyle P and Lunt M (2003). Incidence of cancer among UK Gulf war veterans: cohort study. *British Medical Journal*, **327**, 1373–1375.

Machin D and Campbell MJ (2005). *Design of Studies for Medical Research*. Chichester, John Wiley & Sons.

Machin D, Campbell MJ, Julious SA, Tan S-B and Tan S-H (2008). *Statistical Tables for the Design of Clinical Trials*. Oxford, Blackwell Scientific Publications.

Machin D, Cheung Y-B and Parmar MKB (2006). *Survival Analysis: A Practical Approach*. Chichester, John Wiley & Sons.

Macleod J, Salisbury C, Low N, et al (2005) Coverage and uptake of systematic postal screening for genital *Chlamydia trachomatis* and prevalence of infection in the United Kingdom general population: cross-sectional study. *British Medical Journal*, **330**, 940–942.

Manocha S, Choudhuri G and Tandon BN (1986). A study of dietary intake in pre- and post-menstrual period. *Human Nutrition – Applied Nutrition*, **40**, 213–216.

Matthews JNS, Altman DG, Campbell MJ and Royston JP (1990) Analysis of serial measurements in medical research. *British Medical Journal*, **300**, 230–235.

McKinley RK, Manku-Scott T, Hastings AM, French DP and Baker R (1997) Reliability and validity of a new measure of patient satisfaction with out-of-hours primary medical care in the United Kingdom: development of a patient questionnaire. *British Medical Journal*, **314**, 193–198.

McMaster V, Nichols S and Machin D (1985). Evaluation of breast self-examination teaching materials in a primary care setting. *Journal of the Royal College of General Practitioners*, **35**, 578–580.

Melchart D, Streng A, Hoppe A, Brinkhaus B, Witt C, Wagenpfeil S, Pfaffenrath V, Hammes M, Hummelsberger J, Irnich D, Weidenhammer W, Willich SN and Linde K (2005). Acupuncture in patients with tension-type headache: randomised controlled trial. *British Medical Journal*, **331**, 376–382.

Merza Z, Edwards N, Walters SJ, Newell-Price J and Ross RJM (2003). Patients with chronic pain and abnormal pituitary function require investigation. *Lancet*, **361**, 2203–2204.

Morrell CJ, Walters SJ, Dixon S, Collins KA, Brereton LM, Peters J and Brooker CG (1998). Cost effectiveness of community leg clinics. *British Medical Journal*, **316**, 1487–1491.

Morrell CJ, Spiby H, Stewart P, Walters S and Morgan A (2000). Costs and effectiveness of community postnatal support workers: randomised controlled trial. *British Medical Journal*, **321**, 593–598.

O'Cathain A, Walters SJ, Nicholl JP, Thomas KJ and Kirkham M (2002). Use of evidence based leaflets to promote informed choice in maternity care: randomised controlled trial in everyday practice. *British Medical Journal*, **324**, 643–646.

ONS (2004). Annual Abstract of Statistics, 2004 edition, United Kingdom, No 140. London, HMSO. [4]

Oakeshott P, Kerry S, Hay S and Hay P (1998). Opportunistic screening for chlamydial infection at time of cervical smear testing in general practice: prevalence study. *British Medical Journal*, **316**, 351–352.

Oldham PD and Newell DJ (1977). Fluoridation of water supplies and cancer a possible association? *Applied Statistics*, **26**, 125–135.

O'Sullivan JJ, Derrick G, Griggs P, Foxall R Aitkin M and Wren C (1999). Ambulatory blood pressure in schoolchildren. *Archives of Diseases of Childhood*, **80**, 529–532.

Peacock JL, Bland JM and Anderson HR (1995). Preterm delivery: effects of socioeconomic factors, psychological distress, smoking, alcohol, and caffeine. *British Medical Journal*, **311**, 6531–6535.

Pearson ADJ, Pinkerton CR, Lewis IJ, Imeson J, Ellershaw C and Machin D (Submitted). Randomised trial of high dose rapid schedule with conventional schedule for stage 4 neuroblastoma over the age of one year.

Perneger TV (1998). What's wrong with Bonferroni adjustments? *British Medical Journal*, **316**, 1236–1238.

Persantine-Aspirin Reinfarction Research Study Group (1980). Persantine and aspirin in coronary heart disease. *Circulation*, **62**, 449–461.

Poon C-Y, Goh B-T, Kim M-J, Rajaseharan A, Ahmed S, Thongprasom K, Chaimusik M, Suresh S, Machin D, Wong H-B and Seldrup J (2006). A randomised controlled trial to compare steroid with cyclosporine for the topical treatment of oral lichen planus. *Oral Surgery, Oral Pathology, Oral Radiology and Odontology*, **102**, 47–55.

Prentice AM, Black AE, Coward WA, Davies HL, Goldberg GR, Murgatroyd PR, Ashford J, Sawyer M and Whitehead RG (1986). High levels of energy expenditure in obese women. *British Medical Journal*, **292**, 983–987.

Quist-Paulsen P and Gallefoss F (2003). Randomised controlled trial of smoking cessation intervention after admission for coronary heart disease. *British Medical Journal*, **327**, 1254–1257.

Rigby AS, Armstrong GK, Campbell MJ and Summerton N (2004). A survey of statistics in three UK general practice journals. *BMC Medical Research Methodology*, **4**, 28.

Roche JJW, Wenn RT, Sahota O and Moran CG (2005). Effect of comorbidities and postoperative complications on mortality after hip fracture in elderly people: prospective observational cohort study. *BMJ* doi:10:1136.

Sackett DL, Richardson WS Rosenberg W and Haynes RB (1997). *Evidence-Based Medicine. How to Practice and Teach EBM*. New York, Churchill Livingstone.

Sargent RP, Shepard RM and Glantz SA (2004). Reduced incidence of admissions for myocardial infarction associated with public smoking ban: before and after study. *British Medical Journal*, **328**, 977–983.

Scott RS, Knowles RL and Beaver DW (1984). Treatment of poorly controlled non-insulin-dependent diabetic patients with acarbose. *Australian and New Zealand Journal of Medicine*, **14**, 649–654.

Shaw JL, Sharpe S, Dyson SE, Pownall S, Walters S, Saul C, Enderby P, Healy K and O'Sullivan H (2004). Bronchial auscultation: An effective adjunct to speech and language therapy bedside assessment when detecting dysphagia and aspiration? *Dysphagia*, **19**, 211–218.

Simpson AG (2004). A comparison of the ability of cranial ultrasound, neonatal neurological assessment and observation of spontaneous general movements to predict outcome in preterm infants. PhD Thesis, University of Sheffield.

Streiner G and Norman DL (2003). *Health measurement scales: a practical guide to their development and use*, 3rd edition. Oxford, OUP.

Stulemeijer M, de Jong LW, Fiselier TJ, Hoogveld SW and Bleijenberg G (2005). Cognitive behaviour therapy for adolescents with chronic fatigue syndrome: randomised controlled trial. *British Medical Journal*, **330**, 14–19.

Swinscow TV and Campbell MJ (2002). *Statistics at Square One*, 10th edition. Oxford, Blackwell, BMJ Books.

Taylor B, Miller E, Lingam R, Andrews N, Simmons A and Stowe J (2002). Measles, mumps, and rubella vaccination and bowel problems or development regression in children with autism: population study. *British Medical Journal*, **324**, 393–396.

Thomas KB (1987). General practice consultations: Is there any point in being positive? *British Medical Journal*, **294**, 1200–1202.

Thomas KJ, MacPherson H, Thorpe L, Brazier J, Fitter M, Campbell MJ, Roman M, Walters SJ and Nicholl J (2006). Randomised controlled trial of a short course of traditional acupuncture compared with usual care for persistent non-specific low back pain. *British Medical Journal*, **333**, 623–625.

Tillett HE, Galbraith NS, Overton SE, Porter K (1988). Routine surveillance data on AIDS and HIV infections in the UK: a description of the data available and their use for short-term planning. *Epidemiology and Infection*, **100**, 157–169.

Walters SJ (2003). What is a Cox model? Volume 1, number 10. www.evidence-based-medicine.co.uk.

Wight J, Jakubovic M, Walters S, Maheswaran R, White P and Lennon V (2004). Variation in cadaveric organ donor rates in the UK. *Nephrology Dialysis Transplantation*, **19**, 963–968.

Xu W-H, Zheng W, Xiang Y-B, Ruan Z-X, Cheng J-R, Dai Q, Gao Y-T and Shu X-O (2004). Soya food intake and risk of endometrial cancer among Chinese women in Shanghai: population based case–control study. *British Medical Journal*, **328**, 1285–1291.

Yates J and James D (2006) Predicting the 'strugglers': a case–control study of students at Nottingham University Medical School. *British Medical Journal*, doi:10.1136/bmj.38730.678310.63.

Solutions to exercises

Medical Statistics Fourth Edition, David Machin, Michael J Campbell, Stephen J Walters
© 2007 John Wiley & Sons, Ltd

Chapter 1

1. (i) continuous   (ii) ordinal   (iii) continuous   (iv) continuous
(v) count   (vi) binary.

2. They are both quantitative variables. There are two main differences: (i) Shoe size can, in theory be measured exactly; it is merely convenience to group them into different categories. There is no underlying continuous variable for family size; one cannot have a family with 1.5 children. (ii) The labels for shoe size are not on a ratio scale since there is no shoe size 0. Thus someone with a shoe size 10 (EU scale) does not have feet twice as big as someone with shoe size 5. Family size, on the other hand, is a count variable. A family with two children has twice as many children as a family with one child.

3. One loses information on the spread of the data. You will know how many people have a BMI > 30, but not how many have a BMI $> 25\,\text{kg/m}^2$ say. If you were told a patient was anaemic, you would like to know the proportion of healthy people who are anaemic in the same age/gender group as the patient. It would be useful to know the exact value, to see how far from the cut-off the patient was (although for this to be useful one would also need to know the variability of the data). One might conduct further tests, for example an endoscopy, before treating the patient.

Chapter 2

1. (i) Bar chart of the blood group of 55 women diagnosed as suffering from thromboembolic disease.

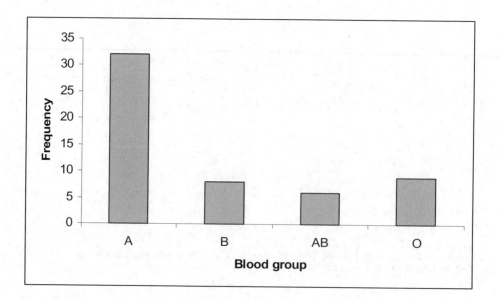

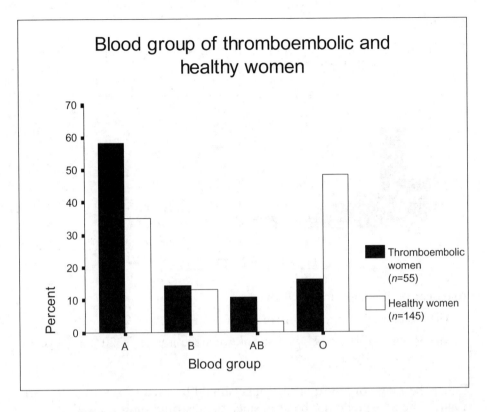

(ii) It would appear that there are more women in the thromboembolic group in blood groups A and AB and fewer in group O.

2. (i) Proportion of women with epidural: Labour in water is 23/49 = 0.47 or 47%: Augmentation is 33/50 = 0.66 or 66%.

(ii) Relative risk of epidural for the Labour in water women compared with those having Augmentation is 0.47/0.66 = 0.71.

(iii) Odds of epidural: Labour in water = 0.47/(1 − 0.47) = 0.89 Odds of epidural: Augmentation is 0.66/(1 − 0.66) = 1.94. *OR* of epidural for the Labour in water women compared with Augmentation women is 0.89/1.94 = 0.46. The *OR* is less than the *RR* and they differ because the event is quite common.

(iv) 'Risk' of epidural on Labour in water is 23/49 = 0.47, 'Risk' of epidural on Augmentation is 33/50 = 0.66. The Absolute Risk Difference for labour in water is $ARR = |0.47 − 0.66| = 0.19$.

3. One would like to know what is the actual risk of recurrence. Over what time frame has the risk been measured? Does it work for all breast cancers or only a specific type and grade? Also what are the types and risks of any side-effects?

Chapter 3

1. (i) Histogram and dot plot of the age (in years) of a sample of 20 motor cyclists killed in road traffic accidents

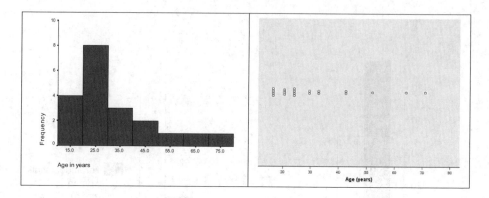

Age distribution is positively skewed

   (ii) Mean = 30.9 years; Median = 24.0 years; Mode = 24.0 years

   (iii) Range is 15 to 71 years; Interquartile range is 20 to 37 years; SD = 15.9 years

Either the range or interquartile range should be used to describe the variability. The SD should *not* be used since the distribution is skewed.

2. (i) Scatter plot of father's height vs. son's height

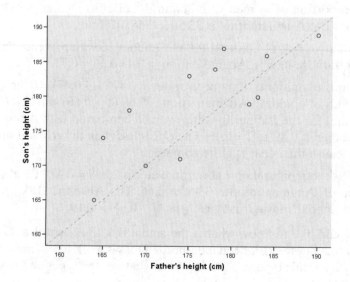

(ii) Yes: there does appear to be a linear relationship: tall fathers seem to have tall sons. Note that father's heights are plotted on the horizontal axis since causality goes from father to son, not vice versa.

Chapter 4

1. The way to answer this sort of question is to set up the 2×2 table supposing we have (say) 100 people in the study. Then we would find that 30 have appendicitis and of these $0.7 \times 30 = 21$ would have a high temperature. We get the following table

		Disease: Acute appendicitis		
		Yes	No	
Test:	High	21	28	49
Temperature	Low	9	42	51
		30	70	100

(a) F (true 21/30)   (b) T   (c) F (true 21/49)   (d) T   (e) F: specificity is independent of prevalence.

2. (a) T   (b) F: Specificity refers to patients without disease   (c) T (d) F: sensitivity is independent of prevalence   (e) T.

3. (a) T   (b) F: in some circumstances it is better to have a test which is more specific   (c) T   (d) T   (e) T.

Chapter 5

1. Using the Binomial distribution formula (5.1)

$$\text{Prob}(4 \text{ 'trivials' out of 5 patients}) = \frac{5!}{4!(5-4)!}0.5^4(1-0.5) = 0.156$$

2. Using the Poisson formula (5.2)

$$\text{Prob}(10 \text{ new cases}) = \frac{\exp(-10)10^{10}}{10!} = 0.1251$$

3. First calculate Z, the number of standard deviations 160 is away from the mean: $(160 - 141.1)/13.62 = 1.39$. Looking for $Z = 1.39$ in the Table T1 gives the probability of being outside the range of the mean ± 1.39 SD to be 0.1645. Therefore the probability of having a systolic blood pressure of 160 mmHg or higher is 0.08225 (or 8%).

4. (i) F   (ii) T   (iii) T.

5. (i) First calculate the number of standard deviations 95 is away from the mean:
   $(95 - 70)/10 = 2.5$. Look for $Z = 2.5$ on the Normal distribution Table T1 which gives the probability of being outside the range of the mean ± 2.5 SD to be 0.0124. Therefore the probability of having a diastolic blood pressure of 95 mmHg or above is 0.0062 (or 0.62%).

   (ii) Calculate the number of standard deviations that 55 is away from the mean $(55 - 70)/10 = -1.5$ (ignore minus sign)

   (iii) $1 - (0.0062 + 0.0668) = 0.9270$

Looking for $Z = 1.5$ in Table T1 gives the probability of being outside the range of the mean ± 1.5 SD to be 0.1336. Therefore the probability of having a diastolic blood pressure of 55 mmHg or less is 0.0668 (or 6.7%)

6. The expected referral rate is 2.8 per 1000 population. Thus in a population of 6000 one would expect 16.8 referrals. Assuming a Poisson distribution, the SD is $\sqrt{16.8} = 4.1$. The GPs observation of 27 is $(27 - 16.8)/4.1 = 2.48$ SDs from the mean. From Table T1 we see that the probability of getting a result this extreme is 0.013, so this GP's rate is unusually high. Note however, this also assumes this GP was chosen at random. If she was picked out of a large number of GPs as being the highest then this probability is not relevant.

Chapter 6

1. (a) F   (b) T   (c) F   (d) T   (e) T.

2. (a) F   (b) T   (c) T   (d) T   (e) F.

3. (a) Sample mean $= (156 + 154 + 140 + 158)/4 = 152.0$ mm. Variance $= [(156 - 152)^2 + (154 - 152)^2 + (140 - 152)^2 + (158 - 152)^2] / (4 - 1) = 66.667$ mm^2. Hence SD $= \sqrt{66.667} = 8.16$ mm.

(b) Dot plot of 10 mean Mid-upper arm circumferences of for samples of size 4.

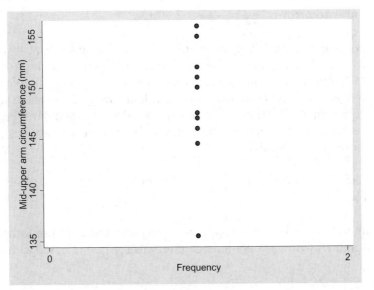

(c) The mean mid-upper arm circumference in mm of sample 10 in Table 6.5 is $\bar{x} = 152.0$ mm with a standard deviation of $s = 8.16$ mm. The standard error of the mean is $\dfrac{s}{\sqrt{n}} = \dfrac{8.16}{\sqrt{4}} = 4.08$ mm .

4. (a) Dot plots of mean mid-upper arm circumferences for 10 random samples of sizes 4 and 16 respectively.

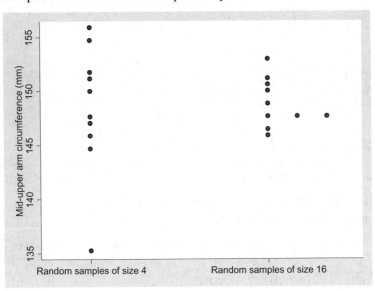

(b) The mean mid-upper arm circumference in mm of sample 4 in Table 6.6 is $\bar{x} = 151.25$ mm with a standard deviation of $s = 11.19$ mm. The standard error is $\dfrac{s}{\sqrt{n}} = \dfrac{11.19}{\sqrt{16}} = 2.80$ mm.

(c) We would expect that means of repeated samples of size 4 will have a Normal distribution with mean = 152 mm and a standard deviation of 4.08 mm. We would expect that means of repeated samples of size 16 will have a Normal distribution with mean = 151 mm and a standard deviation of 2.80 mm. This illustrates that the standard error will decrease as the sample size increases. Hence larger samples provide more precise estimates.

5. (a) The 95% CI = 152.0 − (1.96 × 4.08) to 152.0 + (1.96 × 4.08) or 144 to 160 mm.

Dot plots and 95% CIs for mid-upper arm circumferences for random samples of size 4 and 16 with 95% confidence intervals for two selected samples.

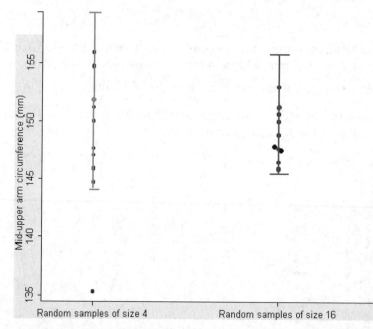

(b) The 95% CI is 151.25 − (1.96 × 2.80) to 151.25 + (1.96 × 2.80) or approximately 146 to 157 mm.

6. The proportion of acute appendicitis cases which are female was: $p = 73/120 = 0.608$ (60.8%) and the standard error $\mathrm{SE}(p) = \sqrt{[\{0.608 \times (1 - 0.608)\}/120]} = 0.045$.

The 95% CI for the true population proportion of female acute appendicitis patients is given by: $0.608 - (1.96 \times 0.045)$ to $0.608 + (1.96 \times 0.045)$ or 0.52 to 0.70.

Chapter 7

1. (a) The null hypothesis is that the percentage of deliveries where there was a failure to respond to signs of foetal distress did not differ between the cerebral palsy babies and the delivery book controls. The alternative hypothesis is that there was a difference between the two groups with respect to failure to respond to signs of foetal distress.

   (b) Failure to respond to signs of foetal distress was noted in 25.8% of the cerebral palsy babies and in 7.1 % of the delivery book babies. The difference between these two percentages was $25.8 - 7.1 = 18.7\%$. This is the actual or absolute difference in the two percentages and so is expressed in percentage points, and is sometimes referred to as the absolute risk difference or absolute risk reduction.

   (c) The 95% *CI* shows that the difference between the two groups is estimated to be at least as large as 10.5% and may be as great as 26.9%. Since the interval excludes 0, there is good evidence for a real difference in the groups in the population from which the samples come.

2. (a) On average the patients in the clinic group had 5.9 more ulcer-free weeks than the control group and the 95% *CI* for this difference ranged from 1.2 to 10.6 weeks. As this confidence interval does not include 0 weeks we can conclude that there was a significant difference between the two groups with respect to the number of ulcer-free weeks over the 12 month study period.

   (b) We know that the 95% *CI* is approximately (mean $- 2 \times SE$) to (mean $+ 2 \times SE$) and so we can use either the lower limit (or the upper limit) of the confidence interval to obtain the SE. For example, SE = (mean $-$ lower limit) / 2 = $(5.9 - 1.2) / 2 = 2.35$ weeks.

   (c) Mean costs were £878 per year for the clinic group and £863 for the control group and the *p*-value for the difference was 0.89. As this value is greater than the critical value of 0.05, we can conclude that there is no evidence of a statistically significant difference between the groups with respect to cost of treatment (technically speaking – there is insufficient evidence to reject the null hypothesis).

   (d) From the information above, it would be reasonable to conclude that community based leg ulcer clinics are more effective than traditional home-based treatment, in terms of the number of ulcer-free weeks. This benefit is achieved at a marginal additional cost. If we divide the mean difference in costs between the two groups by the mean difference between the groups in ulcer-free weeks we get something called the incremental cost-effectiveness ratio. This gives £15/5.9 weeks, and so it costs about £2.50 to achieve an extra-ulcer free week.

3. There were several options here:

(a) The proportion with developmental regression did not change over the 20-year period. The alternative to this is that the proportion did change over the period.

   The proportion with bowel problems did not change over the 20-year period. The alternative to this is that the proportion did change over the study period.

   The proportion reporting bowel problems did not differ between those with developmental regression and those without developmental regression. The alternative to this is that the proportion was different in the two groups.

(b) There was no significant difference in the proportions reporting developmental regression during the 20-year period, as the p-value for this difference was >0.05 (technically speaking – there is insufficient evidence to reject the null hypothesis at the 5% level).

(c) There was no significant difference in the proportions reporting bowel problems during the 20-year study period, as the p-value for this difference was >0.05 (technically speaking – there is insufficient evidence to reject the null hypothesis at the 5% level).

(d) The 95% CI shows that the difference in the percentages with bowel problems between those with developmental regression and those without is estimated to be at least as large as 4.2% and may be as great as 21.5%. Since this interval excludes 0, there is good evidence for a real difference in the population from which the samples come. The p-value for this difference would be <0.05 (in fact it is 0.003).

4. (a) This is the standard error. Estimates of population values vary from sample to sample and therefore have a theoretical distribution: the sampling distribution. The standard error of an estimate is a measure of the variability of this distribution. The standard error is the standard deviation of the sampling distribution of the sample estimate. The standard error therefore provides information about the precision of the estimate and is used to calculate confidence intervals around the estimates. Here the value of 0.68 is the standard error of the percentage of pre-term births. The units of the standard error are the same as for the sample estimate itself; here percentage points. The standard error is used to assess the spread of the mean whilst the standard deviation assesses the spread of the patients.

(b) This is the 95% CI. It is a range of values which we anticipate will contain the true population percentage of pre-term births, for 95% of samples. This is in the sense that if a large number of samples were taken from the same population, then 95% of the calculated confidence intervals would contain the population percentage. This implies that 5% of these samples would *not* contain the true population percentage. Here we deduce that the population value is very likely to lie between 6.1% and 8.8%, but our best estimate of it is 7.5%.

(c) If 90% limits were used the confidence interval would be narrower and fewer (90% rather then 95%) confidence intervals from possible repeats of the study would contain the population incidence. The 90% limits would be 6.4 to 8.6%.

(d) If 99% limits were used the confidence interval would be wider and more (99%) confidence intervals from possible samples would contain the population incidence. Thus there would be less chance of being wrong but the range of possible population values would be greater (the 99% confidence limits would be 5.8 to 9.2%).

(e) The Danish study included many more subjects than the UK study and so the estimate of the pre-term birth incidence is much more precise. Hence, the 95% *CI* is narrower. There were 3% more pre-term in the UK study than in the Danish study and the two 95% CI do not overlap. Hence there is some evidence for a real difference although this (non-overlapping confidence intervals) is not a formal significance test.

Chapter 8

1. (a) H_0: No difference in mean 24-hour total energy expenditure between lean and obese groups of women i.e. $\mu_{Lean} - \mu_{Obese} = 0.0$ MJ/day.

   H_A: There is a difference in mean ulcer-free weeks between intervention and control groups i.e. $\mu_{Lean} - \mu_{Obese} \neq 0.00$ MJ/day.

Note that: In this case the two groups are independent (measurements are not on the same individuals). Therefore we are interested in the difference between the means of each group.

   (b) Independent two-sample *t*-test for comparing means
   Assumptions: Two 'independent' groups, continuous outcome variable, outcome data in both groups are Normally distributed. Outcome data in both groups have similar standard deviations.

$$\text{pooled SD} = \sqrt{\frac{(13-1)1.24^2 + (9-1)1.40^2}{13+9-2}} = 1.306$$

Where n_1 = number of subjects in 1st sample, 13
s_1 = standard deviation of 1st sample, 1.24
n_2 = number of subjects in 2nd sample, 9
s_2 = standard deviation of 2nd sample. 1.40

$$\text{SE of difference} = \text{SE (d)} = 1.306 \times \sqrt{\frac{1}{13} + \frac{1}{9}} = 0.57$$

$$t = \frac{8.07 - 10.30}{0.57} = -3.946$$

on $13 + 9 - 2 = 20\,df$

The probability of the observing this test statistic or more extreme under the null hypothesis is 0.001 using the t distribution on $20\,df$

What does P = 0.001 mean? The results are unlikely when the null hypothesis is true. *Is this result statistically significant?* The result is statistically significant because the P-value is less than the significance level (α) set at 0.05 or 5%.

Decision: There is sufficient evidence to reject the null hypothesis and accept the alternative hypothesis that there is a difference in mean 24-hour total energy expenditure (MJ/day) between the Lean and Obese groups of women.

(c) The 100 $(1 - \alpha)$% confidence interval for the difference in the two population means is

$$d - [t_{1-\alpha} \times \text{SE}(d)] \text{ to } d + [t_{1-\alpha} \times \text{SE}(d)]$$

Where $d = \bar{x}_1 - \bar{x}_2$ and $t_{1-\alpha}$ is taken from the t distribution with $n_1 + n_2 - 2$ degrees of freedom. E.g. $13 + 9 - 2 = 20\,df$, so for a 95% confidence interval $t_{0.05} = 2.086$. The 95% CI for the population difference in the two population means is then given by:

$$-2.23 - (2.086 \times 0.57) \text{ to } -2.23 + (2.086 \times 0.57)$$
$$-3.41 \text{ to } -1.05\,\text{MJ/day}$$

Therefore we are 95% confident that the true population mean difference in 24 hour total energy expenditure (MJ/day) between Lean and Obese women lies somewhere between −3.41 to −1.05 MJ/day, but our best estimate is −2.23 MJ/day. So the result is consistent with women in the obese group having a higher total energy expenditure than women in the lean group.

2. (a) H_0: No difference in outcomes, proportion of CFS, patients feeling better at 6 weeks between the magnesium and placebo treated groups, i.e. $\pi_{Magnesium} - \pi_{Placebo} = 0.0$.

H_A: There is a difference in outcomes, proportion of CFS patients feeling better at 6 weeks between the magnesium and placebo treated groups, i.e. $\pi_{Magnesium} - \pi_{Placebo} \neq 0.00$.

We can test this null hypothesis by a z-test comparison of two proportions or a chi-squared test. We could also use Yates' continuity corrected chi-squared test or Fisher's exact test. All four tests result in $p < 0.001$.

What does P = 0.001 mean? Your results are *unlikely* when the null hypothesis is true.

Is this result statistically significant? The result is *statistically significant* because the *p*-value is less than the significance level (α) set at 0.05 or 5%.

Decision: That there is sufficient evidence to *reject the null hypothesis*. Therefore there is reliable evidence of a difference in the proportion feeling better at 6 weeks between the Magnesium and Placebo treated patient groups.

(b) $p_{Magnesium} = 12/15 = 0.80$
$p_{Placebo} = 3/17 = 0.176$
$p_{Magnesium} - p_{Placebo} = 0.80 - 0.176 = 0.624$
$SE\ (p_{Magnesium} - p_{Placebo}) = 0.139$
95% CI:

$$0.624 - (1.96 \times 0.139) \text{ to } 0.624 + (1.96 \times 0.139)$$
$$0.351 \text{ to } 0.896$$

Therefore we are 95% confident that the true population difference in the proportions of CFS patients feeling better at 6 weeks between the Magnesium and Placebo treated groups lies somewhere between 35% to 90%, but our best estimate is 62%.

So the result is consistent with CFS patients in the Magnesium group having a better outcome, and feeling better than patients in the Placebo group.

3. (a) H_0: No difference (or change) in mean daily dietary energy intake (kJ) over 10 pre-menstrual and 10 post-menstrual days in normally menstruating female subjects i.e. $\mu_{Pre-menstrual} - \mu_{Post-menstrual} = 0.0$ KJ.

H_A: There is a difference (or change) in mean daily dietary energy intake (kJ) over 10 pre-menstrual and 10 post-menstrual days in normally menstruating female subjects $\mu_{Pre-menstrual} - \mu_{Post-menstrual} \neq 0.00$ KJ.

Note that: In this case the two groups are paired and not independent (measurements are made on the same individuals). Therefore we are interested in the mean of the differences not the difference between the two means (not independent groups). We can use a paired t-test to test the null hypothesis.

(b) Assumptions for paired t-test:

The d_is, differences in pre- and post-menstrual dietary intake are plausibly Normally distributed. (Note it is not essential for the original observations to be Normally distributed).
The d_is are independent of each other.

Computer Output

Paired Samples Statistics

		Mean	N	Std deviation	Std. Error Mean
Pair 1	Pre-menstrual dietary intake (kJ/day)	6753.636	11	1142.123	344.3631
	Post-menstrual dietary intake (kJ/day)	5433.182	11	1216.833	366.8888

Paired Samples Test

		Paired Differences							
		Mean	Std deviation	Std. error mean	95%confidence interval of the difference		t	df	Sig. (2-tailed)
					Lower	Upper			
Pair 1	Pre-menstrual dietary intake (kJ/day) – Post-menstrual dietary intake (kJ/day)	1320.455	366.74551	110.5779	1074.072	1566.838	11.941	10	.000

What does P = 0.001 mean? Your results are *unlikely* when the null hypothesis is true.

Is this result statistically significant? The results is *statistically significant* because the P-value is less than the significance level (α) set at 0.05 or 5%.

Decision: That there is sufficient evidence to *reject the null hypothesis* and accept the alternative hypothesis that there is a difference or change in mean daily dietary intake (kJ) between pre- and post-menstrual phases of the cycle in normal menstruating female subjects.

(c) We are 95% confident that the true population difference in mean daily dietary intake between the 10 pre-menstrual and 10 post-menstrual days, in normal healthy women, lies somewhere between 1074 to 1567 kJ, but our best estimate is 1320 kJ. So the result is consistent with normally menstruating females having a higher mean daily dietary intake in the 10 post-menstrual days than the 10 pre-menstrual days of their cycle.

Chapter 9

1. (i) A = 1.198 B = 2.92   (ii) Yes. Assumption is that the effect of medication is the same for both sexes   (iii) 94.18   (iv) 79.41   (v) No, the R-squared value is very small. Only about 5% of the variation is accounted for.

2. (i) A = 0.812, B = 0.861, C = 1.392   (ii) No both P values are above 0.05. The value of C 1.39 means that a person of a given age has an odds ratio (approximate relative risk) of being 40% more likely to consider their health poor.

Chapter 10

1. (a) See Sections 10.1 and 10.4 for definitions of *censored* and *hazard ratio* respectively.

(b)

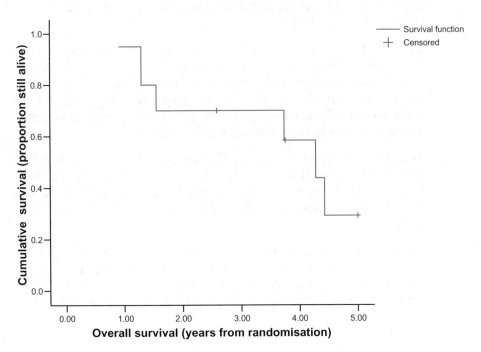

Kaplan–Meier estimate of the overall survival function (*n* = 10 intervention patients)

(c) From the graph the estimated median survival times are 4.3 years and 3.5 years for the Intervention and Control groups respectively. The log rank test is not significant (p-value > 0.05), which implies we cannot reject the null hypothesis that the two groups come from the same population as regards survival times.

(d) Only the terms for gender and histology are statistically significant. In this sample age and treatment group (after allowing for the other covariates) are not associated with survival. Statistical significance alone does not mean one could use the model for prediction. One should compare the observed and predicted outcomes.

(e) The regression coefficient (hazard ratio) for the simple model containing treatment group alone suggests that, the risk of dying in the Intervention Group (coded 1) is 0.92 times (95% CI: 0.74 to 1.13) that of the Control group (coded 0). This is of similar magnitude to the model with other covariates included. As we would expect the p-value from the Cox model ($p = 0.391$) is similar to the results of the log rank test. However, analysis 2 reassures us that there is no difference in overall survival between the two groups even after adjustment for age, gender and histology.

2. (a) People with an acute hip fracture are 60% more likely to die in the first year afterwards if they have respiratory disease. If one takes into account the age and sex of the patient, and their other risk factors, this is reduced to 40%.

(b) Comorbid cardiovascular disease is a significant risk factor in the univariate analysis. The reason why this appears to be not a risk factor in the multivariate analysis might be because people with comorbid cardiovascular disease are likely to be older (and possibly male) than those without. Thus *given* a person's age and sex, comorbid cardiovascular disease is not a significant risk factor.

(c) In addition to possibly the fact that people who get a chest infection may be older than those who do not, it is also likely that they have comorbid respiratory disease, so that *given* their age and respiratory disease, a chest infection is still important, but the hazard is halved.

(d) The main assumption is that the risk factor remains constant over the year. This is likely with the comorbid states and with Parkinson's disease, but a chest infection is likely only to be a risk factor whilst the patient suffers it, and so the risk will revert to unity once the infection is cured.

Chapter 11

1. $\kappa = 0.5$, or only moderate agreement, so one would not substitute one method for the other.

2. $k = 10$, $\sum s_i^2 = 1.04^2 + 1.11^2 + \ldots + 1.03^2 = 11.16$, $\sum s_T^2 = 8.80^2 = 77.44$ and finally $\alpha_{\text{Cronbach}} \dfrac{10}{10-1}\left(1 - \dfrac{11.16}{77.44}\right) = 0.95$. This indicates a high degree of consistency and so may be regarded as satisfactory for clinical application.

Chapter 12

1. (a) Prevalence study   (b) unmatched case–control study   (c) retrospective cohort study   (d) cluster randomised trial   (e) quasi-experimental study.

2. Women who are given HRT may be better educated and informed than women not given it. Women who are better educated tend to have lower risk of heart disease.

3. $OR = 61 \times 324/(62 \times 168) = 1.90$. $SE[\log(OR)] = \sqrt{(1/61 + 1/62 + 1/168 + 1/324)} = 0.20$. Thus 95% CI for $\log(OR)$ is $0.64 - 1.96 \times 0.20$ to $0.64 + 1.96 \times 0.20$ or 0.248 to 1.032. Finally the 95% CI for the OR is $\exp(0.248) = 1.28$ to $\exp(1.032) = 2.81$.

Chapter 14

1. Here $\pi_{\text{Plan}} = 0.2$, $SE_{\text{Plan}} = 0.025$, thus from Section 14.5 $m = 0.2 \times (1 - 0.2) / (0.025^2) = 256$. Allowing for a 20% refusal rate (often quite high in surveys) increases this to $256/0.8 = 320$

2. The previous trial based on 554 patients had a 95% CI for the effect of 4.90 to 5.09. This leads to a $SE = 0.10$, so that a reasonable anticipated value of the standard deviation for the new study is $\sigma_{\text{Plan}} = 0.10 \times \sqrt{554} = 2.35$ or approximately 2.5. The anticipated effect size is $\delta_{\text{Plan}} = 0.5\,\text{mmol}$, then formula 14.1 gives $m = 16 \times (2.5/0.5)^2 = 400$ per group or $N = 800$ subjects in all, a withdrawal rate of 10% would bring this close to 900.

3. $m = 2\theta \dfrac{\sigma_{\text{Plan}}^2}{\delta_{\text{Plan}}^2}$

$\sigma^2{}_{\text{Plan}} = 27^2$, $\delta_{\text{Plan}} = 10$, $\alpha = 0.05$ and $1 - \beta = 0.90$, $\theta = 10.5$ from Table 14.3. $m = (2 \times 10.5) \times (27^2/10^2) = 153.09$

This gives an approximate sample size of 154 in each group (308 in total).

4. We have $\pi_1 = 0.20$ and $\pi_2 = 0.15$, so $\delta = \pi_1 - \pi_2 = 0.20 - 0.15 = 0.05$, and $\alpha = 0.05$, $1 - \beta = 0.08$. Using Table 14.1, to meet the conditions specified for the trial we thus need to have 906 men in each group (1812 in total).

Chapter 15

1. This is a classic regression to the mean phenomenon. Since black-spots are chosen because their accident rates are high, one might expect, by chance that the rates would fall on re-measurement. This is less of a problem if the rates are consistently high for a number of years and then fall after the camera is installed, but one should also consider other aspects, such as whether accidents were falling generally over the period of interest.

2. Since this a randomised controlled trial, with a control group, the regression to the mean phenomenon does not apply to the comparison between groups, since it would be expected to apply equally to both groups. If other aspects of the trial are satisfactory (for example a high proportion of the eligible children took part in the trial, and a high proportion were follow-up in both groups) then that is strong evidence for a casual effect. Whether it can be recommend depends on a number of factors: (i) the *size* of the effect: a very small effect may not be worthwhile; (ii) the *cost* of treatment: an expensive treatment may not be affordable; (iii) side effects: cod liver oil may have untoward gastro-intestinal effects that mean that it is unsuitable for many people.

Statistical Tables

Medical Statistics Fourth Edition, David Machin, Michael J Campbell, Stephen J Walters
© 2007 John Wiley & Sons, Ltd

STATISTICAL TABLES

Table T1 The Normal distribution. The value tabulated is the probability that a Normally distributed random variable with mean zero and standard deviation one will be greater than z or less than −z

z	0.00	0.01	0.02	0.03	0.04	0.05	0.06	0.07	0.08	0.09
0.00	1.0000	0.9920	0.9840	0.9761	0.9681	0.9601	0.9522	0.9442	0.9362	0.9283
0.10	0.9203	0.9124	0.9045	0.8966	0.8887	0.8808	0.8729	0.8650	0.8572	0.8493
0.20	0.8415	0.8337	0.8259	0.8181	0.8103	0.8206	0.7949	0.7872	0.7795	0.7718
0.30	0.7642	0.7566	0.7490	0.7414	0.7339	0.7263	0.7188	0.7114	0.7039	0.6965
0.40	0.6892	0.6818	0.6745	0.6672	0.6599	0.6527	0.6455	0.6384	0.6312	0.6241
0.50	0.6171	0.6101	0.6031	0.5961	0.5892	0.5823	0.5755	0.5687	0.5619	0.5552
0.60	0.5485	0.5419	0.5353	0.5287	0.5222	0.5157	0.5093	0.5029	0.4965	0.4902
0.70	0.4839	0.4777	0.4715	0.4654	0.4593	0.4533	0.4473	0.4413	0.4354	0.4295
0.80	0.4237	0.4179	0.4122	0.4065	0.4009	0.3953	0.3898	0.3843	0.3789	0.3735
0.90	0.3681	0.3628	0.3576	0.3524	0.3472	0.3421	0.3371	0.3320	0.3271	0.3222
1.00	0.3173	0.3125	0.3077	0.3030	0.2983	0.2837	0.2891	0.2846	0.2801	0.2757

z	0.00	0.01	0.02	0.03	0.04	0.05	0.06	0.07	0.08	0.09
1.00	0.3173	0.3125	0.3077	0.3030	0.2983	0.2937	0.2891	0.2846	0.2801	0.2757
1.10	0.2713	0.2670	0.2627	0.2585	0.2543	0.2501	0.2460	0.2420	0.2380	0.2340
1.20	0.2301	0.2203	0.2225	0.2187	0.2150	0.2113	0.2077	0.2041	0.2005	0.1971
1.30	0.1936	0.1902	0.1868	0.1835	0.1802	0.1770	0.1738	0.1707	0.1676	0.1645
1.40	0.1615	0.1585	0.1556	0.1527	0.1499	0.1471	0.1443	0.1416	0.1389	0.1362
1.50	0.1336	0.1310	0.1285	0.1260	0.1236	0.1211	0.1188	0.1164	0.1141	0.1118
1.60	0.1096	0.1074	0.1052	0.1031	0.1010	0.0989	0.0969	0.0949	0.0930	0.0910
1.70	0.0891	0.0873	0.0854	0.0836	0.0819	0.0801	0.0784	0.0767	0.0751	0.0735
1.80	0.0719	0.0703	0.0688	0.0672	0.0658	0.0643	0.0629	0.0615	0.0601	0.0588
1.90	0.0574	0.0561	0.0549	0.0536	0.0524	0.0512	0.0500	0.0488	0.0477	0.0466
2.00	0.0455	0.0444	0.0434	0.0424	0.0414	0.0404	0.0394	0.0385	0.0375	0.0366

z	0.00	0.01	0.02	0.03	0.04	0.05	0.06	0.07	0.08	0.09
2.00	0.0455	0.0444	0.0434	0.0424	0.0414	0.0404	0.0394	0.0385	0.0375	0.0366
2.10	0.0357	0.0349	0.0340	0.0332	0.0324	0.0316	0.0308	0.0300	0.0293	0.0285
2.20	0.0278	0.0271	0.0264	0.0257	0.0251	0.0244	0.0238	0.0232	0.0226	0.0220
2.30	0.0214	0.0209	0.0203	0.0198	0.0193	0.0188	0.0183	0.0178	0.0173	0.0168
2.40	0.0164	0.0160	0.0155	0.0151	0.0147	0.0143	0.0139	0.0135	0.0131	0.0128
2.50	0.0124	0.0121	0.0117	0.0114	0.0111	0.0108	0.0105	0.0102	0.0099	0.0096
2.60	0.0093	0.0091	0.0088	0.0085	0.0083	0.0080	0.0078	0.0076	0.0074	0.0071
2.70	0.0069	0.0067	0.0065	0.0063	0.0061	0.0060	0.0058	0.0056	0.0054	0.0053
2.80	0.0051	0.0050	0.0048	0.0047	0.0045	0.0044	0.0042	0.0041	0.0040	0.0039
2.90	0.0037	0.0036	0.0035	0.0034	0.0033	0.0032	0.0031	0.0030	0.0029	0.0028
3.00	0.0027	0.0026	0.0025	0.0024	0.0024	0.0023	0.0022	0.0021	0.0021	0.0020

Table T2   Random numbers table

Each digit 0–9 is independent of every other digit and is equally likely to occur.

94071	63090	23901	93268	53316	87773
67970	29162	60224	61042	98324	30425
91577	43019	67511	28527	61750	55267
84334	54827	51955	47256	21387	28456
03778	05031	90146	59031	96758	57420
58563	84810	22446	80149	99676	83102
29068	74625	90665	52747	09364	57491
90047	44763	44534	55425	67170	67937
54870	35009	84524	32309	88815	86792
23327	78957	50987	77876	63960	53986
03876	89100	66895	89468	96684	95491
14846	86619	04238	36182	05294	43791
94731	63786	88290	60990	98407	43473
96046	51589	84509	98162	39162	59469
95188	25011	29947	48896	83408	79684

Table T3 Student's t-distribution. The value tabulated is t_α such that if X is distributed as Student's t-distribution with df degrees of freedom, then α is the probability that $X \leqslant -t_{r\alpha}$ or $X \geqslant t_{r\alpha}$

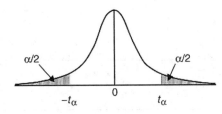

df	α							
	0.20	0.10	0.05	0.04	0.03	0.02	0.01	0.001
1	3.078	6.314	12.706	15.895	21.205	31.821	63.657	636.6
2	1.886	2.920	4.303	4.849	5.643	6.965	9.925	31.60
3	1.634	2.353	3.182	3.482	3.896	4.541	5.842	12.92
4	1.530	2.132	2.776	2.999	3.298	3.747	4.604	8.610
5	1.474	2.015	2.571	2.757	3.003	3.365	4.032	6.869
6	1.439	1.943	2.447	2.612	2.829	3.143	3.707	5.959
7	1.414	1.895	2.365	2.517	2.715	2.998	3.499	5.408
8	1.397	1.860	2.306	2.449	2.634	2.896	3.355	5.041
9	1.383	1.833	2.262	2.398	2.574	2.821	3.250	4.781
10	1.372	1.812	2.228	2.359	2.528	2.764	3.169	4.587
11	1.363	1.796	2.201	2.328	2.491	2.718	3.106	4.437
12	1.356	1.782	2.179	2.303	2.461	2.681	3.055	4.318
13	1.350	1.771	2.160	2.282	2.436	2.650	3.012	4.221
14	1.345	1.761	2.145	2.264	2.415	2.624	2.977	4.140
15	1.340	1.753	2.131	2.249	2.397	2.602	2.947	4.073
16	1.337	1.746	2.120	2.235	2.382	2.583	2.921	4.015
17	1.333	1.740	2.110	2.224	2.368	2.567	2.898	3.965
18	1.330	1.734	2.101	2.214	2.356	2.552	2.878	3.922
19	1.328	1.729	2.093	2.205	2.346	2.539	2.861	3.883
20	1.325	1.725	2.086	2.196	2.336	2.528	2.845	3.850
21	1.323	1.721	2.079	2.189	2.327	2.517	2.830	3.819
22	1.321	1.717	2.074	2.183	2.320	2.508	2.818	3.790
23	1.319	1.714	2.069	2.178	2.313	2.499	2.806	3.763
24	1.318	1.711	2.064	2.172	2.307	2.492	2.797	3.744
25	1.316	1.708	2.059	2.166	2.301	2.485	2.787	3.722
26	1.315	1.706	2.056	2.162	2.396	2.479	2.779	3.706
27	1.314	1.703	2.052	2.158	2.291	2.472	2.770	3.687
28	1.313	1.701	2.048	2.154	2.286	2.467	2.763	3.673
29	1.311	1.699	2.045	2.150	2.282	2.462	2.756	3.657
30	1.310	1.697	2.042	2.147	2.278	2.457	2.750	3.646
∞	1.282	1.645	1.960	2.054	2.170	2.326	2.576	3.291

Table T4   The χ^2 distribution. The value tabulated is $\chi^2\,(\alpha)$, such that if X is distributed as χ^2 with df degrees of freedom, then α is the probability that $X \geq \chi^2$

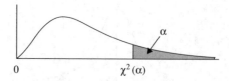

df	α							
	0.2	0.1	0.05	0.04	0.03	0.02	0.01	0.001
1	1.64	2.71	3.84	4.22	4.71	5.41	6.63	10.83
2	3.22	4.61	5.99	6.44	7.01	7.82	9.21	13.82
3	4.64	6.25	7.81	8.31	8.95	9.84	11.34	16.27
4	5.99	7.78	9.49	10.03	10.71	11.67	13.28	18.47
5	7.29	9.24	11.07	11.64	12.37	13.39	15.09	20.52
6	8.56	10.64	12.59	13.20	13.97	15.03	16.81	22.46
7	9.80	12.02	14.07	14.70	15.51	16.62	18.48	24.32
8	11.03	13.36	15.51	16.17	17.01	18.17	20.09	26.13
9	12.24	14.68	16.92	17.61	18.48	19.68	21.67	27.88
10	13.44	15.99	18.31	19.02	19.92	21.16	23.21	29.59
11	14.63	17.28	19.68	20.41	21.34	22.62	24.73	31.26
12	15.81	18.55	21.03	21.79	22.74	24.05	26.22	32.91
13	16.98	19.81	22.36	23.14	24.12	25.47	27.69	34.53
14	18.15	21.06	23.68	24.49	25.49	26.87	29.14	36.12
15	19.31	22.31	25.00	25.82	26.85	28.26	30.58	37.70
16	20.47	23.54	26.30	27.14	28.19	29.63	32.00	39.25
17	21.61	24.77	27.59	28.45	29.52	31.00	33.41	40.79
18	22.76	25.99	28.87	29.75	30.84	32.35	34.81	42.31
19	23.90	27.20	30.14	31.04	32.16	33.69	36.19	43.82
20	25.04	28.41	31.41	32.32	33.46	35.02	37.57	45.32
21	26.17	29.61	32.67	33.60	34.75	36.34	38.91	47.00
22	27.30	30.81	33.92	34.87	36.04	37.65	40.32	48.41
23	28.43	32.01	35.18	36.13	37.33	38.97	41.61	49.81
24	29.55	33.19	36.41	37.39	38.62	40.26	43.02	51.22
25	30.67	34.38	37.65	38.65	39.88	41.55	44.30	52.63
26	31.79	35.56	38.88	39.88	41.14	42.84	45.65	54.03
27	32.91	36.74	40.12	41.14	42.40	44.13	47.00	55.44
28	34.03	37.92	41.35	42.37	43.66	45.42	48.29	56.84
29	35.14	39.09	42.56	43.60	44.92	46.71	49.58	58.25
30	36.25	40.25	43.78	44.83	46.15	47.97	50.87	59.66

Table T5   Normal ordinates for cumulative probabilities. The value tabulated is z such that for a given probability α, a random variable, Normally distributed with mean zero and standard deviation one will be less than z with probability α.

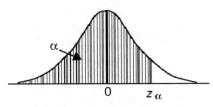

| | | | | | α | | | | |
	0.00	0.01	0.02	0.03	0.04	0.05	0.06	0.07	0.08	0.09
0.00		−2.33	−2.05	−1.88	−1.75	−1.64	−1.56	−1.48	−1.41	−1.34
0.10	−1.28	−1.23	−1.17	−1.13	−1.08	−1.04	−0.99	−0.95	−0.92	−0.88
0.20	−0.84	−0.81	−0.77	−0.74	−0.71	−0.67	−0.64	−0.61	−0.58	−0.55
0.30	−0.52	−0.50	−0.47	−0.44	−0.41	−0.39	−0.36	−0.33	−0.31	−0.28
0.40	−0.25	−0.23	−0.20	−0.18	−0.15	−0.13	−0.10	−0.08	−0.05	−0.03
0.50	0.00	0.03	0.05	0.08	0.10	0.13	0.15	0.18	0.20	0.23
0.60	0.25	0.28	0.31	0.33	0.36	0.39	0.41	0.44	0.47	0.50
0.70	0.52	0.55	0.58	0.61	0.64	0.67	0.71	0.74	0.77	0.81
0.80	0.84	0.88	0.92	0.95	0.99	1.04	1.08	1.13	1.17	1.23
0.90	1.28	1.34	1.41	1.48	1.56	1.64	1.75	1.88	2.05	2.33

Index

Note: boxed text is indicated by **emboldened page numbers**, and Figures and Tables by *italic numbers*